Neil J. Friedman, M.D.
Arrowhead Eye Center
Glendale, Arizona
Formerly Chief Resident
Department of Ophthalmology
New York Eye and Ear Infirmary
New York, New York
Clinical Instructor
Moran Eye Center
University of Utah Health Sciences Center
Salt Lake City, Utah

Roberto Pineda II, M.D.
Department of Ophthalmology
Massachusetts Eye and Ear Infirmary
Boston, Massachusetts

Peter K. Kaiser, M.D.
Division of Ophthalmology
Cleveland Clinic Foundation Eye Institute
Cleveland, Ohio

D1520095

The Massachusetts Eye and Ear Infirmary Illustrated Manual of Ophthalmology

W.B. SAUNDERS COMPANY
A Division of Harcourt Brace & Company
Philadelphia / London / Toronto / Montreal / Sydney / Tokyo

A D

The Curti
Independence
Philadelphia, Pennsylvania 19106

Library of Congress Cataloging-in-Publication Data

Friedman, Neil J.
   The Massachusetts Eye and Ear Infirmary illustrated manual of
ophthalmology / Neil J. Friedman, Roberto Pineda II, Peter K. Kaiser.

p.   cm.

Includes index.

ISBN 0–7216–7025–3

1. Ophthalmology—Handbooks, manuals, etc.   I. Pineda, Roberto II
   II. Kaiser, Peter K.   III. Massachusetts Eye and Ear Infirmary.
   IV. Title.   [DNLM: 1. Eye—anatomy & histology—handbooks.   2. Eye
Diseases—handbooks.   WW 39 F911m 1998]

RE48.9.F75 1998   617.7—dc21

DNLM/DLC   97-37851

THE MASSACHUSETTS EYE AND EAR INFIRMARY
ILLUSTRATED MANUAL OF OPHTHALMOLOGY   ISBN 0–7216–7025–3

Copyright © 1998 by W.B. Saunders Company

Printed in The United States of America

Last digit is the print number: 9   8   7   6   5   4   3   2

Foreword

Writing a concise handbook on a topic can be more challenging and arduous than writing a logorrheal multivolume treatise. What does one include in the shorter version? How much weight is given to various topics? What is the cut-off point for rare conditions? How much detail does one offer regarding therapeutic options and side effects, including the debunking of facile bromides and nostrums? Such matters have been negotiated with utmost success in this handbook of ophthalmology. The style is uniformly readable, the bibliography is up-to-date and carefully selected, and the color illustrations are unique for this kind of publishing format. This handbook deserves a widespread readership, and I am proud and delighted that the name of the Massachusetts Eye and Ear Infirmary is associated with this project.

Three bright and highly resourceful recent resident graduates came together to work on this project. All three have a first-class intellectual pedigree and a Harvard association: Dr. Kaiser went to Harvard Medical School, did his internship in medicine at the Massachusetts General Hospital, his residency at the Infirmary, and completed his training with a retinal fellowship at the Bascom Palmer Eye Institute; Dr. Pineda did his residency and corneal fellowship at the Massachusetts Eye and Ear Infirmary, where he also served as Chief Resident in Ophthalmology; and Dr. Friedman trained at Harvard Medical School, did his residency at the New York Eye and Ear Infirmary, and did his fellowship in refractive and anterior segment surgery at the Cullen Eye Institute.

It was my privilege to serve as Chief of Ophthalmology at the Infirmary while Drs. Kaiser and Pineda were in training; they were model residents and adept in the subject matter at hand. Together with Dr. Friedman, they have pooled their extensive collective knowledge and burgeoning clinical experience to provide all ophthalmologists, particularly residents and fellows in training, with an invaluable ocular florilegium.

Frederick A. Jakobiec, M.D., D.Sc.
Henry Willard Williams Professor of Ophthalmology,
Professor of Pathology, and Chairman,
Department of Ophthalmology,
Harvard Medical School;
Chief of Ophthalmology,
The Massachusetts Eye and Ear Infirmary

One of the special aspects of ophthalmology is its visual nature. Because most ocular pathology is directly visible, accurate diagnosis depends on careful examination of all ocular structures. Therefore, it is important for the examiner to be familiar with the symptoms and signs as well as the appearance of every disorder.

The purpose of this book is twofold: to present concise, useful information on a broad range of ophthalmic disorders, and to direct this information to a wide audience. Thus, we have created a user-friendly diagnostic atlas that also integrates essential therapeutic information. It is geared toward anyone who administers eye care regardless of training, including medical students, residents, primary care and emergency medicine physicians, ophthalmic technicians, optometrists, and ophthalmologists.

We have organized the book into sections corresponding to each ocular structure and the different aspects of a routine eye examination. For most disease processes, we provide the classic symptoms and signs and figures illustrating typical presentations. This allows the pertinent diagnostic information on any given disorder to be quickly and easily accessed without any previous ophthalmic training or knowledge of the entity. Moreover, once a disorder is identified, the epidemiology, work-up, treatment, and prognosis are available to guide its management.

To maintain this easy-to-use format and prevent the text from becoming too unwieldy, only a limited amount of information is presented for each diagnosis. Therefore, we have used an outline format to include all essential data for making a diagnosis and properly managing most common ophthalmic disorders. The summaries should not be considered definitive or exhaustive, which is beyond the scope of this book. Rather, this manual should be used as a diagnostic guide to aid the examiner in making the correct diagnosis as well as to help him or her learn about the disorder and formulate a treatment plan.

One additional word of caution regarding using this text solely as a therapeutic "bible," which is not our intent; rather, the treatment sections include typical strategies and favored options that we have been exposed to during our training. They are meant to be guidelines, not rigid orders. As in any specialty, management choices exist and often change with time; therefore, a certain degree of clinical judgment is necessary, and in difficult or uncertain cases other sources should be consulted. In addition, every effort was made to ensure that the drug selections and dosages were in accordance with current therapeutic guidelines; however, these recommendations are continually evolving. Therefore, we advise referring to the individual package inserts or the *Physicians' Desk Reference* for more specific information and warnings. We have also provided a list of some of the standard textbooks that contain more detailed coverage related to etiology, diagnosis, and management of these disorders.

We wish that a similar book existed during our training, and we hope that you will find it a useful addition to your library, white coat, or black bag.

Neil J. Friedman, M.D.
Roberto Pineda II, M.D.
Peter K. Kaiser, M.D.

Acknowledgments

We gratefully acknowledge the faculty, staff, and our colleagues and peers at the various training programs, including the Bascom Palmer Eye Institute, the Cullen Eye Institute, the Massachusetts Eye and Ear Infirmary, and the New York Eye and Ear Infirmary for their guidance, instruction, and support of this project at all stages of its development. We owe a special debt of gratitude to a number of individuals who helped review chapters and made invaluable comments and suggestions, including David S. Greenfield, M.D., Frederick A. Jakobiec, M.D., Maureen O. Kaiser, D.M.D., Douglas D. Koch, M.D., Andrew G. Lee, M.D., Jeffrey M. Liebmann, M.D., Alice Y. Matoba, M.D., Timothy G. Murray, M.D., Susannah Rowe, M.D., Peter A.D. Rubin, M.D., Mark G. Speaker, M.D., and William B. Trattler, M.D.

In addition, we would like to especially acknowledge the expert assistance of Louise Carr-Holden, Ditte Hesse, Kit Johnson, Bob Masini, Audrey Melacan, and Jim Shigley as well as the dedicated members of their photography departments for all the wonderful pictures, without which this book would not be possible. We would also like to thank the many physicians who contributed photographs to complete the vast collection of ophthalmic disorders found in this manual.

Finally, we are indebted to our families, including Alan, Diane, Lisa, Joe, Roberto, Anne, Gabriela, Nicole, Susannah, Peter, Anafu, Christine, and Maureen for their love, support, and encouragement during the course of this project.

Contents

Chapter 3

Lids/Lashes/Lacrimal,   45

Chapter 4

Conjunctiva/Sclera,   89

Chapter 6

Anterior Chamber,   170

C h a p t e r 7

Iris/Pupils,   187

Chapter 8

Lens,   217

Chapter 9

Vitreous,   240

Chapter 1 0

Retina/Choroid,   246

Chapter 11

Optic Nerve/Glaucoma,   344

Chapter 1 2

Visual Acuity/Refractive/Sudden Visual Loss,   371

Figure Credit Lines

The following illustrations are courtesy of Massachusetts Eye and Ear Infirmary: 1–1, 1–2, 1–3, 1–4, 1–5, 1–6, 1–7, 1–8, 1–10, 1–11, 1–12, 1–13, 1–14, 1–15, 1–16, 1–17, 1–22, 2–1, 2–2, 2–3, 2–6, 2–7, 2–8, 2–11, 2–14, 2–15, 2–16, 3–4, 3–5, 3–6, 3–7, 3–9, 3–10, 3–13, 3–14, 3–16, 3–20, 3–29, 3–31, 3–33, 3–38, 3–39, 3–40, 3–41, 4–2, 4–3, 4–4, 4–6, 4–7, 4–8, 4–9, 4–11, 4–12, 4–13, 4–14, 4–15, 4–17, 4–18, 4–20, 4–21, 4–22, 4–23, 4–24, 4–26, 4–27, 4–28, 4–29, 4–32, 4–36, 4–37, 4–38, 4–41, 4–42, 4–44, 4–45, 4–46, 4–48, 5–1, 5–2, 5–3, 5–11, 5–12, 5–13, 5–14, 5–15, 5–16, 5–17, 5–18, 5–21, 5–22, 5–23, 5–27, 5–28, 5–30, 5–32, 5–33, 5–34, 5–38, 5–41, 5–44, 5–45, 5–47, 5–49, 5–55, 5–56, 5–57, 5–59, 5–62, 5–64, 5–66, 5–67, 5–68, 5–69, 5–70, 5–72, 6–2, 6–3, 6–7, 6–8, 6–11, 7–1, 7–2, 7–3, 7–6, 7–9, 7–11, 7–15, 7–18, 7–20, 7–21, 7–23, 7–26, 7–27, 7–28, 7–29, 7–30, 7–31, 7–32, 7–33, 7–35, 8–1, 8–3, 8–4, 8–5, 8–6, 8–7, 8–9, 8–10, 8–11, 8–13, 8–16, 8–25, 8–29, 8–30, 8–31, 8–33, 9–1, 9–2, 10–3, 10–12, 10–14, 10–16, 10–27, 10–28, 10–30, 10–34, 10–37, 10–39, 10–40, 10–41, 10–48, 10–49, 10–50, 10–51, 10–54, 10–56, 10–57, 10–58, 10–59, 10–62, 10–64, 10–65, 10–66, 10–71, 10–77, 10–78, 10–83, 10–84, 10–85, 10–86, 10–87, 10–89, 10–90, 10–93, 10–95, 10–101, 10–104, 10–107, 10–108, 10–113, 10–114, 10–115, 10–120, 10–122, 10–123, 10–124, 10–126, 10–129, 10–132, 11–2, 11–3, 11–5, 11–7, 11–8, 11–10, 11–17, 11–19, 11–20, 12–2, and 12–3.

The following illustrations are courtesy of New York Eye and Ear Infirmary: 3–2, 3–15, 3–24, 3–26, 3–28, 3–30, 3–32, 4–10, 4–25, 4–33, 4–34, 4–35, 4–40, 4–43, 4–47, 5–8, 5–9, 5–10, 5–29, 5–35, 5–37, 5–39, 5–42, 5–43, 5–46, 5–48, 7–4, 7–8, 7–10, 7–17, 8–8, 8–15, 8–18, 8–21, 8–23, 8–28, 9–3, 9–5, 10–2, 10–6, 10–7, 10–8, 10–11, 10–13, 10–15, 10–19, 10–31, 10–35, 10–43, 10–44, 10–53, 10–61, 10–63, 10–68, 10–76, 10–80, 10–81, 10–88, 10–91, 10–92, 10–94, 10–97, 10–98, 10–102, 10–106, 10–109, 10–112, 10–116, 10–117, 10–118, 10–129, 10–134, and 11–9.

The following illustrations are courtesy of Bascom Palmer Eye Institute: 3–18, 4–1, 4–31, 4–39, 4–49, 5–4, 5–7, 5–20, 5–26, 5–31, 5–36, 5–50, 5–51, 5–54, 5–58, 5–60, 5–63, 6–5, 6–6, 6–9, 6–10, 7–5, 7–7, 7–13, 7–14, 7–34, 8–2, 8–14, 8–22, 8–24, 8–26, 9–4, 10–1, 10–4, 10–5, 10–9, 10–10, 10–17, 10–18, 10–20, 10–21, 10–22, 10–23, 10–24, 10–25, 10–26, 10–29, 10–32, 10–33, 10–36, 10–38, 10–42, 10–45, 10–46, 10–47, 10–52, 10–55, 10–60, 10–67, 10–69, 10–70, 10–72, 10–73, 10–74, 10–75, 10–79, 10–82, 10–96, 10–99, 10–100, 10–103, 10–105, 10–110, 10–111, 10–119, 10–121, 10–125, 10–127, 10–128, 10–130, 10–131, 10–133, 10–135, 10–136, 10–137, 10–138, 10–139, 10–140, 10–141, 10–142, 10–143, 10–144, 11–11, 11–12, 11–14, 11–15, and 11–16.

The following illustrations are courtesy of Cullen Eye Institute: 5–61 and 11–13.

The following illustrations are courtesy of M. Bowes Hamill, M.D.: 3–1, 3–12, 4–5, 4–16, 4–19, 4–30, 4–50, 5–5, 5–6, 5–19, 5–65, 7–22, and 7–25.

The following illustrations are courtesy of Douglas D. Koch, M.D.: 5–24, 5–25, 5–52, 8–12, 8–17, 8–19, 8–20, 8–27, 8–32, 12–4, and 12–5.

The following illustrations are courtesy of Ronald L. Gross, M.D.: 5–53, 6–1, 6–4, 7–16, 7–19, 7–24, and 11–18.

The following illustrations are courtesy of Andrew G. Lee, M.D.: 2–12, 2–13, 2–17, 7–12, 11–1, 11–4, and 11–6.

The following illustration is courtesy of Richard A. Lewis, M.D.: 5–71.

The following illustrations are courtesy of James R. Patrinely, M.D.: 1–9, 1–19, 1–20, 1–21, 3–3, 3–8, 3–11, 3–19, 3–21, 3–22, 3–23, 3–25, 3–27, 3–34, 3–35, 3–36, and 3–37.

The following illustrations are courtesy of Paul G. Steinkuller, M.D.: 1–18, 2–4, 2–5, and 12–1.

The following illustrations are courtesy of Warren Chang, M.D.: 2–9 and 2–10.

The following illustration is courtesy of Alice Y. Matoba, M.D.: 3–17.

Chapter 1

External / Orbit

Trauma

Intraorbital Foreign Body: Retained orbital foreign body with or without associated ocular and optic nerve involvement. Organic and copper foreign bodies are poorly tolerated; brass and bronze (copper content <85%) are better tolerated; inert material such as aluminum, steel, iron, lead, glass, plastic, and stone are generally well tolerated (BBs are mostly lead with some iron). Patients are usually asymptomatic but may report pain or decreased vision. Signs include ecchymosis, lid edema and erythema, conjunctival laceration or hemorrhage, proptosis, limitation of ocular movements; may have positive relative afferent pupillary defect (RAPD); old orbital foreign bodies may have no signs. Prognosis is generally good if the globe and optic nerve are not affected.

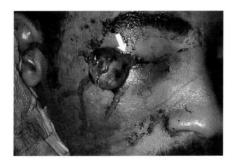 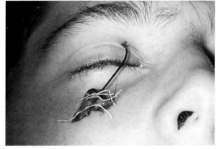

Figure 1–1. Traumatic avulsion of the globe; note optic nerve (arrow).

Figure 1–2. Intraorbital foreign body (fishhook).

- Orbital computed tomography (CT) to determine position of foreign body; magnetic resonance imaging (MRI) is contraindicated
- Consider B-scan ultrasonography if unable to visualize foreign body on CT scan
- Lab tests: culture if infection is suspected

1

- If there is no ocular or optic nerve injury, small inert foreign bodies are usually not removed but observed, with the patient on systemic antibiotics (amoxicillin/clavulanate [Augmentin] 500 mg PO tid for 10 days), with close follow-up the next day
- Tetanus booster (tetanus toxoid 0.5 mL IM) if necessary for prophylaxis (>10 years since last tetanus shot or if status is unknown)
- Indications for surgical removal include fistula formation, infection, optic nerve compression, intolerable foreign body, large foreign body, or easily removable foreign body (usually anterior to the equator of the globe); removal usually performed by orbital plastic surgeon
- Admit patient for systemic antibiotics after surgical removal (see Orbital Cellulitis section)

Orbital Contusion: Periocular bruising usually due to blunt trauma; often with associated injury to the globe, adjacent adnexa, sinuses, and bony socket; the globe and optic nerve may be severely damaged by compressive or contre-coup forces; may have orbital hemorrhage. Patients report pain and decreased vision. Signs include lid edema and ecchymosis, ptosis, limitation of ocular movements. Usually resolves without sequelae if other structures are not involved.

- Orbital CT scan if findings suggest orbital fracture, foreign body, open globe, or retrobulbar hemorrhage
- When the globe is intact and vision unaffected, ice compresses for 15 minutes three times a day for 36 hours to decrease swelling
- Systemic nonsteroidal anti-inflammatory drugs (ibuprofen 400–600 mg PO q4h)
- If other ocular structures are involved, treat accordingly

Orbital Fractures: Fracture of the orbital bones often with concomitant ocular, optic nerve, paranasal sinus, or intracranial injuries. Several types of fractures exist; orbital apex and large orbital roof fractures have a worse prognosis.

Le Fort I: Involves low transverse maxillary bone; no orbital involvement.

Le Fort II: Involves nasal, lacrimal, and maxillary bones (medial orbital wall); may involve nasolacrimal duct.

Le Fort III: Involves orbital floor, lateral and medial wall (craniofacial dysjunction); may involve optic canal.

Medial Orbit: Involves maxilla, lacrimal, and ethmoid bones; associated with depressed nasal bridge, traumatic telecanthus, and orbital floor fracture; complications include severe epistaxis due to anterior ethmoidal artery damage, cerebrospinal fluid (CSF) rhinorrhea, lacrimal system injury, and orbit and lid emphysema.

Orbital Apex: Usually associated with other facial fractures; may involve optic canal and superior orbital fissure; complications include CSF leaks and carotid-cavernous fistula; difficult to manage owing to proximity of structure to multiple cranial nerves and vessels.

Orbital Floor (Blow-Out Fracture): Usually involves maxillary bone and posterior medial floor (weakest point); orbital contents may prolapse or become entrapped in maxillary sinus; complications include diplopia on upgaze and downgaze, enophthalmos, globe ptosis, infraorbital nerve hypesthesia, and orbit and lid emphysema; may have associated medial wall fracture; indirect blow-out fractures usually do not involve orbital rim.

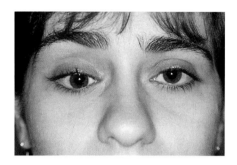

Figure 1–3. Orbital blow-out fracture with enophthalmos and globe dystopia of the right eye (OD).

Orbital Roof: Uncommon fracture from blunt or projectile injuries, may involve frontal sinus, cribriform plate, and brain; complications include CSF rhinorrhea and pneumocephalus.

Zygomatic (Tripod Fracture): Involves three articulations of the zygoma (zygomaticomaxillary suture, zygomaticofrontal suture, zygomatic arch) and the orbital floor; patients report pain, focal tenderness, binocular diplopia, and pain on opening mouth or chewing. Signs include orbital rim discontinuity or "step off," malar flattening, enophthalmos; infraorbital nerve hypesthesia; orbital, conjunctival, or lid emphysema; limitation of ocular movements; epistaxis; rhinorrhea; ecchymosis; and ptosis

- Orbital CT scan (axial and coronal images) better than radiographs; if CT scan unavailable, then perform orbital radiographs with Water's (orbital roof and floor) and Caldwell projections (orbital rim)
- Neurosurgical, otolaryngology, and oral maxillofacial consultation as needed
- **Medial Orbit:** Consider surgical repair if entrapment of medial rectus muscle exists
- **Orbital Apex:** Difficult to manage
  - Obvious bony impingement or optic canal fracture with optic nerve dysfunction requires immediate surgical intervention by an oculoplastic surgeon or neurosurgeon
  - High-dose systemic steroids (methylprednisolone 30 mg/kg IV initial dose for traumatic optic neuropathy); dose, length of treatment, and efficacy controversial
- **Orbital floor:** Instruct patient not to blow nose
  - Nasal decongestant (oxymetazoline HCl [Afrin nasal spray] bid for 10 days)
  - Ice compresses for 24–48 hours
  - Systemic antibiotics (amoxicillin/clavulanate [Augmentin] 250–500 mg PO tid for 10 days)
  - Consider surgical repair after 10–14 days for (1) diplopia within 30 degrees of primary gaze, (2) floor fracture >50% of area, or (3) >2 mm of unacceptable enophthalmos; should be performed by an oculoplastic surgeon

- **Orbital roof:** Requires neurosurgical management; check for rhinorrhea with CSF litmus paper
- **Zygomatic:** No treatment required if not displaced
  - Open reduction with interosseous wiring or mini-plate fixation if displaced; treat any associated floor fracture

Orbital Hemorrhage (Retrobulbar): Accumulation of blood within the orbit from surgery or trauma (orbital compartment syndrome) causing compression of the globe and orbital structures (optic nerve). Patients report pain and decreased vision. Signs include bullous subconjunctival hemorrhage, tense orbit, proptosis, resistance to retropulsion of globe, limitation of ocular movements, lid ecchymosis, and increased intraocular pressure. Immediate recognition and treatment are critical in determining outcome.

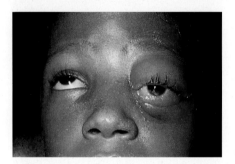

Figure 1–4. Retrobulbar hemorrhage of the left eye; note inability to look up.

OPHTHALMIC EMERGENCY:

- Orbital CT scan once visual status has been determined
- If vision is stable and intraocular pressure is <30 mm Hg, then lower intraocular pressure with systemic acetazolamide (Diamox; 500 mg PO), topical apraclonidine (q15 minutes × 2), and topical β-blocker (timolol 0.5% q15 minutes × 2); add a hyperosmotic agent if necessary (glycerin [Osmoglyn] 500 mL PO or mannitol 20% 1–2 g/kg IV over 1 hour)
- If vision is decreased and intraocular pressure is >30 mm Hg, then perform immediate lateral canthotomy and cantholysis. The lateral canthotomy is performed by compressing the lateral canthus for 30 seconds with a hemostat. Stevens or Westcott scissors are then used to make a lateral incision approximately 10–12 mm long 15 degrees below the horizontal of the lateral canthus. After separation of the conjunctiva and skin, the scissors are then used to cut the inferior crus of the lateral canthal tendon. If the inferior eyelid is not free or mobile, the inferior crus is only partially cut or not cut at all, then the procedure should be reattempted. If the intraocular pressure is still elevated, the superior crus of the lateral canthal tendon should be cut. Finally, if the globe is still tense, an emergent inferior orbital floor decompression can be performed using the hemostat. Pressure is used to control bleeding. The canthotomy and cantholysis can be repaired in 2–3 days.

Carotid Cavernous Fistula

Spontaneous high-flow fistula formation between the cavernous sinus and internal carotid artery (carotid-cavernous fistula). Usually occurs in patients with atherosclerosis and hypertension; can also be due to trauma (basal skull fracture). Patients often hear a "swishing" noise (venous souffle). Signs may include orbital bruit, pulsating proptosis, chemosis, epibulbar injection and vascular tortuosity (corkscrew vessels), congested retinal vessels, and increased intraocular pressure. Alternatively, small meningeal arterial branches may cause low-flow fistula formation with the dural walls of the cavernous sinus (dural-sinus fistula); slower onset compared to the carotid-cavernous variant with only mild proptosis and orbital congestion, often with spontaneous closure.

- Orbital CT scan or MRI: enlargement of superior ophthalmic vein
- Arteriography is usually required to identify the fistula

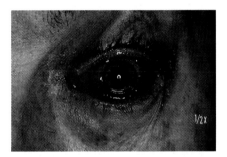

Figure 1–5. Carotid-cavernous fistula with conjunctival injection and chemosis.

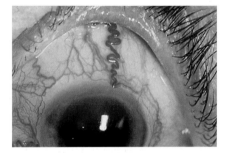

Figure 1–6. Carotid-cavernous fistula with dilated, corkscrew, episcleral and conjunctival vessels.

- Consider treatment with selective embolization or ligation for severely symptomatic patients

Phthisis Bulbi

Progressive functional decompensation, after either accidental or surgical trauma, through a degenerative process, the endstage of which is called phthisis bulbi. Three stages exist: (1) atrophia bulbi without shrinkage: globe shape and size are normal, but with cataract, retinal detachment, synechiae, and/or cyclitic membrane; (2) atrophia bulbi with shrinkage: soft and smaller globe with decreased intraocular pressure, collapse of the anterior chamber, edematous cornea with vascularization, fibrosis, and opacification; (3) atrophia bulbi with disorganization (phthisis bulbi): globe approximately two-thirds normal size with thickened sclera, intraocular disorganization, and calcification of cornea, lens, and retina. Bone may be present in the uveal tract. These eyes usually have no vision, spontaneous hemorrhages or inflammation can occur, and they carry an increased risk of intraocular malignancies.

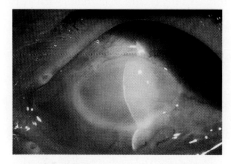

Figure 1–7. Phthisis bulbi.

- B-scan ultrasonography should be performed annually to rule out intraocular malignancy
- Topical steroid (prednisolone acetate 1% qid) and cycloplegic (atropine 1% tid) for pain
- Consider retrobulbar alcohol or chlorpromazine (Thorazine) injection for severe ocular pain
- May require enucleation for blind, painful eye if medical therapy fails

Idiopathic Orbital Inflammation (IOI) (Orbital Pseudotumor)

Definition

Acute or chronic idiopathic inflammatory disorder of the orbital tissues sometimes collectively termed orbital pseudotumor. Tolosa-Hunt syndrome is a form of orbital pseudotumor involving the orbital apex and/or cavernous sinus that produces a painful ophthalmoplegia.

Epidemiology

Occurs in all age groups; bilateral disease is common in children; bilateral disease in adults requires evaluation for systemic vasculitis (eg, Wegener's granulomatosis, polyarteritis nodosa) or lymphoproliferative disorders.

Symptoms

Acute onset of orbital pain, decreased vision, binocular diplopia, red-eye, headaches, and constitutional symptoms (constitutional symptoms are present in 50% of children with idiopathic orbital inflammation).

Signs

Lid edema and erythema, lacrimal gland enlargement, limitation of extraocular movements, proptosis, decreased orbital retropulsion, induced hyperopia, chemosis, reduced corneal sensation (due to cranial nerve V_1 involvement), increased intraocular pressure; papillitis or iritis may occur in children.

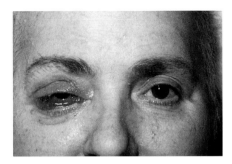

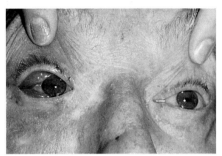

Figure 1–8. Idiopathic orbital inflammation affecting the right orbit.

Figure 1–9. Idiopathic orbital inflammation with lacrimal gland involvement.

Differential Diagnosis

Thyroid ophthalmopathy, orbital cellulitis, orbital tumors, lacrimal gland tumors, orbital vasculitis, trauma, phycomycosis, arteriovenous fistula, cavernous sinus thrombosis, cranial nerve palsy.

Evaluation

- Complete ophthalmic history with attention to previous episodes and history of cancer or other systemic disease
- Complete eye exam with attention to pupils, motility, Hertel exophthalmometry, lids, cornea, tonometry, and ophthalmoscopy
- Lab tests for bilateral or unusual cases (vasculitis suspected): complete blood count (CBC) with differential, erythrocyte sedimentation rate (ESR), antinuclear antibodies (ANA), blood urea nitrogen (BUN), creatinine, fasting blood glucose, antineutrophil cytoplasmic antibodies (ANCA), and urinalysis
- Orbital CT scan: thickened, enhancing sclera (ring sign), extraocular muscle enlargement with involvement of the tendons, and/or lacrimal gland involvement
- Consider orbital biopsy for steroid-unresponsive or unusual cases

Management

- Systemic steroids (prednisone 80–100 mg PO qd for 1–2 weeks, then taper slowly); check purified protein derivative (PPD), blood glucose, and chest radiographs before starting systemic steroids

Management Continued

- Add H$_2$-blocker (ranitidine HCl [Zantac] 150 mg PO bid) when giving systemic steroids
- Low-dose orbital radiotherapy in non–steroid-responsive or steroid-intolerant individuals; orbital biopsy should be performed in steroid-resistant patients to establish diagnosis prior to radiotherapy
- Consider immunosuppressive therapy (cyclophosphamide); should be administered by a specialist trained in inflammatory diseases
- Orbital decompression is rarely indicated and only considered in the presence of compressive optic neuropathy

Prognosis

Generally good for acute disease although recurrence is common. The sclerosing form of this disorder has a more insidious onset and is often less responsive to treatment.

Thyroid Ophthalmopathy (Graves' Orbitopathy)

Definition

An immune-mediated disorder linked to the thyroid gland, causing a spectrum of ocular abnormalities.

Epidemiology

Most common cause of unilateral or bilateral proptosis in adults; female predilection (8:1); 80% of patients have abnormal thyroid function tests; hyperthyroidism (particularly Graves' disease) is the most common state, but patients may be euthyroid or even hypothyroid; associated with myasthenia gravis.

Symptoms

Asymptomatic; may have red-eye, foreign body sensation, tearing, decreased vision, dyschromatopsia, diplopia; may notice prominent ("bulging") eyes.

Signs

Proptosis, lid lag (von Graefe's sign), lid retraction, lid edema, lagophthalmos, reduced blinking, limitation of extraocular movements (most commonly involved extraocular muscle is inferior rectus, then medial rectus), resistance to retropulsion of globe, scleral show, conjunctival injection, corneal exposure with superficial punctate keratopathy (especially inferiorly); may have decreased visual acuity and color vision, positive RAPD, and visual field defect if optic nerve compression (<5%).

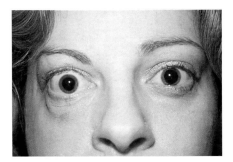 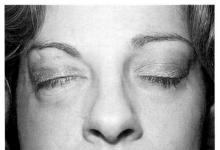

Figure 1–10. Thyroid ophthalmopathy with proptosis, lid retraction, and scleral show of the right eye.

Figure 1–11. Same patient as shown in Figure 1–10, demonstrating lagophthalmos of the right eye on eyelid closure.

Differential Diagnosis

Myasthenia gravis, idiopathic orbital inflammation, retrobulbar mass, orbital and lacrimal gland tumors, orbital vasculitis, trauma, phycomycosis, arteriovenous fistula, cavernous sinus thrombosis, gaze palsy, dorsal midbrain syndrome, aberrant regeneration of cranial nerve III.

Evaluation

- Complete ophthalmic history with attention to history of thyroid disease or cancer
- Complete eye exam with attention to cranial nerves, acuity, color vision, pupils, motility, forced ductions, lids, Hertel exophthalmometry, cornea, tonometry, and ophthalmoscopy
- Check visual fields if compressive optic neuropathy is suspected
- Lab tests: thyroid function tests (thyroid stimulating hormone [TSH], thyroxine [total and free T_4], and triiodothyronine [T_3])
- Orbital CT scan: extraocular muscle enlargement with sparing of the tendons (tendons are involved in idiopathic orbital inflammation)
- Medical consultation

Management

- Topical lubrication with nonpreserved artificial tears (see Appendix) up to q1h and ointment (Refresh P.M.) at bedtime if signs of exposure keratopathy exist
- Consider lid taping or goggles at bedtime, punctal occlusion, tarsorrhaphy if exposure symptoms are severe
- Consider lateral tarsorrhaphy, systemic steroids (prednisone 80–100 mg PO qd for 2–3 days), and orbital decompression for progressive corneal exposure and eyelid retraction

Management Continued

- Systemic steroids (prednisone 80–100 mg PO qd for 1–2 weeks, then taper) for acute diplopia and congestive orbitopathy; may benefit from prism glasses
- Immediate treatment with systemic steroids (prednisone 100 mg PO qd for 2–7 days), radiotherapy (15–30 Gy), and/or posterior orbital decompression for compressive optic neuropathy
- Consider muscle surgery, orbital decompression, and/or lid surgery as clinical situation dictates; should be performed by an oculoplastic surgeon; if multiple treatments are required, the recommended order is: (1) ocular lubrication, (2) systemic steroids, (3) orbital decompression, (4) extraocular muscle surgery, (5) eyelid recession, and (6) orbital radiotherapy
- Treat underlying thyroid disease (treatment of systemic disease does not have any effect on ocular abnormalities)

Prognosis

Generally good; may require multiple surgeries if extensive orbital involvement exists.

Acne Rosacea

Rosacea is an idiopathic, chronic midline facial inflammatory disorder of adults with frequent ocular manifestations (>50% of patients with rosacea develop ocular involvement); slight female predilection, but men are affected more severely. Patients are often of Northern European descent and have erythema, pustules, papules, and telangiectasis of the nose, chin, forehead and cheeks; rhinophyma occurs late. Common ocular findings include blepharitis, chalazia, conjunctival injection, and keratoconjunctivitis sicca; may develop superficial punctate keratitis, sterile peripheral infiltrates, corneal neovascularization, corneal thinning, and even corneal perforation. Rosacea is a clinical diagnosis.

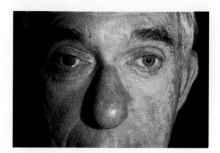

Figure 1–12. Acne rosacea demonstrating malar and brow distribution and bulbous nose.

- Treat with systemic antibiotics (tetracycline 250 mg PO qid or doxycycline 50–100 mg PO bid for 4–6 weeks, then taper to qd maintenance dose indefinitely)
- Topical metronidazole (Metrogel) is also effective for facial skin eruptions
- Lid hygiene and warm compresses for blepharitis and meibomitis (see Chap. 3)
- Consider topical steroid (prednisolone acetate 1% qid for 1–2 weeks) for moderate to severe rosacea keratitis with corneal neovascularization

Preseptal Cellulitis

Definition

Infection and inflammation located anterior to the orbital septum and limited to the superficial periorbital tissues and eyelids; the globe is not involved.

Etiology

Usually follows periorbital trauma or dermal infection; suspect *Staphylococcus aureus* in traumatic cases, and *Haemophilus influenzae* in children <5 years old.

Symptoms

Lid edema, erythema, and pain; low-grade fever.

Signs

Normal visual acuity; full ocular motility without pain; lid edema, erythema, and tenderness; no proptosis; may have skin wound.

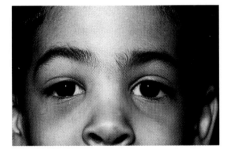 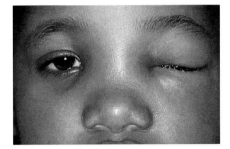

Figure 1–13. Preseptal cellulitis with mild right lid erythema.

Figure 1–14. Preseptal cellulitis with left lid edema and erythema.

Differential Diagnosis

Orbital cellulitis, idiopathic orbital inflammation, orbital tumors, lacrimal gland tumors, conjunctivitis, trauma.

Evaluation

- Complete ophthalmic history with attention to trauma, sinus disease, recent dental work or infections, history of diabetes or immunosuppression
- Complete eye exam with attention to acuity, color vision, pupils, motility, Hertel exophthalmometry, lids, conjunctiva, cornea, and ophthalmoscopy
- Check vital signs, head and neck lymph nodes, meningeal signs (nuchal rigidity), and sensorium
- Orbital and sinus CT scan: paranasal sinus opacification
- Lab tests: CBC with differential, blood cultures; wound culture if appropriate

---

Management

- **Mild preseptal cellulitis:**
  - Systemic antibiotics (10-day course):
    - Amoxicillin/clavulanate (Augmentin; 250–500 mg PO tid) *or*
    - Cefaclor (Ceclor; 250–500 mg PO tid)
    - Trimethoprim/sulfamethoxazole ([Bactrim] 1 double-strength tablet PO bid) or erythromycin in penicillin-allergic patients
  - Warm compresses tid
  - Topical antibiotics (bacitracin or erythromycin ointment qid) for concurrent conjunctivitis
  - Consider surgical drainage of abscess (avoid orbital septum and levator aponeurosis)
- **Moderate to severe preseptal cellulitis:**
  - Systemic antibiotics:
    - Cefuroxime (1 g IV q8h)
    - Ampicillin/sulbactam (Unasyn; 1.5–3 g IV q6h)
  - Systemic intravenous treatment also indicated for septic patients, outpatient noncompliance, children <5 years old, and failed oral antibiotic treatment after 48 hours.
- Daily follow-up in both forms until improvement noted

Prognosis

Usually good when treated early.

Orbital Cellulitis

Definition

Infection posterior to the orbital septum, involving the globe.

Etiology

Often due to pre-existing paranasal sinusitis (particularly ethmoids); other causes include dacryocystitis, dacryoadenitis, dental or intracranial infections, trauma, and postorbital surgery; *Streptococcus* species and *Staphylococcus* species are common isolates; *Haemophilus influenzae* should be considered in children <5 years old. Fungi in the group Phycomycetes are the most common cause of fungal orbital infection (*Absidia, Mucor,* or *Rhizopus*), causing necrosis, vascular thrombosis, and orbital invasion; usually seen in patients with diabetes mellitus, metabolic acidosis, malignancy, or immunosuppression; can be fatal due to spread along ophthalmic artery to cranium.

Symptoms

Decreased vision, pain, red-eye, headache, and fever.

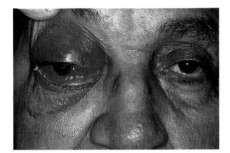

Figure 1–15. Orbital cellulitis.

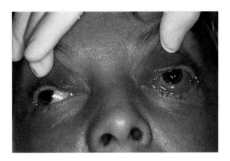

Figure 1–16. Mucormycosis; note inability to look right.

Signs

Decreased visual acuity, fever, lid edema, erythema, and tenderness; limitation of and/or painful ocular movements, proptosis (most common cause of proptosis in children), positive RAPD, conjunctival injection and chemosis, and optic disc swelling; fungal infection usually presents with proptosis and orbital apex syndrome (see Chap. 2).

Differential Diagnosis   *A Pseudotumor*

Thyroid ophthalmopathy, idiopathic orbital inflammation, orbital tumors, lacrimal gland tumors, orbital vasculitis, trauma, arteriovenous fistula, cavernous sinus thrombosis, cranial nerve palsy.

Evaluation

- Complete ophthalmic history with attention to trauma, sinus disease, recent dental work or infections, history of diabetes or immunosuppression
- Complete eye exam with attention to acuity, color vision, pupils, motility, Hertel exophthalmometry, conjunctiva, cornea, and ophthalmoscopy
- Check vital signs, head and neck lymph nodes, meningeal signs (nuchal rigidity), and sensorium
- Orbital and sinus CT scan: paranasal sinus opacification
- Lab tests: CBC with differential, blood cultures (usually negative in phycomycosis); wound culture if present; consider biopsy to rule out phycomycosis (nonseptate, branching hyphae)

Management

- Systemic antibiotics (1-week course):
    Nafcillin (1–2 g IV q4h) and Ceftriaxone (1–2 g IV q12–24h) *or*
    Ampillicin/sulbactam (Unasyn; 1.5–3 g IV q6h)
- Topical antibiotics (bacitracin or erythromycin ointment qid) for conjunctivitis or corneal exposure
- Surgical drainage of orbital or subperiosteal abscess if poor response to systemic antibiotics and no improvement on serial CT scans
- Consultation with otolaryngology specialist if sinus surgery necessary
- Daily follow-up required to monitor visual acuity, color vision (red desaturation), ocular movements, proptosis, intraocular pressure, cornea, and optic nerve
- Oral antibiotics (10-day course) after improvement on IV therapy:
    Amoxicillin/clavulanate (Augmentin; 250–500 mg PO tid) *or*
    Cefaclor (Ceclor; 250–500 mg PO tid)
    Trimethoprim/sulfamethoxazole (Bactrim 1 double-strength tablet PO bid) or erythromycin in penicillin-allergic patients
- **Phycomycosis:** may be fatal if not treated in 2 weeks
    - Local surgical excision of all necrotic tissue
    - Systemic antifungals (amphotericin B 0.25–1.0 mg/kg IV divided equally q6h); do not delay therapy to wait for biopsy or results
    - Management of the underlying medical disorder

Prognosis

Depends on organism and extent of inflammation; may develop orbital apex syndrome, cavernous sinus thrombosis, and/or meningitis, which produce permanent neurologic deficits; mucormycosis is potentially lethal.

Pediatric Orbital Tumors

Capillary Hemangioma: Common benign orbital hamartoma of infancy; appears as an enlarging, red, dimpled, nodular ("strawberry nevus") or blue eyelid mass that blanches with pressure; occurs in the first year of life and slowly involutes by 5 years of age; usually located superonasally; eyelid involvement may induce astigmatism or ptosis and cause anisometropia, strabismus, and/or amblyopia; may also cause proptosis with crying; may be associated with thrombocytopenia (Kasabach-Merritt syndrome) or high-output cardiac failure.

- Orbital CT scan: encapsulated or infiltrative mass
- No treatment recommended if mild and not involving globe
- If anisometropia, strabismus, or amblyopia exists, local steroid injection (triamcinolone acetonide 40 mg) is often first choice; consider systemic steroids, interferon, laser therapy, radiation therapy, or surgical excision; should be performed by an oculoplastic surgeon

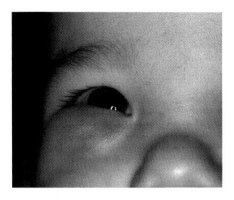

Figure 1–17. Capillary hemangioma involving right lower eyelid.

Dermoid Cyst: Common, benign, palpable, smooth, painless choristoma composed of connective tissue and containing dermal adnexal structures including sebaceous glands and hair follicles; usually manifests in childhood and may slowly enlarge; usually located superotemporally; may be anterior or posterior to orbital septum, often adjacent to orbital bony suture lines (eg, zygomaticofrontal).

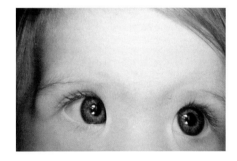

Figure 1–18. Dermoid cyst of the right eye; also note epicanthus causing pseudostrabismus.

- Orbital CT scan: well circumscribed mass with bony molding
- Complete surgical excision should be performed by an oculoplastic surgeon; avoid rupturing cyst to prevent acute inflammatory process

Juvenile Xanthogranuloma (JXG): Nevoxanthoendothelioma, composed of histiocytes and Touton giant cells, that rarely involves the orbit; presents between birth and 1 year of age; associated with yellow-orange cutaneous lesions, and may cause destruction of bone; spontaneous resolution often occurs

- No treatment recommended because spontaneous regression often occurs
- Consider local steroid injection (controversial)
- Surgical excision rarely indicated

Leukemia: Advanced leukemia, particularly the acute lymphocytic type, may present with proptosis; granulocytic sarcoma (chloroma), an uncommon subtype of myelogenous leukemia, may also produce orbital proptosis often prior to hematogenous or bone marrow signs; both forms usually occur in 1st decade.

- Pediatric consultation for systemic evaluation
- Treatment with systemic chemotherapy should be performed by a tumor specialist

Lymphangioma: Rare, benign, bluish choristoma characterized by lymphatic-filled spaces lined by flat endothelial cells; presents in the 1st year of life with an infiltrative growth pattern or with abrupt onset due to hemorrhage within the tumor ("chocolate cyst"); may enlarge during upper respiratory tract infections; strabismus and amblyopia are common complications; spontaneous regression often occurs.

- Orbital CT scan: infiltrative growth pattern
- Complete surgical excision indicated for ocular damage or severe cosmetic deformities; should be performed by an oculoplastic surgeon
- Orbital needle aspiration of hemorrhage or surgical exploration for acute orbital hemorrhage with compressive optic neuropathy; tumor reccurrence common

Neuroblastoma: Most common pediatric orbital metastatic tumor; occurs in children <7 years old; usually arises from a primary tumor in the abdomen, mediastinum, or neck; patients typically have sudden ecchymotic proptosis ("raccoon eyes") that may be bilateral; associated with lateral orbital wall destruction and displacement of the globe.

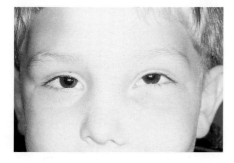

Figure 1–19. Neuroblastoma.

- Pediatric consultation for systemic evaluation
- Treatment with local radiotherapy and systemic chemotherapy should be performed by a tumor specialist

Rhabdomyosarcoma: Most common primary pediatric orbital malignancy and most common pediatric soft tissue malignancy; 90% of cases occur in patients <15 years old, usually between 7 and 8 years of age; male predilection; presents with rapid onset of unilateral proptosis, eyelid edema, and discoloration; may have history of trauma; predilection for superonasal orbit; CT scan commonly demonstrates bony orbital destruction; arises from primitive mesenchyme, not extraocular muscles; biopsy necessary for diagnosis; histologically four forms: (1) alveolar (most malignant, worst prognosis, inferior orbit, second most common); (2) botryoid (grape-like with spread from paranasal sinus involvement); (3) embryonal (most common); and (4) pleomorphic (rarest, most differentiated, seen in older patients, best prognosis); 90–95% 5-year survival rate if limited to orbit.

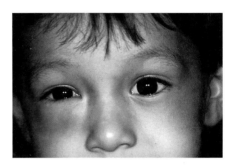

Figure 1–20. Rhabdomyosarcoma of the right eye.

- Emergent diagnostic biopsy with immunohistochemical staining in all cases; should be coordinated with pediatric oncologist
- Pediatric consultation for systemic evaluation
- Treatment with local radiotherapy (45–60 Gy over 6 weeks) and systemic chemotherapy should be performed by a tumor specialist

Adult Orbital Tumors

Cavernous Hemangioma: Most common benign adult orbital tumor; usually occurs in 30- to 50-year-old females; signs include slowly progressive proptosis and compressive optic neuropathy; may have induced hyperopia, strabismus, increased intraocular pressure, and chorioretinal folds; may enlarge during pregnancy.

- A-scan ultrasonography: high internal reflectivity
- Orbital CT scan: well-circumscribed intraconal lesion
- Orbital MRI: tumor appears hypointense on T1- and hyperintense on T2-weighted images
- Complete surgical excision indicated for compressive optic neuropathy; should be performed by an oculoplastic surgeon

Fibrous Histiocytoma: Most common mesenchymal orbital tumor; firm, well-defined lesion that is usually located in the superonasal quadrant; occurs in middle-aged adults; less than 10% have metastatic potential; often confused with hemangiopericytoma; histologically, cells have a cartwheel or storiform pattern.

- Complete surgical excision should be performed by an oculoplastic surgeon; recurrence is often more aggressive with possible malignant transformation

Fibro-Osseous Tumors: Fibrous dysplasia (nonmalignant bony proliferation often involving single or multiple facial and orbital bones, seen in Albright's syndrome); osteoma (benign bone tumor frequently involving frontal and ethmoidal sinuses); other tumors include chondrosarcoma, osteosarcoma, cholesterol granuloma, and aneurysmal bone cyst.

- Osteoma can usually be completely excised; others require systemic therapy; should be performed by a tumor specialist

Histiocytic Tumors: Rare group of tumors composed of Langerhans' cell histiocytosis; several types including eosinophilic granuloma (best prognosis), Hand-Schüller-Christian disease (rare; classic triad of proptosis, lytic skull lesions, and diabetes insipidus), and Letterer-Siwe disease (occurs in infancy with systemic spread, worst prognosis); electron microscopy reveals characteristic Birbeck's (Langerhans') granules.

- Local incision and curettage, intralesional steroid injection, or radiotherapy for eosinophilic granuloma
- Systemic corticosteroids and chemotherapy for Hand-Schüller-Christian disease and Letterer-Siwe disease

Lymphoid Tumors: Occurs in patients 50–70 years old, rare in children; spectrum of disease from benign reactive lymphoid hyperplasia and atypical lymphoid hyperplasia to malignant lymphoma. The former is a benign local tumor of unknown etiology composed of mature lymphocytes (T-helper cells predominate) and reactive germinal centers, while the latter may be focal or systemic with atypical or immature lymphocytes (monoclonal B-cells predominate), mitotic figures, nuclear cleavage, and a follicular or diffuse pattern. Lymphoid lesions cause painless proptosis with associated conjunctival, epibulbar, or lacrimal gland lesions (40% in palpebral lobe); orbital lesions usually involve superior orbit behind the septum; may have strabismus or visual abnormalities; extraorbital spread occurs in 50% of poorly differentiated tumors; requires tissue biopsy for diagnosis.

- Orbital CT scan: infiltrative but molding solid tumor; bony changes are usually absent (cannot distinguish among the various types)
- Tissue biopsy and immunohistochemical studies on fresh specimens required for diagnosis
- Hematology and oncology consultation for systemic evaluation
- Lab tests: CBC with differential, serum protein electrophoresis, ANA, rheumatoid factor (RF), erythrocyte sedimentation rate (ESR), bone marrow biopsy, chest and abdominal CT scan, bone scan
- Low-dose, fractionated radiotherapy for localized orbital lesions (15–20 Gy for benign lesions; 20–30 Gy for malignancy) and chemotherapy with or without adjunctive ocular radiotherapy for systemic disease; should be performed by a tumor specialist

Metastatic Tumors: 10% of orbital tumors, most commonly breast and lung (bronchogenic) cancer; prostate and gastrointestinal cancers also metastasize to orbit; patients have rapid-onset, painful proptosis, limitation of extraocular movements, inflammation, and bony erosion; scirrhous breast cancer may cause enophthalmos owing to orbital fibrosis.

- Local radiotherapy for palliative therapy should be performed by a tumor specialist; carcinoid may be treated with wide orbital excision
- Hematology and oncology consultation

Mucocele: Cystic sinus mass due to obstructed excretory ducts, lined by pseudostratified ciliated columnar epithelium and filled with mucoid material; may invade the orbit wall through bony erosion; patients usually have a history of chronic sinusitis (frontal and ethmoidal sinuses); associated with cystic fibrosis; must be differentiated from encephalocele and meningocele.

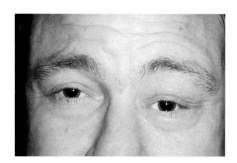

Figure 1–21. Mucocele with globe dystopia of the left eye.

- Head and orbital CT scan: orbital lesion and orbital wall defect with sinus opacification
- Complete surgical excision should be performed by an oculoplastic surgeon; add pre- and postoperative systemic antibiotics (ampillicin/sulbactam [Unasyn] 1.5–3 g IV q6h)

Neurilemoma (Schwannoma): Rare tumor (1% of all orbital tumors) that occurs in young to middle-aged individuals; patients have gradual proptosis and downward globe displacement; associated with neurofibromatosis type 1; histologic exam demonstrates two patterns of Schwann cell proliferation enveloped by perineurium: Antoni A (solid, nuclear palisading Verocay bodies) and Antoni B (loose, myxoid areas).

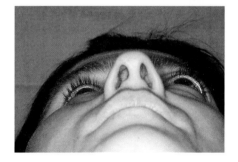

Figure 1–22. Neurilemoma (Schwannoma) producing proptosis of the left eye.

- Orbital CT scan: well-circumscribed partially cystic lesion
- Complete surgical excision should be performed by an oculoplastic surgeon; recurrence and malignant transformation are rare

Ocular Motility / Cranial Nerves

Strabismus

Definition

Ocular misalignment, which may be congenital or acquired; horizontal or vertical; comitant (same angle of deviation in all positions of gaze) or incomitant (angle of deviation varies in different positions of gaze).

Esotropia (ET): Eye turns inward; most common ocular deviation (>50%).

Congenital: Presents by age 6 months with a large, constant angle of deviation (80% >50 prism diopters [PD]); normal refractive error; positive family history is common; may be associated with inferior oblique overaction, dissociated vertical deviation (DVD), latent nystagmus, and persistent smooth pursuit asymmetry.

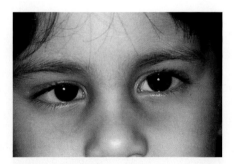

Figure 2–1. Esotropia of the right eye.

- Treat amblyopia with occlusive therapy of fixating/dominant eye (see later) before performing surgery
- Correct any hyperopia >+3.00 diopters (D)
- Muscle surgery should be performed early (6 months to 2 years): bilateral medial rectus recession or unilateral recession of medial rectus and resection of lateral rectus; most require more than one surgery to correct

Accommodative: Develops between age 6 months and 6 years of age, usually around age 2 1/2, with variable angle of deviation (eyes straight as infant because they do not accommodate); initially intermittent when child is tired or sick; three types:

Refractive: Usually hyperopic (average +4.75D), normal accommodative convergence/accommodation (AC/A) ratio (4–6 PD), esotropia at distance (ET) similar to that at near (ET′); (ET = ET′)

Nonrefractive: high AC/A ratio; esotropia at near greater than at distance (ET′ > ET)

Mixed: Not correctable with refraction or bifocals

- Give full cycloplegic refraction if child is <6 years old, and as much as tolerated if >6 years old; if esotropia corrects to within 8 PD, then no further treatment necessary
- With high AC/A ratio and residual ET′, prescribe executive-style, flat-top bifocal segment that bisects the pupil (+2.50D to +3.00D) or try miotics, especially in infants too young for glasses (echothiophate iodide 0.125% qd; be careful not to use with succinylcholine for general anesthesia); both can be used in refractory cases
- Muscle surgery as above should be performed if residual esotropia >10 PD

Nonaccommodative: Due to stress, sensory deprivation, divergence insufficiency (ET ≥ ET′), spasm of near reflex, consecutive (after exotropia surgery), or cranial nerve VI palsy.

- Usually no treatment required; muscle surgery can be considered in symptomatic refractory cases

Cyclic: Very rare form (1:3000); occurs between 2 and 6 years of age; child is usually orthophoric (eyes straight) but develops esotropia for 24- to 48-hour periods; can progress to constant esotropia.

- Correct any hyperopia > +3.00D
- Muscle surgery as above can be performed when deviation stabilizes

Exotropia (XT): Eye turns outward; may be intermittent (usually at age 2 years, amblyopia rare) or constant (rarely congenital, consecutive [after esotropia surgery], due to decompensated intermittent XT or from sensory deprivation [in children >5 years of age]); amblyopia rare due to formation of anomalous retinal correspondence.

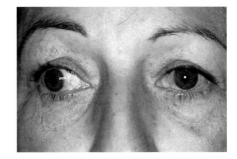

Figure 2–2. Exotropia of the right eye.

Basic: Exotropia at distance (XT) equal to that at near (XT′); normal AC/A ratio, normal fusional convergence.

Convergence Insufficiency: Inability to maintain convergence as object is brought in from distance to near (increased near point of convergence); exotropia at near greater than at distance (XT′ > XT); reduced fusional convergence amplitudes; rare before 10 years of age; slight female predilection; symptoms often begin during teen years with asthenopia, difficulty reading, blurred near vision, diplopia, and fatigue; may be associated with accommodative insufficiency, ciliary body dysfunction, and head trauma.

- Orthoptic exercises: near-point pencil push-ups (bring pencil in slowly from distance until breakpoint reached, then repeat 10–15 times) or prism convergence exercises (increase amount of base-out prism until breakpoint reached, then repeat starting with low prism power, 10–15 times)
- Muscle surgery: bilateral medial rectus resection (rarely required)

Pseudo-Divergence Excess: XT > XT′ except after prolonged patching (patch test) when near deviation increases (full latent deviation); near deviation also increases with +3.00D lens; may have high AC/A ratio.

True Divergence Excess: XT > XT′ even after patch test, may have high AC/A ratio.

- Correct any refractive error and add additional minus, especially with high AC/A ratio
- Consider base-in prism lenses
- Muscle surgery if the patient manifests exotropia >50% of the time and is >4 years old: bilateral lateral rectus recession; postoperative diplopia can be managed with prisms unless it lasts >8 weeks, then re-operate

Hypertropia (HT): Eye turns upward; vertical deviations are usually designated by the hypertropic eye, but if the process is clearly causing one eye to turn downward, this eye is designated hypotropic.

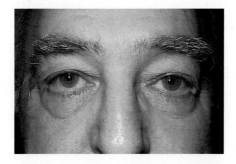

Figure 2–3. Hypertropia of the right eye.

A-pattern: Amount of horizontal deviation changes between upgaze (larger esotropia in upgaze) and downgaze (larger exotropia in downgaze); more common with exotropia; clinically significant if difference is ≥10 PD; associated with superior oblique muscle overaction; patients often have chin-up position.

- Muscle surgery if clinically significant: weakening of superior oblique muscles (bilateral superior oblique tenotomies) if overaction exists or transposition of horizontal muscles (medial recti moved up, lateral recti moved down) if no oblique overaction

V-pattern: Amount of horizontal deviation changes between upgaze (larger exotropia in upgaze) and downgaze (larger esotropia in downgaze); more common with esotropia; clinically significant if difference is ≥15 PD; associated with inferior oblique muscle overaction, increased lateral rectus muscle innervation, underaction of superior rectus muscle, Apert's syndrome, and Crouzon's syndrome; patients often have chin-down position.

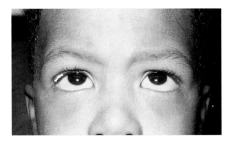

Figure 2–4. V-pattern esotropia demonstrating reduced esotropia in upgaze.

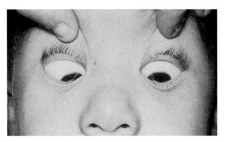

Figure 2–5. Same patient as shown in Figure 2–4, demonstrating increased esotropia in downgaze.

- Muscle surgery if deviation is clinically significant: weakening of inferior oblique muscles if overaction exists or transposition of horizontal muscles (medial recti moved down, lateral recti moved up) if no oblique overaction

Brown's Syndrome: Congenital or acquired anomaly of the superior oblique tendon sheath, causing an inability to elevate the affected eye especially in adduction; elevation in abduction is normal or slightly decreased; usually hypotropia with chin-up position; positive forced duction testing that is worse on retropulsion and when moving eye up and in (differentiates from inferior rectus restriction, which is worse with proptosing eye); V-pattern (differentiates from superior oblique overaction, which is A-pattern), no superior oblique overaction, downshoot in adduction, and widened palpebral fissures on adduction in severe cases; 10% bilateral, female predilection (3:2), and affects right eye (OD) more often than left eye (OS); acquired forms are associated with rheumatoid arthritis, juvenile rheumatoid arthritis, sinusitis, sinus surgery, muscle surgery, retinal detachment surgery, scleroderma, hypogammaglobulinemia, post partum, and trauma.

- No treatment usually required, especially for acquired forms, which often spontaneously improve
- Consider injection of steroids near trochlea or oral steroids if inflammatory etiology exists
- Muscle surgery for abnormal head position or large hypotropia in primary position: superior oblique muscle tenotomy/tenectomy or silicon rubber expander with or without ipsilateral inferior oblique muscle recession

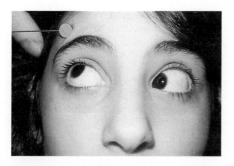

Figure 2–6. Brown's syndrome, demonstrating inability to elevate left eye in adduction.

Dissociated Vertical Deviation (DVD): Updrift and/or torsional movement of nonfixating eye when fixating eye is covered; Bielschowsky phenomenon (downdrift of occluded eye as increasing neutral density filters are placed over fixating eye); usually bilateral, asymmetric, and asymptomatic; does not obey Hering's law (equal innervation to yoke muscles); associated with congenital esotropia (75%) more than exotropia and with exotropia more than hypertropia; also seen with latent nystagmus and after esotropia surgery.

- No treatment usually required
- Muscle surgery if symptomatic: recession of superior rectus muscles. May be combined with posterior fixation of superior rectus or inferior rectus resection.

Duane's Retraction Syndrome: Congenital anomalous innervation of lateral rectus muscle by cranial nerve III due to agenesis of cranial nerve VI; 20% bilateral, female predilection (3:2), affects OS more often than OD (3:1); three types (1 more common than 3, and 3 more common than 2):

(1) limited abduction; esotropia in primary position
(2) limited adduction; exotropia in primary position
(3) limited abduction and adduction.

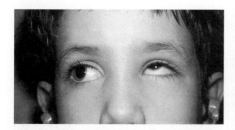

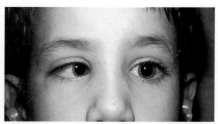

Figure 2–7. Duane's retraction syndrome type 3, demonstrating limited adduction, upshoot, and narrowing of the palpebral fissure of the left eye.

Figure 2–8. Same patient as shown in Figure 2–7, demonstrating limited abduction of the left eye.

Narrowing of palpebral fissure on adduction and widening on abduction in all 3 types; upshoots and downshoots (leash phenomenon) common; may have head-turn to fuse; amblyopia rare.

- No treatment usually required
- Muscle surgery if there is significant ocular misalignment in primary position, abnormal head position, or significant upshoot or downshoot: medial rectus muscle recession in type 1 or lateral rectus muscle recession in type 2; never perform lateral rectus muscle resection. Significant globe retraction: medial and lateral muscle recession. Leash phenomenon: split lateral rectus or tandem procedure.

Möbius' Syndrome: Congenital bilateral aplasia of cranial nerve VI and VII nuclei (cranial nerves V, IX, and XII may also be affected); inability to abduct either eye past midline; associated with esotropia, epiphora, exposure keratitis, and mask-like facies; patient may have limb deformities and/or absence of pectoralis muscle (Poland's syndrome). Can also get gaze palsies if paramedian pontine reticular formation (PPRF) involved.

Monocular Elevation Deficiency (Double Elevator Palsy): Supranuclear palsy causing total inability to elevate eye (may have good Bell's reflex); hypotropia in primary position, ptosis and pseudoptosis common, may have chin-up head position to fuse.

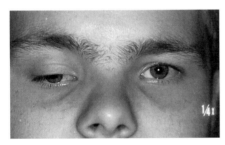 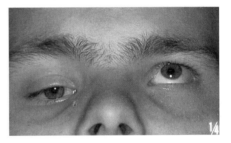

Figure 2–9. Monocular elevation deficiency (double elevator palsy) demonstrating ptosis and hypotropia of the right eye.

Figure 2–10. Same patient as shown in Figure 2–9 demonstrating inability to elevate right eye.

Restrictive: Various disorders that cause tethering of one or more extraocular muscles; restriction of eye movement in the direction of action of the affected muscle (these processes cause incomitant strabismus). Commonly seen in thyroid ophthalmopathy (see Chap. 1), orbital floor fracture (see Chap. 1), and congenital fibrosis syndrome.

Figure 2–11. Restrictive strabismus due to an orbital fracture of the left eye with inferior rectus entrapment; also note enophthalmos.

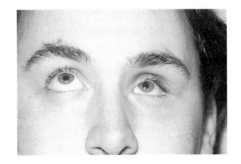

Five types of congenital fibrosis syndrome:

(1) Generalized fibrosis (autosomal dominant [AD] more common than autosomal recessive [AR], and AR more common than idiopathic): All muscles in both eyes affected, inferior rectus usually affected the worst
(2) Congenital fibrosis of inferior rectus: Only inferior rectus affected
(3) Strabismus fixus (sporadic): Horizontal muscles affected in both eyes; medial rectus more often than lateral rectus
(4) Vertical retraction syndrome: Vertical muscles affected in both eyes; superior rectus more often than inferior rectus
(5) Congenital unilateral fibrosis (sporadic): All muscles affected in one eye; also associated with enophthalmos and ptosis

Skew Deviation: Comitant or incomitant acquired vertical misalignment of the eyes due to supranuclear dysfunction from brain stem or cerebellar process; hypotropic eye is ipsilateral to lesion.

Symptoms

Asymptomatic; may have eye-turn, head-turn, head-tilt, decreased vision, diplopia (especially in adults), headaches, asthenopia, and eye fatigue.

Signs

Normal or decreased visual acuity (amblyopia), strabismus, limitation of ocular movements, reduced stereopsis; may have other ocular pathology (ie, cataract, aphakia, retinal detachment, optic atrophy, macular scar, phthisis) causing a secondary sensory strabismus (usually esotropia in children <5 years old, exotropia in older children and adults).

Differential Diagnosis

Pseudostrabismus (epicanthal fold), negative angle kappa (pseudo-esotropia), positive angle kappa (pseudo-exotropia), and secondary to dragged macula (eg, retinopathy of prematurity, toxocariasis), cranial nerve palsy, and myasthenia gravis.

Evaluation

■ Complete ophthalmic history and eye exam with attention to visual acuity (see Chap. 12 for age-adjusted eye charts), refraction, cycloplegic refraction, pupils, motility (versions, ductions, cover and alternate cover test), measure deviation (Hirschberg's, Krimsky's, and/or prism cover tests), measure torsional component (double Maddox rod test), stereopsis (Titmus stereoacuity test, Randot's Dot E stereotest), suppression/anomalous retinal correspondence (Worth's 4-dot, 4 PD base-out prism, Maddox rod, red glass, Bagolini's striated lens, and/or after-image tests), fusion (amblyoscope, Hess' screen tests), forced ductions, and ophthalmoscopy
■ Orbital computed tomography (CT) in cases of muscle restriction
■ Lab tests: thyroid function tests (triiodothyronine [T_3], thyroxine [T_4], thyrotropin [TSH]) in cases of muscle restriction, and anti-acetylcholine (ACh) receptor antibody titers if myasthenia gravis is suspected
■ Consider edrophonium chloride (Tensilon) test to rule out myasthenia gravis

- Neurology consultation if cranial nerves are involved
- Medical consultation for dysthyroid and myasthenia patients

Management

- Correct any refractive component
- In children, patching/occlusion therapy for amblyopia (see Chap. 12); initially patch dominant/fixating eye during all waking hours, then taper as amblyopia improves; timing of re-examination is based on patient's age (1 week per each year of age; eg, 2 weeks for 2-year-old, 4 weeks for 4-year-old; patching not recommended for infants less than 1 year old)
- Consider muscle surgery based on the indications outlined earlier

Prognosis

Usually good; depends on etiology.

Nystagmus

Definition

Involuntary, rhythmic oscillation of eyes; may be horizontal, vertical, rotary, or a combination; fast or slow; symmetric or asymmetric; pendular (equal speed in both directions) or jerk (direction designated by the fast phase component).

Etiology

Congenital: Nystagmus is different depending on gaze; may have null point (nystagmus slows or stops in certain eye positions); mapped to chromosome 6p.

Afferent/Sensory Deprivation Nystagmus: Pendular nystagmus due to sensory deprivation; associated with ocular albinism, aniridia, achromatopsia, congenital stationary night blindness, congenital optic nerve anomaly, Leber's congenital amaurosis, and congenital cataracts.

Efferent/Motor Nystagmus: Due to ocular motor disturbance; present at or shortly after birth, may be hereditary; usually horizontal; may have null point and head-turn (to move eyes in direction of null point); decreases with convergence and stops during sleep; same plane in all positions of gaze, no oscillopsia; may have head oscillations, a latent component, and inversion with horizontal optokinetic (OKN) testing.

Convergence-Retraction: Co-contraction of extraocular muscles causes jerk convergence-retraction of eyes, especially on convergence or upgaze; seen in dorsal midbrain syndrome; also associated with aqueductal stenosis, pinealoma, trauma, brain stem arteriovenous malformation, multiple sclerosis, or basilar artery cerebrovascular accident.

Dissociated: Nystagmus is different in the two eyes; usually due to posterior fossa disease.

Downbeat: Nystagmus with rapid downbeat and slow upbeat; null point is usually in upgaze; associated with cervicomedullary junctional lesions including Arnold-Chiari malformation, syringomyelia, multiple sclerosis, cerebrovascular accidents, and drug intoxication.

Drug-Induced: Associated with use of anticonvulsants (phenytoin, carbamazepine), barbiturates, tranquilizers, and phenothiazines; often gaze-evoked.

Latent: Bilateral jerk nystagmus when one eye is covered (jerk component away from covered eye) that resolves when eye is uncovered; form of congenital nystagmus; may be associated with congenital esotropia and dissociated vertical deviation (DVD); binocular visual acuity is better than monocular.

Nonspecific Gaze-Evoked: Nystagmus in direction of gaze, no nystagmus in primary position; often due to medications (anticonvulsants, sedatives) or brain stem or posterior fossa lesions.

Opsoclonus (Saccadomania): Rapid, unpredictable, multidirectional eye movements; absent during sleep; associated with neuroblastoma or after post-viral encephalopathies in children; seen with visceral carcinomas in adults.

Periodic Alternating: Very rare, horizontal jerk nystagmus with spontaneous direction changes every 60–90 seconds with 10- to 15-second periods of no nystagmus; cycling persists despite fixating on targets; may be congenital or due to vestibulocerebellar disease; also associated with cervicomedullary junction lesions; may respond to treatment with baclofen.

Physiologic: Occurs normally in a variety of situations including end gaze, optokinetic (OKN), caloric, and rotational.

See-Saw: One eye rises and incyclotorts while other eye falls and excyclotorts, then the process alternates; may have internuclear ophthalmoplegia (INO); usually due to suprasellar or diencephalon lesions; also after cerebrovascular accidents or trauma; or congenital.

Spasmus Nutans: Triad of nystagmus (monocular, asymmetric, fine, very rapid, horizontal, and variable), head-nodding, and torticollis (head-turning); develops between 4 and 12 months of age, disappears by 3 years of age; otherwise neurologically intact; similar eye movements can be seen with chiasmal gliomas; therefore, check relative afferent pupillary defect (RAPD) and optic nerve carefully and perform neuroimaging; spasmus nutans is a diagnosis of exclusion.

Upbeat: Nystagmus occurs in primary position; usually due to anterior vermis and lower brain stem lesion; also associated with Wernicke's syndrome or drug intoxication.

Vestibular: Usually horizontal with rotary component (fast component toward normal side, slow component toward abnormal side); may have associated vertigo, tinnitus, and deafness; due to lesion of end organ, peripheral nerve (fixation inhibits nystagmus), or central (fixation does not inhibit nystagmus).

Voluntary: Usually hysterical or malingering; unable to sustain nystagmus >30 seconds.

Symptoms

Asymptomatic, may have decreased vision, oscillopsia (in acquired nystagmus), and other neurologic deficits.

Signs

Variable decreased visual acuity, ocular oscillations; may have better near than distance visual acuity, astigmatism, head-turn, other ocular or systemic pathology (eg, aniridia, bilateral media opacities, macular scars, optic atrophy, foveal hypoplasia, albinism).

Differential Diagnosis

See above; multiple sclerosis.

Evaluation

- Complete ophthalmic history, with attention to drug or toxin ingestion, and eye exam, with attention to monocular and binocular visual acuity, retinoscopy, pupils, motility, and ophthalmoscopy
- Neurology consultation
- Head CT scan or magnetic resonance imaging (MRI) to rule out intracranial process

Management

- No effective treatment in most forms
- Consider baclofen (5–80 mg PO tid) for periodic alternating nystagmus
- Consider muscle surgery with Kestenbaum's procedure for congenital nystagmus if patient has head-turn to keep eyes in null point
- Discontinue inciting agent if condition is due to drug or toxin ingestion

Prognosis

Usually benign; depends on etiology.

Third Nerve Palsy

Definition

Paresis of cranial nerve (CN) III (oculomotor) caused by a variety of processes anywhere along its course from the midbrain to the orbit; can be complete or partial (superior division innervates superior rectus and levator; inferior division innervates medial rectus, inferior rectus, inferior oblique, and parasympathetic fibers to iris sphincter and ciliary muscle); can be isolated with or without pupil involvement.

Etiology

Depends on age: Congenital due to birth trauma or neurologic syndrome; in children due to infection, post-viral illness, trauma, or tumors (pontine glioma); in adults, most commonly due to ischemia or microvascular problems (20–45%; eg, hypertension or diabetes mellitus); also associated with aneurysm (15–20%), trauma (10–15%), and tumors (10–15%); 10–30% are of undetermined cause; rarely associated with ophthalmoplegic migraine. Aberrant regeneration may occur after intracavernous aneurysm, trauma, and tumors, but never after ischemic or microvascular causes; pupil-sparing usually microvascular or ischemic (80% are pupil-sparing); 95% of compressive lesions involve the pupil; important to localize level of pathology:

Nuclear: Very rare, usually due to microvascular infarctions; signs include bilateral ptosis and contralateral superior rectus involvement

Fascicular: Usually due to vascular or metastatic lesions; associated with several syndromes including Benedikt's syndrome (CN III palsy with contralateral hemitremor, hemiballismus, and loss of sensation), Nothnagel's syndrome (CN III palsy and ipsilateral cerebellar ataxia and dysmetria), Claude's syndrome (combination of Benedikt's and Nothnagel's syndromes), and Weber's syndrome (CN III palsy and contralateral hemiparesis)

Subarachnoid Space: Usually involves pupil and is due to aneurysms (notably posterior communicating artery aneurysm), trauma, or uncal herniation; rarely microvascular disease and infections

Intracavernous Space: Usually due to cavernous sinus fistula, aneurysms, tumors, Tolosa-Hunt syndrome, infections (eg, herpes zoster), or pituitary apoplexy; usually associated with CN IV, V, and VI findings and sympathetic abnormalities (see Multiple Cranial Nerve Palsies section); pupil usually spared (90%)

Orbital Space: Usually due to trauma, infections, and trauma; often associated with CN II, IV, V, and VI findings (see Multiple Cranial Nerve Palsies section); CN III splits before superior orbital fissure, so partial (superior or inferior division) palsies may occur

Symptoms

Binocular diplopia (disappears with one eye closed), eye-turn; may have pain, headache, or droopy eyelid.

Signs

Ptosis, ophthalmoplegia except lateral gaze, negative forced ductions, and exotropia and hypotropia in primary gaze (eye is down and out); may have dilated pupil, positive relative afferent pupillary defect (RAPD); in cases of aberrant regeneration: lid-gaze dyskinesis (inferior rectus or medial rectus fibers to levator causing upper lid retraction on downgaze [pseudo–von Graefe's sign] or on adduction), pupil-gaze dyskinesis (inferior rectus or medial rectus fibers to iris sphincter causing pupil constriction on downgaze or on adduction); depending on syndrome causing the paresis may have other neurologic deficits or cranial nerve palsies.

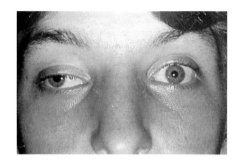

Figure 2–12. Third nerve palsy with right ptosis, pupillary dilation, exotropia, and hypotropia.

Differential Diagnosis

Myasthenia gravis, thyroid ophthalmopathy, migraine, chronic progressive external ophthalmoplegia.

Evaluation

- Complete ophthalmic history, neurologic exam with attention to cranial nerve exam, and eye exam with attention to pupils, lids, proptosis, motility, and forced ductions
- Head and orbital CT scan and/or MRI/magnetic resonance angiography (MRA) if pupil involved in any patient, if associated with other neurologic abnormalities, if pupil spared in young patients (<45 years old), if signs of aberrant regeneration are present, or if no improvement of isolated pupil-sparing microvascular cases after 3 months is evident; can defer neuroimaging in older patients with known microvascular disease if pupil spared
- Lab tests: fasting blood glucose, complete blood count (CBC), erythrocyte sedimentation rate (ESR), venereal disease research laboratory (VDRL), fluorescent treponemal antibody absorption (FTA-ABS), antinuclear antibody (ANA)
- Check blood pressure
- Consider cerebral angiography to rule out aneurysm (neurosurgical emergency) if pupil involved and MRA inconclusive
- Consider lumbar puncture if subarachnoid hemorrhage suspected
- Consider edrophonium chloride (Tensilon) test to rule out myasthenia gravis
- Neurology or neurosurgical consultation (especially if pupil involved)

Management

- Treatment depends on etiology
- Follow isolated pupil-sparing lesions closely for pupil involvement during 1st week
- Occlusion with Transpore clear surgical tape or clear nail polish across one spectacle lens to help alleviate diplopia in adults
- Aneurysms, tumors, and trauma may require neurosurgery
- Treat underlying medical condition

Prognosis

Depends on etiology; usually poor except microvascular palsies, which tend to resolve within 1–2 months (6 months maximum)

Fourth Nerve Palsy

Definition

Paresis of CN IV (trochlear) caused by a variety of processes anywhere along its course from the midbrain to the orbit

Etiology

Most commonly trauma (30–40%; especially closed-head trauma with contrecoup forces) and microvascular disease (20%; eg, hypertension or diabetes mellitus); also can be congenital (with long-standing head-tilt), idiopathic (30%), or rarely due to a tumor, hemorrhage, or aneurysm; bilateral seen after severe head trauma (damage at anterior medullary velum); important to localize level of pathology:

Nuclear: Rare, due to trauma, vascular lesion (eg, hemorrhage, infarction), or demyelinating disease; signs include contralateral superior oblique palsy

Fascicular: Rare, same associations as nuclear; may get contralateral Horner's syndrome; trauma (especially near anterior medullary velum) usually causes bilateral CN IV palsies

Subarachnoid Space: Usually due to closed-head trauma; rarely tumor or infection

Intracavernous Space: Due to trauma, tumors, and inflammation; usually associated with CN III, V, and VI findings and sympathetic abnormalities (see Multiple Cranial Nerve Palsies section)

Symptoms

Binocular vertical diplopia; may have tilted vision, blurred vision, head-tilt toward contralateral side, or eye-turn.

Signs

Positive three-step test, ipsilateral hypertropia (greatest on contralateral gaze and ipsilateral head-tilt), excyclotorsion (if >10 degrees, likely bilateral), large vertical fusional amplitude in congenital cases (10–15 prism diopters); chin-down position; negative forced ductions; bilateral cases have V-pattern esotropia, left hypertropia on right gaze, and right hypertropia on left gaze; other neurologic deficits if CN IV paresis is not isolated.

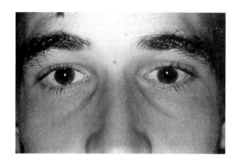

Figure 2–13. Fourth nerve palsy with right hypertropia.

Differential Diagnosis

Myasthenia gravis, thyroid ophthalmopathy, orbital disease, CN III palsy, Brown's syndrome, skew deviation, superior oblique myokymia.

Evaluation

- Complete ophthalmic history, neurologic exam with attention to cranial nerve exam, and eye exam with attention to motility, head posture (check old photographs for long-standing head-tilt in congenital cases), vertical fusion, double Maddox rod test (measure torsional component; bilateral superior oblique paresis >10 degrees of torsion), and forced ductions
- Perform Parks-Bielschowsky three-step test to determine paretic muscle:

  Step 1: Which eye is hypertropic in primary gaze (eg, if right hypertropia then problem is with right inferior rectus/superior oblique or left superior rectus/inferior oblique)

  Step 2: Which direction of gaze makes the hypertropia worse (eg, if left gaze then problem is with right superior oblique/inferior oblique or left superior rectus/inferior rectus)

  Step 3 (Bielschowsky head-tilt test): Head-tilt toward which side makes the hypertropia worse (eg, if right head-tilt, then problem is with right superior oblique/superior rectus or left inferior oblique/inferior rectus)

  After three steps, the paretic muscle will be identified (eg, right hypertropia in primary position, worse on left gaze and right head tilt = right superior oblique)

- Lab tests: fasting blood glucose, CBC, ESR, VDRL, FTA-ABS, ANA
- Check blood pressure

- Head and orbital CT scan and/or MRI/MRA if history of head trauma, history of cancer, signs of meningitis, young age, associated with other neurologic abnormalities, or no improvement of isolated microvascular cases after 3–4 months; isolated and microvascular cases in adults >40 years do not initially require neuroimaging
- Consider lumbar puncture
- Consider edrophonium chloride (Tensilon) test to rule out myasthenia gravis
- Neurology consultation

Management

- Treatment depends on etiology
- Occlusion with Transpore clear surgical tape, clear nail polish across one spectacle lens, or prism glasses to help alleviate diplopia in adults
- Consider muscle surgery in long-standing, stable cranial nerve IV palsy
- Aneurysms, tumors, and trauma may require neurosurgery
- Treat underlying medical condition

Prognosis

Depends on etiology; microvascular palsies tend to resolve within 3 months.

Sixth Nerve Palsy

Definition

Paresis of cranial nerve VI caused by a variety of processes anywhere along its course from the pons to the orbit.

Etiology

Depends on age: In children (0–15 years old), most commonly tumors (eg, pontine glioma) or post-viral; in young adults (15–40 years old), usually miscellaneous or undetermined (8–30%); in adults (>40 years old), usually due to trauma and microvascular disease (eg, hypertension, diabetes mellitus); also associated with multiple sclerosis, cerebrovascular accidents, increased intracranial pressure, and rarely tumors (eg, nasopharyngeal carcinoma); important to localize level of pathology:

Nuclear: Due to pontine infarcts, pontine gliomas, cerebellar tumors, microvascular disease, and Wernicke-Korsakoff syndrome; causes an ipsilateral, horizontal gaze palsy (cannot look to side of lesion)

Fascicular: Usually due to tumors, microvascular disease, or demyelinating disease; can cause Foville's syndrome (dorsal pons lesions with horizontal gaze palsy, ipsilateral CN V, VI, VII, VIII palsies, and ipsilateral Horner's syndrome) and Millard-Gubler syndrome (ventral pons lesion with ipsilateral CN VI and VII palsies and contralateral hemiparesis)

Subarachnoid Space: Usually due to elevated intracranial pressure (30% of patients with idiopathic intracranial hypertension have CN VI palsy); also basilar tumors (eg, acoustic neuroma, chordomas), basilar artery aneurysm, hemorrhage, inflammations, or meningeal infections

Petrous Space: Due to trauma (eg, basal skull fracture) and infections; can cause Gradenigo's syndrome (infection of petrous bone secondary to otitis media causing ipsilateral CN VI and VII paresis, ipsilateral Horner's syndrome, ipsilateral trigeminal pain, and ipsilateral deafness; seen in children) or pseudo-Gradenigo's syndrome (nasopharyngeal carcinoma may cause severe otitis media with findings similar to those of Gradenigo's syndrome)

Intracavernous Space: Usually due to trauma, vascular lesion, inflammation, or tumors; associated with CN III, IV, and V findings and sympathetic abnormalities (see Multiple Cranial Nerve Palsies section); isolated palsy is rare

Symptoms

Horizontal binocular diplopia (worse at distance than near, and in direction of gaze of paretic muscle); may have eye-turn.

Signs

Esotropia or lateral rectus muscle palsy; negative forced ductions; other neurologic deficits if CN VI paresis is not isolated.

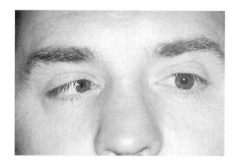

Figure 2–14. Sixth nerve palsy demonstrating deficient abduction of the left eye.

Differential Diagnosis

Thyroid ophthalmopathy, myasthenia gravis, orbital inflammatory pseudotumor, Duane's retraction syndrome type I, Möbius' syndrome (CN VI and VII palsy), orbital fracture with medial rectus entrapment, spasm of near reflex.

Evaluation

- Complete ophthalmic history, neurologic exam with attention to cranial nerve exam, and eye exam with attention to motility, forced ductions, and ophthalmoscopy

■ Head and orbital CT scan and/or MRI/MRA if in child, history of pain, history of head trauma, history of cancer, signs of meningitis, associated with other neurologic abnormalities, or no improvement of isolated microvascular cases after 3–6 months; isolated and microvascular cases in adults >40 years old do not initially require neuroimaging
■ Lab tests: fasting blood glucose, CBC, ESR, VDRL, FTA-ABS, ANA
■ Check blood pressure
■ Consider lumbar puncture if elevated intracranial pressure suspected
■ Consider edrophonium chloride (Tensilon) test to rule out myasthenia gravis
■ Neurology consultation

Management

■ Treatment depends on etiology
■ Occlusion with Transpore clear surgical tape or clear nail polish across one spectacle lens to help alleviate diplopia in adults
■ Consider muscle surgery in long-standing, stable cases
■ Aneurysms, tumors, and trauma may require neurosurgery
■ Treat underlying medical condition

Prognosis

Depends on etiology; microvascular palsies tend to resolve within 3 months.

Multiple Cranial Nerve Palsies

Definition

Multiple cranial nerve abnormalities appearing simultaneously; lesions can be located in the brain stem, subarachnoid space, cavernous sinus, or orbital space.

Etiology

Important to localize level of pathology:

Brain Stem: Due to midbrain or pons vascular lesions and tumors involving cranial nerve nuclei that are in close proximity

Subarachnoid Space: Usually due to infections or midline tumors

Cavernous Sinus Syndrome: Multiple cranial nerve pareses (CN III, IV, VI, V_1, V_2) and sympathetic involvement due to parasellar lesions, which affect these motor nerves in various combinations in the sinus or superior orbital fissure; may have Horner's syndrome due to oculosympathetic paresis; caused by aneurysms (eg, posterior cerebral artery, intracavernous carotid artery), arteriovenous fistulas (eg, carotid-cavernous fistula, dural-sinus fistula), tumors (eg, leukemia, lymphoma, meningioma, pituitary adenoma, chordoma), inflammations (eg, Wegener's granulomatosis, sarcoidosis, Tolosa-Hunt syndrome), and infections (eg, cavernous sinus thrombosis, herpes zoster, tuberculosis, syphilis, mucormycosis)

Orbital Apex Syndrome: Multiple motor cranial nerve palsies (as above except no CN V_2 involvement) and optic nerve (CN II) dysfunction; etiologies similar to those mentioned above

Symptoms

Pain, diplopia, droopy eyelid, variable decreased vision.

Signs

Normal or decreased visual acuity (orbital apex syndrome), ptosis, strabismus, limitation of ocular motility, decreased facial sensation in CN V_1/V_2 distribution, positive relative afferent pupillary defect (RAPD), miosis (Horner's syndrome), and trigeminal (facial) pain; pupil usually spared; may have proptosis, conjunctival injection, chemosis, increased intraocular pressure, bruit, and retinopathy in cases of high-flow arteriovenous fistulas; fever, lid edema, and signs of facial infection in cases of cavernous sinus thrombosis.

Differential Diagnosis

Thyroid ophthalmopathy, myasthenia gravis, giant cell arteritis, Miller-Fisher variant of Guillain-Barré syndrome, chronic progressive external ophthalmoplegia, orbital disease (see Chap. 1).

Evaluation

- Complete ophthalmic history, neurologic exam with attention to cranial nerve exam, and eye exam with attention to facial sensation, ocular auscultation, pupils, motility, Hertel exophthalmometry, tonometry, and ophthalmoscopy
- Lab tests: fasting blood glucose, CBC with differential, ESR, VDRL, FTA-ABS, ANA; consider blood cultures if infectious etiology suspected
- Head, orbital, and sinus CT scan and/or MRI/MRA
- Consider lumbar puncture
- Consider cerebral angiography to rule out aneurysm or arteriovenous fistula
- Consider edrophonium chloride (Tensilon) test to rule out myasthenia gravis
- Neurology, neurosurgical, and/or medical consultations as needed

Management

- Treatment depends on etiology
- Aneurysms, tumors, and trauma may require neurosurgery
- Systemic steroids (prednisone 60–100 mg PO qd) for Tolosa-Hunt syndrome; check purified protein derivative (PPD), blood glucose, and chest radiographs before starting systemic steroids

Management *Continued*

- Add H_2-blocker (ranitidine [Zantac] 150 mg PO bid) when administering systemic steroids
- Systemic antibiotics (vancomycin 1 g IV q12h and ceftazidime 1 g IV q8h) for cavernous sinus thrombosis; penicillin G (2.4 million U IV q4h for 10–14 days, then 2.4 million U IM q week for 3 weeks) for syphilis
- Systemic antifungals (amphotericin B 0.25–1.0 mg/kg IV over 6h) for mucormycosis
- Treat underlying medical condition

Prognosis

Usually poor.

Chronic Progressive External Ophthalmoplegia (CPEO)

Definition

Slowly progressive, bilateral, external ophthalmoplegia affecting all directions of gaze.

Etiology

Isolated or hereditary myopathy; several rare syndromes:

Kearns-Sayre Syndrome (mitochondrial DNA): Triad of chronic progressive external ophthalmoplegia (CPEO), pigmentary retinopathy (see Chap. 10), and cardiac conduction defects (arrhythmias, heart block, cardiomyopathy); also associated with mental retardation, short stature, deafness, vestibular problems, and elevated cerebrospinal fluid (CSF) protein

MELAS: CPEO with mitochondrial encephalopathy, lactic acidosis, and stroke (MELAS)

MERRF: CPEO with myoclonus, epilepsy, and "ragged red" fibers (MERRF)

Myotonic Dystrophy (AD): CPEO, bilateral ptosis, lid lag, orbicularis oculi weakness, miotic pupils, Christmas tree cataracts, and pigmentary retinopathy with associated muscular dystrophy (worse in morning), cardiomyopathy, baldness, testicular atrophy, and mental retardation; mapped to chromosome 19q

Oculopharyngeal Muscular Dystrophy (AD): CPEO with dysphagia; usually French-Canadian lineage; mapped to chromosome 14q

Symptoms

Variable decreased vision, droopy eyelids, foreign body sensation, tearing.

Signs

Normal or decreased visual acuity, limitation of eye movements (even with doll's head maneuvers and caloric stimulation), ptosis, orbicularis oculi weakness, superficial punctate keratitis (especially inferiorly), retinal pigment epithelial (RPE) changes or pigmentary retinopathy (see Chap. 10); pupils usually spared.

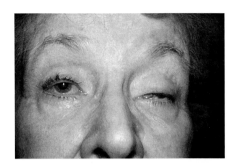

Figure 2–15. Chronic progressive external ophthalmoplegia demonstrating ptosis and limited elevation in both eyes.

Differential Diagnosis

Downgaze palsy (lesion of rostral interstitial nucleus of the medial longitudinal fasciculus [riMLF]), upgaze palsy, progressive supranuclear palsy, dorsal midbrain syndrome, oculogyric crisis, myasthenia gravis.

Evaluation

- Complete ophthalmic history, neurologic exam with attention to cranial nerve exam, and eye exam with attention to motility, doll's head maneuvers, caloric stimulation, lids, pupils, and ophthalmoscopy
- Consider muscle biopsy to check for "ragged red" abnormal muscle fibers or electromyography for definitive diagnosis
- Consider edrophonium chloride (Tensilon) test to rule out myasthenia gravis
- Consider lumbar puncture (Kearns-Sayre syndrome)
- Medical consultation for complete cardiac evaluation including electrocardiogram (Kearns-Sayre syndrome, myotonic dystrophy) and swallowing studies (oculopharyngeal dystrophy)

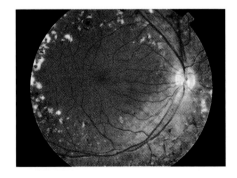

Figure 2–16. Retinal pigmentary changes in a patient with Kearns-Sayre syndrome.

Management

- No treatment effective
- Topical lubrication with nonpreserved artificial tears (see Appendix) up to q1h and ointment (Refresh P.M.) at bedtime if signs of exposure keratopathy exist
- Occlusion with Transpore clear surgical tape or clear nail polish across one spectacle lens to help alleviate diplopia in adults
- Kearns-Sayre syndrome and myotonic dystrophy require cardiology consultation; may require pacemaker

Prognosis

Depends on syndrome; usually poor.

Horizontal Gaze Palsy

Definition

Internuclear Ophthalmoplegia (INO): Lesion of medial longitudinal fasciculus (MLF) in brain stem causing gaze defects in both eyes by blocking connection between contralateral cranial nerve VI nucleus and the ipsilateral cranial nerve III nucleus; ipsilateral deficiency of adduction and contralateral abduction nystagmus (named after side of MLF lesion); convergence can be absent (mesencephalic lesion; anterior lesion) or intact (lesion posterior in the MLF); may be unilateral or bilateral (appears exotropic; WEBINO = "wall-eyed" bilateral INO).

One-and-a-Half Syndrome: So-called "INO Plus" with lesion of paramedian pontine reticular formation (PPRF, the horizontal gaze center) or cranial nerve VI nucleus, and the ipsilateral MLF causing conjugate gaze palsy to ipsilateral side (one) and internuclear ophthalmoplegia or inability to adduct on gaze to contralateral side (half).

Etiology

Depends on age: <50 years old usually multiple sclerosis (unilateral INO) or tumor (pontine glioma for one-and-a-half syndrome); bilateral in children, often due to brain stem glioma; >50 years old usually vascular disease (cerebrovascular accident affecting frontal lobes, arteriovenous malformation, aneurysm, basilar artery occlusion), multiple sclerosis, or tumor (pontine metastases).

Symptoms

Binocular horizontal diplopia.

Signs

Limitation of eye movements (cannot adduct on side of lesion in INO; can only abduct on side contralateral to lesion in one-and-a-half syndrome); nystagmus in abducting contralateral eye (INO); may have upbeat nystagmus.

Differential Diagnosis

Medial rectus palsy, myasthenia gravis.

Evaluation

- Complete ophthalmic history, neurologic exam with attention to cranial nerve exam, and eye exam with attention to motility, doll's head maneuvers, and caloric stimulation
- Head and orbital CT scan and/or MRI/MRA with attention to brain stem and midbrain
- Consider edrophonium chloride (Tensilon) test to rule out myasthenia gravis
- Consider neurology or neurosurgical consultation

Management

- Treatment depends on etiology
- Aneurysms, tumors, and trauma may require neurosurgery
- Treat underlying neurologic or medical condition

Prognosis

Usually poor.

Vertical Gaze Palsy

Definition

Progressive Supranuclear Palsy (PSP, Steele-Richardson-Olszewski Syndrome): Degenerative neurologic disorder that causes progressive, bilateral, external ophthalmoplegia affecting all directions of gaze; usually starts with vertical gaze (downgaze first).

Dorsal Midbrain Syndrome (Parinaud's Syndrome): Supranuclear palsy of vertical gaze (upgaze first) due to lesions of the dorsal midbrain.

Etiology

Most commonly due to pineal tumor, also seen with cerebrovascular accidents, hydrocephalus, arteriovenous malformation, trauma, multiple sclerosis, or syphilis.

Symptoms

Blurred vision, binocular diplopia (at near with dorsal midbrain syndrome); may have trouble reading, foreign body sensation, tearing, and/or dementia (PSP).

Signs

PSP: Progressive limitation of voluntary eye movements (but doll's head maneuvers give full range of motion); may have nuchal rigidity and seborrhea, progressive dementia, dysarthria, hypometric saccades.

Dorsal Midbrain Syndrome: Supranuclear paresis of upgaze (therefore vestibular, doll's head maneuvers, and Bell's phenomenon intact), light-near dissociation, papilledema, convergence-retraction nystagmus (on attempted upgaze), lid retraction (Collier's sign), spasm of convergence and accommodation (causing induced myopia), skew deviation, superficial punctate keratitis (especially inferiorly).

Differential Diagnosis

Downgaze palsy (lesion of rostral interstitial nucleus of the medial longitudinal fasciculus [riMLF]), upgaze palsy, chronic progressive external ophthalmoplegia, oculogyric crisis, myasthenia gravis.

Evaluation

- Complete ophthalmic history, neurologic exam with attention to cranial nerve exam, and eye exam with attention to motility, lids, accommodation, pupils, cornea, and ophthalmoscopy
- Head and orbital CT scan and/or MRI/MRA with attention to brain stem and midbrain
- Consider edrophonium chloride (Tensilon) test to rule out myasthenia gravis
- Consider neurology or neurosurgical consultation

Management

- Treatment depends on etiology
- Topical lubrication with nonpreserved artificial tears (see Appendix) up to q1h and ointment (Refresh P.M.) at bedtime if signs of exposure keratopathy exist
- Aneurysms, tumors, and trauma may require neurosurgery
- Treat underlying neurologic or medical condition

Prognosis

Poor; usually death within 5 years in PSP.

Myasthenia Gravis

Definition

Systemic disease of the neuromuscular junction causing muscle weakness; hallmark is variability and fatigue; detectable levels of antibodies to acetylcholine (ACh) receptors found in 30%.

Etiology

Autoantibodies to acetylcholine receptors in voluntary striated muscles seen in 70–90% of patients; does not affect pupils or ciliary muscle.

Epidemiology

Female predilection; positive family history in 5%; 90% have eye involvement (levator and extraocular muscles), 75% as initial manifestation, 20% ocular only; increased incidence of thyroid disease, thymoma (15%), and autoimmune diseases including scleroderma, lupus erythematosus, rheumatoid arthritis, Hashimoto's thyroiditis, multiple sclerosis, and thyroid ophthalmopathy.

Symptoms

Asymptomatic; may have diplopia (especially when tired), droopy eyelids, dysarthria, dysphagia.

Signs

Variable, asymmetric ptosis (worse with fatigue, sustained upgaze, and at end of day), variable limitation of extraocular movements (mimics any motility disturbance), strabismus, gaze-evoked nystagmus, orbicularis oculi weakness; Cogan's lid twitch (upper eyelid twitch when patient looks up to primary position after looking down for 10–15 seconds); may have an internuclear ophthalmoplegia (INO).

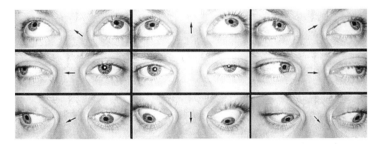

Figure 2–17. Myasthenia gravis with left ptosis and adduction deficit.

Differential Diagnosis

Gaze palsy, multiple sclerosis, thyroid ophthalmopathy, chronic progressive external ophthalmoplegia, inflammatory orbital pseudotumor.

Evaluation

- Complete ophthalmic history, neurologic exam with attention to cranial nerve exam, and eye exam with attention to motility, lids, pupils, and cornea
- Lab tests: anti-ACh receptor antibodies, thyroid function tests (T_3, T_4, TSH), rheumatoid factor (RF), ANA
- Edrophonium chloride (Tensilon) test: Test dose of Tensilon 2 mg IV with 1 mL saline flush then observe for improvement in diplopia and lid signs over next minute; if no improvement, increase Tensilon dose to 4 mg IV with 1 mL saline flush and observe for improvement in diplopia and lid signs; repeat two times; if no improvement in diplopia and lid signs after 3–4 minutes, the test is negative; a negative test result does not rule out myasthenia gravis. **Note:** test should be performed with cardiac monitoring because of cardiovascular effects of Tensilon; if bradycardia, angina, or bronchospasm develop, inject atropine (0.4 mg IV) immediately; consider pretreatment with atropine 0.4 mg IV
- Consider electromyography of peripheral muscles for definitive diagnosis
- Chest radiographs or chest CT scan to rule out thymoma
- Neurology and/or medical consultation

Management

- No treatment required if symptoms are mild
- Oral anticholinesterase (pyridostigmine 60–120 mg PO qid) for moderate symptoms
- Consider systemic steroids (prednisone 20–100 mg PO qd); check purified protein derivative (PPD), blood glucose, and chest radiographs before starting systemic steroids
- Add H_2-blocker (ranitidine [Zantac] 150 mg PO bid) when taking systemic steroids
- Occlusion with Transpore clear surgical tape or clear nail polish across one spectacle lens to help alleviate diplopia in adults
- Surgery for thymoma if present
- Treat underlying medical condition

Prognosis

Variable, chronic, progressive; good if ocular only.

Lids / Lashes / Lacrimal

Trauma

Avulsion: Tearing or shearing injury to the eyelid resulting in partial or complete severance of eyelid tissue. Surgical repair of eyelid defect depends upon the degree of tissue loss and damage; all procedures should be performed by an oculoplastic surgeon:

- **Upper lid defects:**
  (1) Small (<25%): direct closure
  (2) Moderate (25–50%): Tenzel semicircular flap advancement or lateral segment lid advancement
  (3) Large (>50%): Cutler-Beard procedure, or full-thickness lower eyelid flap advancement
- **Lower lid defects:**
  (1) Small: direct closure
  (2) Moderate: Tenzel semicircular flap advancement or full thickness composite graft from contralateral lid
  (3) Large: modified Hughes' procedure, upper eyelid tarsal conjunctival flap advancement into posterior lamellar defect, Mustarde's rotational cheek flap, or anterior lamella reconstruction with retroauricular free skin graft or skin flap advancement
- Beware of lid-sharing procedures in children because occlusion amblyopia may result

Canalicular Laceration: Laceration involving the canaliculus (tear duct) at the nasal lid margin between the punctum and the medial canthus of either eyelid; often identified on inspection as a pouting gray structure, or with probing and irrigation of the lacrimal system; good prognosis if repaired early with stent.

- Surgical repair with stent (silicone intubation) placement in the nasolacrimal duct system; should be performed by an oculoplastic surgeon
- Upper canalicular repair is controversial

Contusion: Bruising of eyelid with edema and ecchymosis, usually secondary to blunt injury; ocular involvement is common; usually excellent prognosis if no ocular or bony injuries.

- Cold compresses for 10–15 minutes qid for 24–48 hours
- Rule out and treat open globe (see Chap. 4) or other associated ocular trauma

Laceration: Cut in the eyelid involving skin and deeper structures (muscle and fat), usually due to penetrating trauma. Lid lacerations are divided into (1) non–lid margin involvement, (2) lid margin involvement, and (3) canthal angle involvement (tendon and lacrimal gland system). Early, clean wounds are usually repaired successfully, but can be complicated by lid notching, entropion, ectropion, or cicatrix; dirty wounds are also at risk for infection.

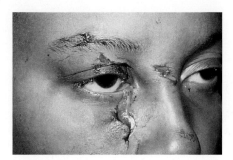

Figure 3–1. Upper and lower eyelid lacerations.

- Tetanus booster (tetanus toxoid 0.5 mL IM) if necessary for tetanus prophylaxis (>10 years since last tetanus shot or if status is unknown); consider rabies with animal bites
- If orbital septum violated with fat prolapse, evaluate for presence of retained foreign body and/or levator muscle damage
- **Surgical repair of eyelid without margin involvement:** Débridement of wound and saline irrigation with a large-gauge needle after local anesthesia is administered. Small-caliber suture repair (6-0 to 7-0 nylon, silk, or Vicryl) of superficial layers (skin and orbicularis) with wound edge eversion. Deep lacerations require two-layer closure, first with 6-0 Polydac or Vicryl to close tarsus (deep layer), followed by repair of the superficial layer
- **Surgical repair of eyelid with margin involvement:** Same as eyelid without margin involvement except eyelid margin is closed first using three-suture eyelid margin closure (6-0 or 7-0 silk): (1) gray line (just anterior to meibomian glands) suture placed 2 mm on either side of laceration, and 2 mm deep; leave suture very long; (2) tarsal suture placed anterior, parallel, and similar to gray line suture with long ends; and (3) posterior lash line suture placed anterior, parallel, and similar to tarsal suture. Include long ends of all three sutures on stretch into skin suture adjacent to lid margin to avoid corneal and conjunctival irritation from the suture ends
- **Surgical repair with canthal angle involvement** (should be performed by an oculoplastic surgeon): open granulation or full-thickness skin grafts for the medial canthus; semicircular advancement flaps or tarsal and conjunctival transposition flaps for lateral canthus
- Topical antibiotic ointment (bacitracin or erythromycin bid to tid) to wound
- For dirty wounds, systemic antibiotics (dicloxacillin 250–500 mg PO qid for 7–10 days, consider penicillin V 500 mg PO qid for animal or human bites)

- Early removal of superficial layer sutures after 3–7 days
- Eyelid margin sutures are removed after 9–14 days

Contact Dermatitis

Definition

Acute dermatitis resulting from chemical or mechanical irritants, or from immunologic hypersensitivity to an allergic stimulus.

Symptoms

Swelling, redness, itching, tearing, foreign body sensation, and ocular and eyelid discomfort.

Signs

Erythematous, flaking, or crusting rash accompanied by edema; may have vesicular or weeping lesions; lichenified plaques suggest chronic exposure to irritant.

Differential Diagnosis

Herpes simplex, herpes zoster, preseptal cellulitis; chemical, ultraviolet, or thermal burns.

Evaluation

- Complete history with attention to exposure to irritants such as soaps, fragrances, cosmetics, hairspray, nail polish, jewelry, medications, poison ivy; and chemical, ultraviolet, or thermal exposure
- Complete eye exam with attention to lids and conjunctiva

Management

- Identify and remove inciting agent(s); may require allergic patch testing to determine causative allergens
- Gentle saline compresses bid to qid and topical antibiotic ointment (erythromycin or bacitracin bid) to crusted or weeping lesions
- Consider mild steroid cream (<1% hydrocortisone cream bid to tid for 7–10 days) on eyelids; avoid lid margins and ocular exposure (for this reason, it is safer to use an ophthalmic preparation, eg, FML ointment)
- Oral antihistamine (diphenhydramine 25–50 mg PO tid to qid) for severe or widespread lesions or excessive itching
- Consider short-term oral steroids (prednisone 40–80 mg PO qd tapered over 10–14 days) for severe cases; check purified protein derivative (PPD), blood glucose, and chest radiographs before starting systemic steroids
- Add H_2-blocker (Zantac 150 mg PO bid) when taking systemic steroids

Prognosis

Usually good; resolution occurs 1–2 weeks after removal of inciting agent; rebound can occur if steroids tapered too rapidly.

Vitiligo/Poliosis

Total absence of melanin in hair follicles of the eyelashes or eyebrow (poliosis) and in skin (vitiligo), leading to focal patches of white hair or skin; associated with severe dermatitis, Vogt-Koyanagi-Harada syndrome, tuberous sclerosis, localized irradiation, sympathetic ophthalmia, and Waardenburg's syndrome (congenital poliosis, deafness, iris heterochromia, and hypertelorism).

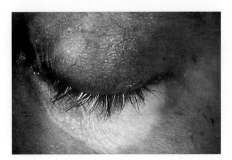

Figure 3–2. Vitiligo and poliosis in a patient with Vogt-Koyanagi-Harada syndrome.

■ Treat underlying medical condition

Blepharospasm

Definition

Essential Blepharospasm: Bilateral, episodic spasms of the orbicularis oculi muscles leading to uncontrolled blinking; thought to be caused by disorder of the basal ganglia; usually with gradual onset in the 5th to 7th decade.

Meige's Syndrome: Essential blepharospasm with facial grimacing; may have cog-wheeling in the neck and extremities.

Symptoms

Uncontrollable blinking, squeezing, or twitching of eyelids or facial muscles.

Signs

Spasms of orbicularis oculi or facial muscles; may prevent examiner from prying open lids during episodes; may be absent during sleep.

Differential Diagnosis

Reflex blepharospasm (caused by eyelid irritation, dry eye, or meningeal irritation), hemifacial spasm, facial myokymia, Tourette's syndrome, tic douloureux (trigeminal neuralgia), Parkinson's disease, Huntington's disease, basal ganglia infarct.

Evaluation

- Complete ophthalmic history with attention to causes of ocular irritation, stress and caffeine use, and history of neurologic disorders
- Complete eye exam with attention to cranial nerves, motility, and lids
- Head and orbital computed tomography (CT) or magnetic resonance imaging (MRI) with attention to the posterior fossa

Management

- Injection of botulinum type A toxin (BTX, Botox) into the orbicularis muscle to weaken contractions; repeat injections are often required every 2–8 weeks as the therapeutic effect declines; transient ptosis and diplopia are uncommon side effects
- Medical therapy with haloperidol, clonazepam, bromocriptine, or baclofen has limited success

Prognosis

Good with appropriate therapy; in most cases, repeat injections are needed indefinitely.

Ptosis

Definition

Drooping of the upper eyelid(s).

Etiology

Acquired Aponeurotic: Disinsertion, central dehiscence, or attenuation of the levator aponeurosis causing poor levator function. Most common form of ptosis, often associated with advanced age, eye surgery or trauma, pregnancy, chronic eyelid swelling, and blepharochalasis.

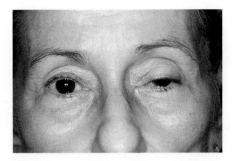

Figure 3–3. Acquired ptosis of the left eye.

Acquired Mechanical: Poor upper eyelid elevation due to mass effect of tumors, or to tethering of the eyelid by scarring (cicatricial ptosis).

Acquired Myogenic: Poor levator or Müller's muscle function, due to disorders of neuromuscular junction including myasthenia gravis, chronic progressive external ophthalmoplegia, myotonic dystrophy, and oculopharyngeal dystrophy (rare).

Acquired Neurogenic: Defects in innervation to cranial nerve III (oculomotor palsy) or sympathetic input to Müller's muscle (Horner's syndrome).

Congenital: Poor levator function from birth; usually unilateral, nonhereditary, and myogenic with fibrosis and fat infiltration of levator muscle; rarely from aponeurosis dehiscence (possibly birth trauma), congenital Horner's syndrome (ptosis, miosis, anhidrosis) with poor Müller's muscle function from decreased sympathetic tone, or congenital neurogenic with Marcus Gunn jaw-winking syndrome from aberrant connections between cranial nerve V (innervating the pterygoid muscles) and the levator muscle.

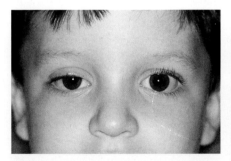

Figure 3–4. Congenital ptosis of the right eye.

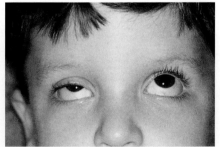

Figure 3–5. Same patient as shown in Figure 3–4 demonstrating poor levator function with upgaze of the right eye.

Symptoms

Decreased vision, brow ache, loss of depth perception.

Signs

Drooping of upper eyelid(s) with impaired elevation on upgaze, recruitment of brow muscles with brow furrows, higher lid crease and apparently smaller eye on ptotic side, abnormally high contralateral eyelid (Hering's law); in downgaze, affected lid may be *higher* than contralateral lid in congenital ptosis (lid lag), and *lower* in acquired cases; may have decreased visual acuity when visual axis obscured or head tilt with chin-up position when bilateral; other associated abnormalities in congenital ptosis include lagophthalmos, decreased superior rectus function, high astigmatism, anisometropia, strabismus, amblyopia, epicanthus, and blepharophimosis.

Differential Diagnosis

Dermatochalasis (excess skin of upper eyelids), lid swelling, enophthalmos (eg, orbital floor fracture), hypotropia, contralateral eyelid retraction causing asymmetry (eg, thyroid ophthalmopathy), small eye (eg, phthisis bulbi, microphthalmia, anophthalmia).

Evaluation

- Complete ophthalmic history with attention to age of onset, previous surgeries or trauma, degree of functional impairment and time of day when worst, associated symptoms such as generalized fatigue, breathing problems, diplopia
- Complete eye exam with attention to amblyopia in children, visual acuity with and without lid taping, palpebral fissure (PF) height, margin-reflex distance (MRD), upper lid crease height (high in aponeurotic), and levator function (LF) (normal in aponeurotic, decreased in congenital), pupils, motility, Bell's phenomenon, corneal sensation, and cornea
- Consider edrophonium chloride (Tensilon) test to rule out myasthenia gravis
- Consider phenylephrine 2.5% to stimulate Müller's muscle (positive test-achieve good vertical height with MRD of >4); rule out Horner's syndrome with topical cocaine 4–10% and/or hydroxyamphetamine 1% (see Chap. 7)
- Check visual fields with and without lid taping (ptosis fields) to document visual impairment prior to surgery

Management

- Eyelid crutches attached to glasses or lid taping may be used as temporizing measures
- **With good levator function:** levator aponeurosis advancement, levator resection, Fasanella-Servat tarsoconjunctival resection
- **With inadequate levator function:** fascia lata–frontalis sling or other procedure utilizing accessory muscles of lid elevation

Management Continued

- Superior tarsal (Müller's muscle) resection in Horner's syndrome with positive phenylephrine test or mild ptosis with good levator function
- All surgery should be performed by an oculoplastic surgeon
- Avoid surgery or undercorrect when poor Bell's reflex or decreased corneal sensation exists
- Treat underlying medical problems

Prognosis

Prognosis for acquired mechanical and aponeurotic ptosis is excellent; congenital is fair to excellent; myogenic and neurogenic are variable.

Ectropion

Definition

Eversion of the eyelid margin.

Etiology

Cicatricial: Due to burns (thermal or chemical), trauma (surgical or mechanical), or chronic inflammation with anterior lamellar contraction.

Congenital: Due to vertical shortening of anterior lamella (skin and orbicularis oculi), rarely isolated, may be associated with blepharophimosis syndrome.

Inflammatory: Due to chronic eyelid skin inflammation (atopic dermatitis, herpes zoster infections, rosacea).

Involutional: Due to horizontal lid laxity and tissue relaxation, followed by lid elongation, sagging, and conjunctival hypertrophy; usually involves lower eyelid, most frequent cause of ectropion in adults.

Mechanical: Due to lid edema, bulky lid tumors, orbital fat herniation, or lid-riding spectacles.

Paralytic: Usually follows cranial nerve VII palsy; often temporary.

Symptoms

Asymptomatic; may have eyelid or ocular irritation, tearing.

Signs

Eversion of eyelid margin, lid keratinization, conjunctival injection and hypertrophy, superficial punctate keratitis.

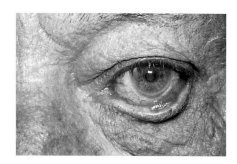

Figure 3–6. Ectropion.

Evaluation

- Complete ophthalmic history with attention to history of burns, trauma, surgery, or facial droop (cranial nerve VII [Bell's] palsy)
- Complete eye exam with attention to orbicularis function, lateral canthal tendon laxity, lids, herniated fat and scarring, conjunctiva, and cornea

Management

- Treat ectropion-related corneal and conjunctival exposure with topical lubrication with nonpreserved artificial tears (see Appendix) up to q1h and ointment (Refresh P.M.) at bedtime
- All surgery should be performed by an oculoplastic surgeon
- **Cicatricial:** Three-step procedure: (1) cicatrix release and relaxation; (2) horizontal lid tightening with lateral tarsal strip; and (3) anterior lamella lengthening with full-thickness skin graft
- **Congenital:** Mild ectropion often requires no treatment. Moderate or severe ectropion treated like cicatricial ectropion with horizontal lid tightening and full-thickness skin graft to vertically lengthen anterior lamella
- **Inflammatory:** Treat underlying dermatologic condition. Temporizing measures include taping temporal side of eyelid, using moisture chambers, and topical lubrication with nonpreserved artificial tears (see Appendix) up to q1h
- **Involutional:** Three procedures may be used individually or in combination: (1) medial spindle procedure for punctal ectropion; (2) horizontal lid shortening using lateral tarsal strip procedure, lateral lid wedge resection, or canthal tendon plication; and (3) lower lid retractor reinsertion
- **Mechanical:** Treat mechanical force causing ectropion (tumor or fat removal, eyeglass adjustment, etc.)

Management Continued

- **Paralytic:** Often resolves spontaneously within 6 months if due to Bell's palsy. Temporizing measures include taping temporal side of eyelid, using moisture chambers, and topical lubrication with nonpreserved artificial tears (see Appendix) up to q1h; rarely, if chronic, consider canthoplasties, lateral tarsorrhaphy, brow suspensions, and horizontal lid tightening procedures

Prognosis

Usually good with surgical treatment; cicatricial or inflammatory ectropion are prone to recurrence; paralytic ectropion may resolve spontaneously within 6 months after Bell's palsy.

Entropion

Definition

Inversion of the eyelid margin; may affect either eyelid, although the lower lid is more frequently affected.

Etiology

Cicatricial: Due to posterior lamella (tarsus and conjunctiva) shortening with lid inversion and rubbing of lashes and lid margin on globe; associated with Stevens-Johnson syndrome, ocular cicatricial pemphigoid, trachoma, herpes zoster, ocular surgery, and ocular trauma.

Congenital: Due to structural tarsal plate defects, shortened posterior lamellae, or eyelid retractor dysgenesis; usually affects upper eyelid.

Involutional: Most common cause of entropion in older patients, usually affects lower lid; predisposing factors include: horizontal lid laxity, over-riding preseptal orbicularis, disinserted or atrophied lid retractors, and involutional enophthalmos.

Spastic: Due to ocular inflammation or irritation; often seen following ocular surgery in patients with early underlying involutional changes.

Symptoms

Tearing, foreign body sensation, red eye.

Signs

Inturned eyelid margin, keratinized eyelid margins (cicatricial), poor eyelid tone (involutional; can pull lid out >6mm), horizontal lid laxity, over-riding preseptal orbicularis, enophthalmos, symblepharon (cicatricial), conjunctival injection, superficial punctate keratitis.

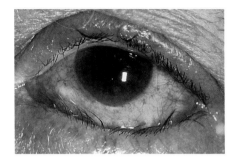

Figure 3–7. Entropion.

Differential Diagnosis

Trichiasis, distichiasis, blepharospasm.

Evaluation

- Complete ophthalmic history with attention to history of eye surgery, trauma, previous eye infections, burns
- Complete eye exam with attention to lid tone (snapback test), lower lid margin (sagging), medial and lateral canthal tendons, inferior fornix (unusually deep), digital eversion test at the inferior border of tarsus to distinguish involutional from cicatricial entropion (involutional corrects, cicatricial does not)

Management

- If corneal involvement exists, topical antibiotic ointment (erythromycin or bacitracin bid to qid)
- All surgery should be performed by an oculoplastic surgeon
- **Cicatricial:** Excision of scar and consider anterior lamellar resection or recession for minimal involvement; tarsal fracture procedure for lower lid involvement; tarsal graft from preserved sclera, ear cartilage, or hard palate if the tarsus is badly damaged; may also require conjunctival and mucous membrane grafts in severe cases
- **Congenital:** Rarely improves and often requires surgical treatment to correct underlying anatomic defect
- **Spastic:** Break entropion/irritation cycle by taping inturned lid to evert margin, thermal cautery, or Quickert suture techniques to temporarily evert lid; often requires more definitive procedure as involutional changes progress (see below)
- **Involutional:** Three procedures may be used individually or in combination: (1) temporizing measure with lid taping below lower lid, Quickert suture or thermal cautery; (2) horizontal lid tightening with lateral tarsal strip procedure; and (3) lid retractor repair with full-thickness transverse blepharoplasty and eyelid margin rotation (Wies' procedure) or retractor reinsertion

Prognosis

Good prognosis except for autoimmune or inflammatory related cicatricial entropion.

Floppy Eyelid Syndrome

Definition

Chronic papillary conjunctivitis with lax tarsi, spontaneous eyelid eversion, and loss of eyelid-globe contact when lying prone; often occurs in obese men with sleep apnea.

Etiology

Nocturnal lid eversion with rubbing of the tarsal conjunctiva against adjacent bedding.

Symptoms

Chronically red and irritated eyes particularly upon awakening, mild mucous discharge.

Signs

Loose, rubbery eyelids (particularly upper lids), very easily everted, palpebral conjunctival papillae, conjunctival injection, superficial punctate keratitis.

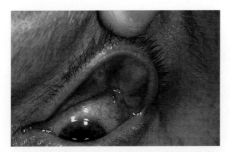

Figure 3–8. Floppy eyelid syndrome demonstrating extreme laxity of upper eyelid.

Differential Diagnosis

Giant papillary conjunctivitis, adult inclusion conjunctivitis, superior limbic keratoconjunctivitis, vernal keratoconjunctivitis, atopic keratoconjunctivitis, medicamentosa.

Evaluation

■ Complete ophthalmic history and eye exam with attention to eyelid laxity, palpebral conjunctiva, and corneal surface staining with fluorescein

Management

- Topical lubrication with nonpreserved artificial tears (see Appendix) up to q1h
- If corneal involvement exists, add topical antibiotic (erythromycin bid to qid for 5–7 days)
- Recommend that patient sleep on back or side
- Tape or patch eyelids closed while sleeping and consider metal eye shield to prevent lid eversion
- Consider lid tightening procedure or eyelid wedge resection to prevent spontaneous eversion; should be performed by an oculoplastic surgeon

Prognosis

Good with proper treatment.

Trichiasis

Definition

Eyelashes directed toward the eye either due to eyelash growth misdirection or eyelid margin inturning.

Etiology

Entropion, cicatricial eye disease, chronic eyelid inflammation, or idiopathic.

Symptoms

Red eye, foreign body sensation, and tearing.

Signs

Eyelashes directed toward and rubbing against the eye, conjunctival injection, superficial punctate keratitis; may have corneal scarring in chronic cases.

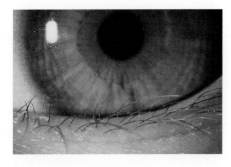

Figure 3–9. Trichiasis.

Differential Diagnosis

Distichiasis.

Evaluation

■ Complete ophthalmic history and eye exam with attention to lids, lashes, tarsal plate, palpebral conjunctiva, and cornea.

Management

- Topical lubrication with nonpreserved artificial tears (see Appendix) up to q1h
- If corneal involvement exists, add topical antibiotic (erythromycin or bacitracin bid to qid for 5–7 days)
- Mechanical epilation using fine forceps if only a few lashes are misdirected
- For segmental trichiasis, consider cryotherapy using a double freeze/thaw technique, lashes then mechanically removed using fine forceps; complications include lid edema, eyelid notching, and skin depigmentation
- Consider electrolysis for recurrent areas; use limited application because of the potential of scarring adjacent follicles and eyelid tissue
- Consider full-thickness wedge resection with primary closure for segmental trichiasis or entropion repair (see entropion section); should be performed by an oculoplastic surgeon

Prognosis

Usually good, frequent recurrences.

Blepharitis/Meibomitis

Definition

Inflammation of the eyelid margins (blepharitis) and inspissation of the oil-producing sebaceous glands of the lids (meibomitis); often occur together; extremely common in adult population and often coexists with dry eyes.

Etiology

Chronic *Staphylococcus* or *Demodex* infection, seborrhea, and eczema; angular blepharitis is associated with *Moraxella* infection.

Symptoms

Itching, red eye, burning, tearing, mild pain, foreign body sensation; often worse on awakening and late in the day.

Signs

Thickened and erythematous eyelid margins with telangiectatic blood vessels, crusting along eyelashes ("scurf" and "collarettes" in blepharitis); swollen, pitted, or blocked meibomian glands (meibomitis); may have "toothpaste sign" (gentle pressure on lids expresses columns of thick, white sebaceous material).

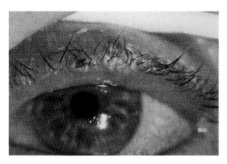

Figure 3–10. Blepharitis with thickened eyelid margins, flakes, and collarettes.

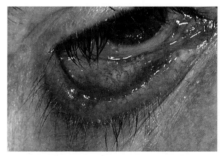

Figure 3–11. Meibomitis.

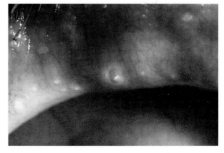

Figure 3–12. Meibomitis with obstructed, pouting meibomian gland orifices.

Differential Diagnosis

Acne rosacea, dry eye syndrome, herpes simplex virus, corneal foreign body, allergic or infectious conjunctivitis, chalazion/hordeolum (stye), sebaceous cell carcinoma, squamous or basal cell carcinoma, discoid lupus, medicamentosa, ocular cicatricial pemphigoid.

Evaluation

- Complete history with attention to history of skin cancer, sexually transmitted diseases, cold sores, allergies, eye medications, and chronic/recurrent disease; unilateral, chronic, or refractory symptoms suggest malignancy
- Complete eye exam with attention to lids, lashes, conjunctiva, and cornea
- Biopsy if lesions are suspicious for malignancy (ulcerated, yellow, chronic, scarred, or unilateral lid lesions, often with concomitant corneal pathology)
- Lab tests: chlamydia cultures (if there is associated chronic follicular conjunctivitis or suspicion of sexually transmitted disease)

Management

- Warm compresses for 10 minutes in both eyes qd to qid
- Daily lid scrubs with a cotton ball or cotton-tipped applicator using a 50:50 mixture of baby shampoo and warm water; stroke from the base of the lash outward
- Topical antibiotic ointment (bacitracin or erythromycin) at bedtime for 1–2 weeks
- Consider doxycycline 50–100 mg PO qd for recalcitrant cases
- Treat associated pathology such as rosacea or dry eye

Prognosis

Good; recurrence common; maintenance treatment often required indefinitely.

Chalazion/Hordeolum (Stye)

Definition

Hordeolum: Blocked, infected eyelid gland; most commonly meibomian glands (internal hordeolum) or the glands of Zeis or Moll (external hordeolum); associated with *Staphylococcus aureus*.

Chalazion: Obstruction and inflammation of meibomian gland with leakage of sebum into surrounding tissue and resultant lipogranuloma formation; often evolving from an internal hordeolum; associated with widespread meibomitis and/or rosacea.

Symptoms

Painful, hot, swollen, red eyelid lump; chronic chalazia become non-tender.

Signs

Erythematous subcutaneous nodule, sometimes tender with visible pointing or drainage; usually solitary, but can be multiple or bilateral; occasionally, severe swelling prevents visualization or palpation of a discrete nodule; may have signs of blepharitis/meibomitis.

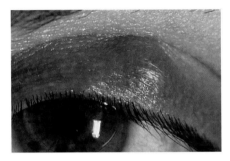

Figure 3–13. Chalazion.

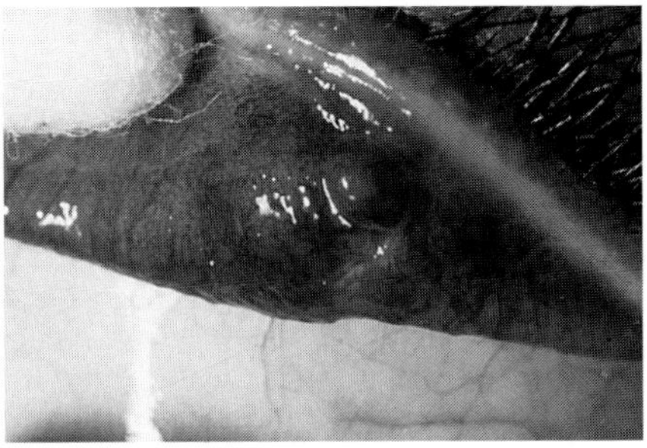

Figure 3–14. Same patient as shown in Figure 3–13 with everted lid.

Differential Diagnosis

Preseptal cellulitis, orbital cellulitis, sebaceous cell carcinoma, pyogenic granuloma.

Evaluation

- Complete ophthalmic history and eye exam with attention to previous episodes, fever, rosacea, meibomian gland evaluation, eyelid eversion, lashes, motility, and cornea.

Management

- Warm compresses with gentle massage for 10 minutes qid
- Topical antibiotic ointment (erythromycin or bacitracin bid to tid) in the inferior fornix if lesion is draining
- Consider incision and curettage after 1 month if no improvement
- Consider intralesional steroid injection (triamcinolone acetate 40 mg/mL; inject 0.5 mL with 30 gauge needle) for chalazia near lacrimal system or if only partially responsive to incision and curettage
- Recurrent lesion **must** be biopsied to rule out malignancy
- Treat underlying meibomitis and rosacea

Prognosis

Good; may take weeks to months to fully resolve; recurrence is common (20%); conservative treatment is recommended; surgical drainage can lead to scarring and further episodes; steroid injection can lead to depigmentation (especially in darkly pigmented individuals).

Lid Infections

Demodicosis: Hair follicle infection by *Demodex folliculorum*; associated with blepharitis; usually asymptomatic; examination of epilated hair follicles reveals sleeves of thin, semitransparent crusting at the base of the lashes.

- Lid scrubs with 50:50 mixture of baby shampoo and warm water followed by topical antibiotic ointment (erythromycin or bacitracin bid for 7–14 days).

Herpes Simplex Virus (HSV): Primary infection due to herpes simplex virus; often mild and unrecognized; patients may note pain, itching, and redness; appear as small crops of seropurulent vesicles on the eyelid that eventually rupture and crust over; marginal ulcerative blepharitis, follicular conjunctivitis, punctate or dendritic keratitis, and preauricular lymphadenopathy may also occur.

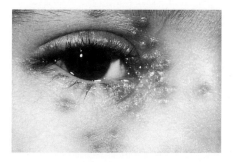

Figure 3–15. Primary herpes simplex virus with lid vesicles.

- Cold compresses bid to qid to affected skin area
- Topical antivirals (trifluridine 0.1% 9 times/day or vidarabine 3% 5 times/day for 14 days) for patients with blepharoconjunctivitis or corneal involvement
- Systemic antiviral (acyclovir [Zovirax] 400 mg PO 5 times/day for 10 days or famciclovir [Famvir] 500 mg PO tid for 7 days) when patient has constitutional symptoms

Herpes Zoster Virus (HZV): Maculopapular skin eruption, followed by vesicular ulceration and crusting due to reactivation of latent varicella zoster virus in the first division of cranial nerve V; usually involves upper lid and does not cross the midline; patients may have fever, lymphadenopathy, headache, malaise, nausea, tingling, paresthesias, and burning over cranial nerve V_1 dermatome; scarring may result with entropion, ectropion, lash loss (madarosis), canalicular and punctal stenosis, and lid retraction with exposure keratitis.

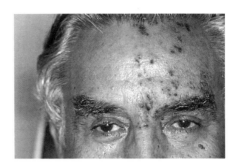

Figure 3–16. Herpes zoster virus demonstrating unilateral dermatomal distribution.

- Cool saline or aluminum sulfate–calcium acetate (Domeboro) compresses bid to tid
- Topical antibiotic ointment (erythromycin or bacitracin bid to tid) to affected skin
- Systemic antiviral (acyclovir [Zovirax] 800 mg PO 5 times/day for 10 days or famciclovir [Famvir] 500 mg PO tid for 7 days); if immunocompromised, acyclovir 10–12 mg/kg/day, IV divided, q8h for 10–14 days
- Treat post-herpetic neuralgia with Zostrix (capsaicin 0.025% tid to qid) cream to affected skin or amitriptyline (25 mg PO tid).

Leprosy: Chronic infectious disease caused by *Mycobacterium leprae*, a pleomorphic, acid-fast bacillus. Of the four variants, tuberculoid and lepromatous leprosy can have eyelid involvement, including loss of eyelashes and eyebrows, trichiasis, paralytic ectropion, lagophthalmos with exposure keratitis, and reduced blink rate; may develop corneal ulceration and perforation.

- Systemic multidrug treatment with dapsone (100 mg PO qd) and rifampin (600 mg PO qd); consider adding clofazimine (100 mg PO qd)
- Reduce corneal exposure with tarsorrhaphy or lateral tarsal strip procedure

Molluscum Contagiosum: Infection due to DNA poxvirus; spread by direct contact; usually asymptomatic; appears as a shiny dome-shaped waxy papule with central umbilication on the lid or lid margin; may be associated with chronic follicular conjunctivitis, superficial pannus, and superficial punctate keratitis; although disease is self-limited, resolution may take years; disseminated disease seen in AIDS patients.

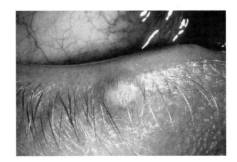

Figure 3–17. Molluscum contagiosum demonstrating characteristic umbilicated lesion.

- Incision and curettage of lesion with No. 11 Bard-Parker blade and chalazion curette, cryotherapy, or simple excision

Phthiriasis/Pediculosis: Infestation of eyelashes with lice (*Phthirus pubis*); usually sexually transmitted or from very close contact with an infected individual; patients note itching and burning; signs include small, pearly, white nits (eggs) attached to lashes, adult lice, preauricular lymphadenopathy, blood-tinged lids and lashes, blepharoconjunctivitis, conjunctival follicles, and conjunctival injection.

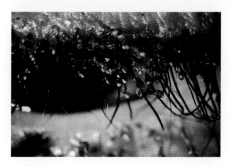

Figure 3–18. Infestation of eyelashes with *Phthirus pubis.*

- Mechanical removal of lice and nits with fine forceps
- Topical ointment (erythromycin, Lacri-Lube [white petrolatum, mineral oil, lanolin], or petroleum jelly tid for 14 days) to suffocate lice
- Physostigmine 0.25% ointment × 1, repeat in 1 week, *or*
- Fluorescein 20% 1–2 drops to lid margins *plus*
- Delousing creams and shampoo *(not for ocular use)*: permethrin cream rinse 1% (Nix), lindane 1%, gamma benzene hexachloride (Kwell), or pyrethrins liquid with piperonyl butoxide (RID, A-200 pyrinate liquid) (**Warning:** Kwell and RID not recommended for pregnant women and children)
- Discard or thoroughly wash in hot cycle all bedding, linens, and clothing
- Treat sexual partner

Verruca Vulgaris (Papilloma): Viral-related growth with potential for malignant transformation; usually asymptomatic; appears as a pedunculated or sessile hyperemic mass on eyelid or tarsal conjunctiva with minimal surrounding inflammation; associated with human papillomavirus (strains 6, 11, and 16); frequently resolves spontaneously.

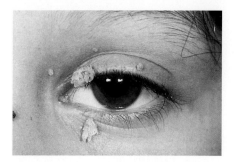

Figure 3–19. Verruca vulgaris.

- Observation if small and no inflammation
- Consider excision or cryotherapy for large or inflamed lesions

Congenital Anomalies

Ankyloblepharon: Partial or complete eyelid fusion; severe forms may be associated with craniofacial abnormalities; prognosis usually good unless severe associated defects.

- Simple cases treated with incision of skin webs after clamping with hemostat for 10–15 seconds; severe cases may necessitate major surgical revision by an oculoplastic surgeon

Blepharophimosis: Tight, foreshortened (vertically and horizontally) palpebral fissures with poor eyelid function and no levator fold; may be part of congenital syndrome (autosomal dominant [AD]): blepharophimosis, blepharoptosis, epicanthus inversus, and telecanthus; prognosis depends on extent of syndrome and need for additional surgery; mapped to chromosome 3q.

- Surgery is usually performed at 4–5 years of age to allow nasal bridge to fully develop
- Congenital syndrome: Consider two-stage oculoplastic repair with medial canthoplasty via Y-V plasty and transnasal wiring, followed by frontalis suspension for ptosis 3 to 4 months later; should be performed by an oculoplastic surgeon

Capillary Hemangioma: Most common benign pediatric eyelid tumor, usually presents at birth or in first few months of life with a bluish subcutaneous mass and normal overlying dermis, or as a superficial strawberry nevus representing hamartomatous growth of capillary blood vessels; spontaneous involution usually occurs by age 5; slight female predilection; possible amblyopia due to occlusion of the visual axis; induced astigmatism, myopia, and/or strabismus may occur; inappropriate early surgical intervention may lead to disfigurement and scarring; prognosis usually good if visual axis clear and no amblyopia.

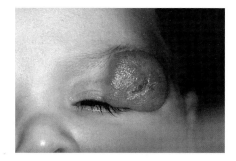

Figure 3–20. Capillary hemangioma.

- Routine follow-up visits to monitor for amblyopia
- Conservative management unless vision threatened by amblyopia, strabismus, occlusion of visual axis, anisometropia, or astigmatism; then consider intra-lesion steroid injection, interferon (Luperon), laser therapy, and/or surgical excision

Coloboma: Full thickness defect due to maldevelopment of the eyelid margin, usually superonasally; inferolateral defects are often bilateral and associated with systemic anomalies such as mandibulofacial dysostosis (AD) (Treacher Collins syndrome); corneal exposure and dryness may occur; small defects (<25%) have good prognosis; prognosis of medium and larger defects depends on location and associated abnormalities.

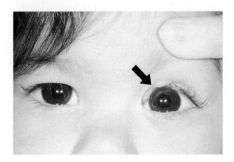

Figure 3–21. Coloboma of left upper eyelid (arrow).

- Topical lubrication with nonpreserved artificial tears or ointments (see Appendix) up to q1h
- Surgical repair should be performed by an oculoplastic surgeon: small defects (<25%) via direct layered closure, medium defects (25–50%) via Tensel flap with or without lateral cantholysis, large defects (>50%) via myocutaneous flap or full-thickness lid rotation flap
- Beware of lid-sharing procedures in children because occlusion amblyopia may result

Cryptophthalmos: Congenital defects of the first, second, and third wave of neural crest migration leading to abnormal lid and anterior eye structure development, including partial or complete absence of eyebrow, palpebral fissure, eyelashes, and conjunctiva; may have hidden or buried eye with smooth skin stretching from brow to cheek; posterior structures are usually normal; prognosis often poor due to underlying structural ocular defects.

- Given severe ocular defects of underlying eye, surgery is usually of no benefit, although success in mild cases has been reported

Distichiasis: Eyelashes growing posterior to or out of the meibomian gland orifices; may be congenital or acquired, sometimes hereditary; lashes are usually shorter, softer, and finer than normal cilia; usually well tolerated. In congenital distichiasis, the embryonic pilosebaceous units inappropriately develop into hair follicles; treat with caution since treatment can be more damaging than disease.

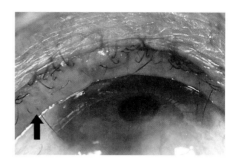

Figure 3–22. Distichiasis with lashes originating from meibomian gland orifice (arrow).

- Topical lubrication with nonpreserved artificial tears or ointments (see Appendix) and/or soft contact lens in mild cases
- Epilation, cryotherapy, electrolysis, laser thermal ablation in more severe cases of corneal involvement

Epiblepharon: Redundant skin and orbicularis muscle leading to inward rotation of the eyelid margin's turning lashes against the globe; usually resolves spontaneously; more common in Asians; prognosis excellent even if surgery necessary.

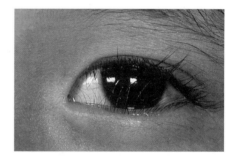

Figure 3–23. Epiblepharon.

- No treatment recommended, usually resolves spontaneously after several years
- If corneal involvement exists, excise redundant skin and muscle immediately adjacent to lid margin and reapproximate the skin edges

Epicanthus: Crescentic vertical skin folds in the medial canthal area overlying the medial canthal tendon; caused by immature facial bones or redundant skin and underlying tissue; may be most prominent superiorly (epicanthus tarsalis), inferiorly (epicanthus inversus), or equally distributed (epicanthus palpebralis); epicanthus tarsalis frequently associated with Asian eyelids, while epicanthus inversus associated with blepharophimosis syndrome; good prognosis.

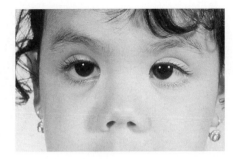

Figure 3–24. Epicanthus demonstrating pseudostrabismus.

- If due to facial bone immaturity, delay treatment
- When treatment required, Z-plasty or Y-V plasty often effective; eyelid crease construction may be required; should be performed by an oculoplastic surgeon

Euryblepharon: Horizontal widening of the palpebral fissure, often temporally; usually involves the lower eyelid with an anti-mongoloid appearance due to inferior insertion of the lateral canthal tendon; patients have a poor blink, poor lid closure, and lagophthalmos with exposure keratitis; usually good prognosis.

- Topical lubrication with nonpreserved artificial tears (see Appendix) in mild cases
- If symptoms severe and corneal pathology exists, full-thickness eyelid resection with repositioning of lateral canthal tendon may be required. If necessary, vertical eyelid lengthening can be achieved with skin grafts; should be performed by an oculoplastic surgeon

Microblepharon: Rare, bilateral, vertical foreshortening of the eyelids, sometimes causing exposure and dry eye symptoms; may be related to cryptophthalmos; usually stable with good prognosis if no exposure keratitis exists.

- Topical lubrication with nonpreserved artificial tears (see Appendix) in mild cases
- Pedicle rotation skin flaps from cheek or brow, eyelid-sharing procedures, or full-thickness skin grafts for severe exposure with a normal globe; should be performed by an oculoplastic surgeon
- Beware of lid-sharing procedures in children because occlusion amblyopia may result

Telecanthus: Increased distance between medial canthi caused by long medial canthal tendons; unlike in hypertelorism, the distance between the medial walls of the orbits is normal; most frequent ocular finding in fetal alcohol syndrome; also associated with Waardenburg's syndrome and blepharophimosis syndrome; good prognosis.

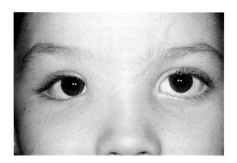

Figure 3–25. Telecanthus.

■ Transnasal wiring to shorten distance between medial canthi and remove excess medial canthal skin; should be performed by an oculoplastic surgeon

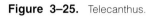

Neurofibromatosis (NF)

Definition

Neurofibromatosis is one of the classic phakomatoses and is an autosomal dominant (AD) disorder of the neuroectodermal system, affecting primarily neural crest–derived tissue (Schwann cells and melanocytes), manifesting with neural, cutaneous, and ocular hamartomas. The disorder displays highly variable expressivity; two types:

NF-1 (von Recklinghausen's disease): Located on chromosome 17q with a prevalence of 1 in 3000; 50% of cases represent new mutations. Diagnostic criteria requires two or more of the following:

(1) Six or more café-au-lait spots 15 mm or larger in adults, 5 mm or larger in children
(2) Two or more neurofibromas; or one plexiform neurofibroma
(3) Axillary or inguinal freckling
(4) Optic nerve or tract glioma
(5) Two or more Lisch nodules
(6) Characteristic osseous lesion (ie, sphenoid dysplasia)
(7) First-degree relative with NF-1 by these criteria

NF-2 (Bilateral Acoustic Neurofibromatosis): Located on chromosome 22q with a prevalence of 1 in 50,000. Diagnostic criteria include:

(1) Bilateral acoustic neuromas
(2) First-degree relative with NF-2 and either a single acoustic neuroma or two of the following: glioma, neurilemoma, meningioma, neurofibroma, or a premature posterior subcapsular cataract

Signs

NF-1: Café-au-lait spots, neurofibromas (fibroma molluscum), plexiform neurofibromas (bag of worms), intertriginous freckling, central nervous system (CNS) and spinal cord gliomas, meningiomas, nerve root neurofibromas, intracranial calcifications, mild intellectual deficit, kyphoscoliosis and pseudoarthroses, gastrointestinal (GI) neurofibromas, pheochromocytoma, plus various other malignant tumors.

NF-1 Ocular Findings: Lisch nodules (iris melanocytic hamartomas), eyelid café-au-lait spots, neurofibromas, and plexiform neurofibroma; at times ipsilateral glaucoma, proptosis secondary to tumors or bony defects, conjunctival neurofibromas, enlarged corneal nerves, diffuse uveal thickening, choroidal hamartomas, retinal astrocytic and combined hamartomas, optic nerve glioma.

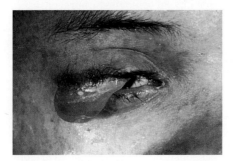

Figure 3–26. Eyelid neurofibroma.

NF-2: Paucity of cutaneous lesions (few or small café-au-lait spots), bilateral acoustic neuromas, CNS and spinal cord gliomas, meningiomas, nerve root neurofibromas, intracranial calcifications, pheochromocytoma, plus various other malignant tumors.

NF-2 Ocular Findings: No Lisch nodules, premature posterior subcapsular cataracts (40%), combined retinal hamartomas, optic nerve meningioma, and glioma.

Evaluation

- Complete ophthalmic history and eye examination with attention to family history (examine family members), color vision, pupils, lids, corneas, tonometry, iris, lens, ophthalmoscopy, visual field testing, general dermatologic evaluation (especially intertriginous regions), and neurologic screening
- Brain and orbital MRI and/or CT scan
- Lab tests: complete blood count (CBC), electrolytes, and urine catecholamines (vanillylmandelic acid [VMA], metanephrines)
- Audiography for NF-2 patients
- Intelligence testing

Management

- Genetic counseling
- Routine (q6–12 months) eye examinations to monitor for glaucoma, cataracts, and ocular malignancies
- Surgical removal of eyelid fibromas possible, but recurrence rate is high

Prognosis

Increased morbidity if associated with CNS or other malignant neoplasm.

Benign Lid Tumors

Actinic Keratosis: Most common precancerous skin lesion; 25% develop squamous cell carcinoma; round, scaly, flat, or papillary keratotic growths with surrounding erythema; seen in sun-exposed areas; occurs in older adults with fair complexions; male predilection; histologically, cellular atypia with mitotic figures and hyperkeratosis.

- Periocular lesions require incisional or excisional biopsy to rule out malignant lesions
- Cryotherapy or additional surgery can be performed once diagnosis is confirmed

Acquired Nevus: Darkly pigmented lesion that contains modified melanocytes called nevocellular nevus cells; classified according to location in skin: junctional (epidermis), compound (epidermis and dermis), or dermal (dermis); may contain hair; malignant transformation rare, although the Halo nevus, a type of compound nevus, is associated with remote cutaneous malignant melanoma. The Spitz nevus, another type of compound nevus, may be confused histologically with malignant melanoma in children and young adults.

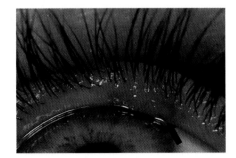

Figure 3–27. Nevus (arrow).

- No treatment usually required
- Consider excision for cosmesis, chronic irritation, or evidence of malignant transformation

Ephelis (Freckle): Focal regions of cutaneous melanocytic overactivity; cells slightly larger than normal; seen in sun-exposed areas; occurs in individuals with fair complexions; no malignant potential.

- No treatment recommended

Epidermal Inclusion Cyst: Firm, freely mobile, subepithelial lesion (1–5 mm in diameter); cyst contains cheesy keratin material produced by cyst lining; thought to arise from occluded surface epithelium or pilosebaceous follicles; multiple epidermal inclusion cysts may be associated with Gardner's syndrome or Torre's syndrome.

- Complete surgical excision

Inverted Follicular Keratosis: Small, solitary, benign lesion with a nodular or verrucous appearance; occurs in older adults; male predilection; may arise over months and is thought to have a viral etiology; histologically, lobular acanthosis of the epithelium with squamous and basal cell proliferation; represents a type of irritated seborrheic keratosis (see farther on).

- Complete surgical excision

Keratoacanthoma: Rapidly growing lesion usually seen in sun-exposed areas with a central ulcerated, keratin-filled crater and hyperkeratotic margins; occurs in older adults; lid or lash involvement may cause permanent damage; spontaneous resolution is common over 4–6 months; histologically, form of pseudoepitheliomatous hyperplasia; may have viral origin; multiple keratoacanthomas seen in Ferguson-Smith syndrome and Muir-Torre syndrome (multiple internal neoplasms, sebaceous lesions, and keratoacanthomas).

- May observe for spontaneous resolution if <6 months
- Complete surgical excision

Milia: Multiple, umbilicated, well-circumscribed, pinhead-sized, elevated, round, white nodules (1–3 mm in diameter); may arise spontaneously, or after trauma, radiation, herpes zoster ophthalmicus, or epidermolysis bullosa; thought to represent retention follicular cysts caused by blockage of pilosebaceous units.

- Complete surgical excision, electrolysis, or diathermy

Nevus of Ota (Oculodermal Melanocytosis): Unilateral, blue-gray, pigmented macule; usually in the distribution of the first and second division of cranial nerve V with ipsilateral melanocytosis of the sclera and uveal tract; 10% bilateral; melanosis of the ipsilateral orbit and leptomeninges may occur; histologically, composed of dermal fusiform dendritic melanocytes. May present at birth or in the 1st year of life; risk of malignant transformation is very low; however, cutaneous and ocular melanoma can occur, especially in Caucasians.

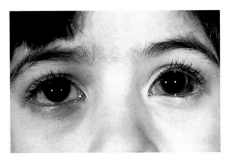

Figure 3–28. Nevus of Ota of the left eye (see Fig. 4–34).

- No treatment usually required
- Periodic examinations to monitor for evidence of malignant transformation

Sebaceous (Pilar) Cyst: Yellow, elevated, smooth, subcutaneous tumor with central comedo plug caused by sebaceous or meibomian gland obstruction; occurs in the elderly; less common than epithelial inclusion cysts; may be associated with chalazia.

- Complete surgical excision with inclusion of epithelial lining

Seborrheic Keratosis: Waxy, pigmented, hyperkeratotic, plaque-like, crusty lesion often seen in the elderly; histologically, composed of intradermal proliferation of basal epithelioid cells; irritation is frequent; no malignant potential.

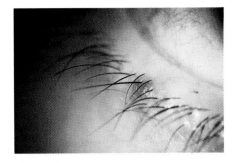

Figure 3–29. Seborrheic keratosis.

- Shave excision or curettage for small lesions
- Complete surgical excision for larger lesions

Squamous Papilloma: Most common benign eyelid growth; found in older adults; benign hyperplasia of the squamous epithelium; may be sessile or pedunculated with color similar to that of skin; grows slowly and in groups; histologically, papillomas display epithelial hyperkeratosis and acanthosis around a central vascular core.

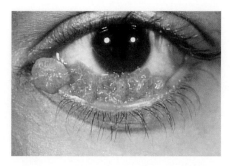

Figure 3–30. Squamous papilloma.

■ Complete surgical excision, cryotherapy, or carbon dioxide laser ablation

Malignant Lid Tumors

Basal Cell Carcinoma (BCC): Firm, pearly nodule or flatter, less well defined lesion with central ulceration, telangiectasia, madarosis (lash loss), and inflammation; associated with ultraviolet radiation exposure; constitutes 90% of all malignant eyelid tumors; occurs in older adults; usually seen on lower lid and medially; locally invasive, but rarely metastatic. Two growth patterns: (1) nodular, cystic, ulcerative (less invasive); and (2) morpheaform, sclerosing (more invasive). Associated with nevoid basal cell carcinoma syndrome, linear unilateral basal cell nevus, and Bazex syndrome; excellent prognosis with appropriate treatment, but 2–10% local recurrence; metastasis in 0.02 to 0.1%.

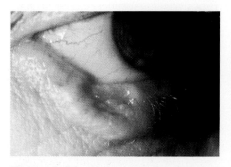

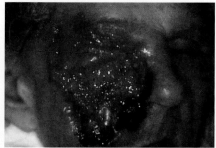

Figure 3–31. Basal cell carcinoma demonstrating central ulceration with pearly, nodular border containing telangiectatic vessels.

Figure 3–32. Advanced invasive basal cell carcinoma.

■ Protect against further sun damage
■ Complete surgical excision using micrographic (Moh's surgery) resection techniques and frozen or permanent section controls
■ May require surgical reconstruction when margins are free of tumor

- Consider additional cryotherapy, carbon dioxide laser treatment, photodynamic therapy, and/or immunotherapy
- Radiotherapy (nodular only) or chemotherapy can be utilized for nonsurgical candidates

Kaposi's Sarcoma of the Eyelid: Soft tissue sarcoma usually associated with AIDS, may also rarely occur in Africans and older men of Mediterranean descent; very malignant in immunocompromised patients; appears as violaceous nodules on the eyelids that are non-tender and progress over several months; may have associated distortion of the eyelid with entropion, edema, and misdirected lashes.

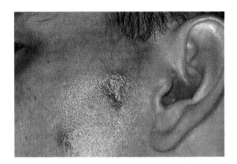

Figure 3–33. Kaposi's sarcoma.

- Complete surgical excision
- May require cryotherapy, radiotherapy, chemotherapy, and/or immunotherapy

Malignant Melanoma: Tan, black, or gray nodule or plaque with irregular, notched borders; often rapidly growing with color changes. Most lethal primary skin tumor, but rare in eyelids. Three patterns: (1) nodular melanoma; (2) superficial spreading melanoma (onset usually 20–60 years of age); and (3) lentigo maligna melanoma (usually in the elderly); acral lentiginous melanoma not seen in the eyelids; orderly growth with Stage 1: localized disease without lymph node spread; Stage 2: palpable regional lymph nodes (preauricular from upper lid, submandibular from lower lid); and Stage 3: distant metastases; choroidal melanoma may reach lids via extrascleral extension into orbit; fair prognosis for Stage 1, poor for Stages 2 and 3.

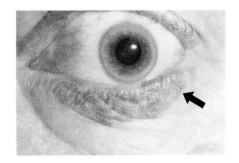

Figure 3–34. Malignant melanoma (arrow).

■ Excision with or without wide margins, neck dissection

Merkel Cell Tumor: Rare, rapidly growing, solitary, violaceous, vascularized, occasionally ulcerated tumor of the amino precursor uptake and decarboxylation (APUD) system; usually seen in sun-exposed areas; onset in 7th decade; reported only in Caucasians; potential for recurrence and lymphatic spread with lymph node enlargement; generally poor prognosis due to early spread after local excision alone, 39% recur locally and 46% recur regionally; after adjuvant radiation therapy or node dissection, 26% recur locally and 22% regionally; 67% tumor mortality for locoregional spread.

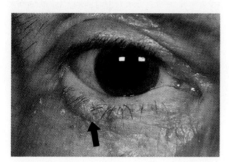

Figure 3–35. Merkel cell tumor (arrow).

■ Wide local excision (immunohistochemical stains for enkephalin, calcitonin, somatostatin, corticotropin, and neuron-specific enolase)
■ Lymph node resection
■ Supplemental radiation therapy

Metastatic Tumors: Metastatic eyelid lesions are very rare; female predilection; occurs in older adults; primary sites include breast and lung (most common) carcinoma, cutaneous malignancies, gastrointestinal and genitourinary carcinomas. Three patterns: (1) single non-tender nodule, (2) painless diffuse induration, (3) ulcerating lesion of eyelid skin or conjunctiva; evidence of primary tumor elsewhere, lymph node enlargement; usually poor prognosis but variable.

■ Local excision or radiation therapy
■ Systemic treatment for primary tumor

Sebaceous Cell Carcinoma: Highly malignant neoplasm of the sebaceous glands in the caruncle or lids; occurs in older patients; often masquerades as chronic blepharitis (20–50% of patients) or recurrent chalazion; usually seen on upper lid; constitutes 1–15% of malignant eyelid tumors; female predilection; usually in the 7th decade of life; sometimes related to previous (often remote) radiotherapy; undergoes pagetoid spread; suspicious signs include recurrent chalazia, thickened, reddened lid margins, madarosis, chronic unilateral blepharitis or blepharoconjunctivitis, and lymph node enlargement; poor prognosis when symptomatic for greater than 6 months (38% mortality vs 14% for less than 6 months), size >2 cm

(60% mortality vs 18% when <1 cm), upper and lower lid involvement (83% mortality), poor differentiation, and local vascular or lymphatic infiltration.

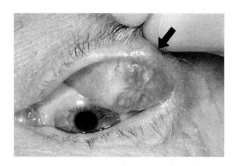

Figure 3–36. Sebaceous cell carcinoma (arrow).

- Surgical incisional or excisional biopsy with intraoperative frozen sections and wide margins
- Conjunctival and nasal mucosal map biopsy
- Exenteration (including lacrimal apparatus) with orbital involvement
- Palliative radiation

Squamous Cell Carcinoma (SCC): Flat or slightly elevated, scaly, ulcerated, erythematous plaque, often arising from actinic keratosis, may also arise from Bowen's disease and radiation dermatosis; constitutes <5% of malignant eyelid tumors; usually seen on lower lid with lid margin involvement; associated with solar or radiation injury, or other irritative insults; less common but faster growing than basal cell carcinoma; potentially metastatic and locally invasive, regional lymph node spread from eyelids occurs in 13–24% of cases; prognosis varies with tumor size, degree of differentiation, underlying etiology, and depth of tumor invasion.

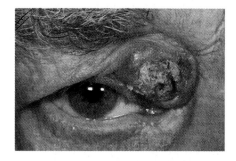

Figure 3–37. Squamous cell carcinoma.

- Protect against further sun damage
- Incisional or excisional biopsy with wide surgical margins
- Adjunctive radiation, cryotherapy, and/or chemotherapy

Canaliculitis

Definition

Inflammation of the canaliculus (duct between the punctum and lacrimal sac) often resulting in recurrent conjunctivitis due to viral (herpes simplex), bacterial, or fungal infections; usually insidious onset.

Etiology

Actinomyces israelii (streptothrix), a filamentous gram-positive rod, is the most common cause; other organisms include *Candida albicans, Aspergillus, Nocardia asteroides*, and herpes simplex/zoster virus; more common in middle-aged women.

Symptoms

Medial eyelid tenderness, tearing, and redness.

Signs

Erythema and swelling of punctum and adjacent tissue, follicular conjunctivitis around medial canthus, expression of discharge from punctum, concretions in canaliculus, grating sensation on lacrimal duct probing, dilated canaliculus on dacryocystography.

Differential Diagnosis

Conjunctivitis, dacryocystitis, nasal lacrimal duct obstruction, carunculitis.

Evaluation

- Complete ophthalmic history and eye exam with attention to history of recurrent conjunctivitis, examination of lids, punctum, lacrimal system, and conjunctiva
- Compression medial to the punctum observing for discharge
- Lab tests: culture and Gram stain (*Actinomyces* branching filaments and sulfur granules on Gram stain)
- Probing and possible irrigation to determine patency of canalicular system
- Consider dacryocystography to confirm a dilated canaliculus, concretions, or normal outflow function in the lower excretory system

Management

- Warm compresses to canalicular region bid to qid
- Canalicular concretion removal either by manual expression (topical anesthetic to conjunctival sac, then massage canaliculus between two cotton tip applicators in attempt to express concretion through punctum) or more commonly through marsupialization of the canaliculus

> **Management** *Continued*
>
> - ***Actinomyces israelii:*** Canalicular irrigation with antibiotic solution (penicillin G 100,000 U/mL) and systemic antibiotic (penicillin V 500 mg PO qid for 7 days)
> - ***Candida albicans:*** Systemic antifungal (fluconazole 600 mg PO qd for 7–10 days)
> - ***Aspergillus:*** Topical antifungal (amphotericin B 0.15% tid) and systemic antifungal (itraconazole 200 mg PO bid for 7–10 days)
> - ***Nocardia asteroides:*** Topical antibiotic (sulfacetamide tid) and systemic antibiotic (trimethoprim-sulfamethoxazole [Bactrim] one double-strength tablet PO qd for 7–10 days)
> - **Herpes simplex/zoster virus:** Topical antiviral (trifluridine 0.1% 5 times/day for 2 weeks); if stenosis present may need silicone intubation

Prognosis

Often good; depends on infecting organism.

Dacryoadenitis

Definition

Acute: Acute inflammation of the lacrimal gland usually of viral, bacterial, or rarely parasitic etiology.

Chronic: Chronic inflammation of the lacrimal gland (more common than acute form).

Etiology

Acute: Most commonly due to infection (*Staphylococcus* species, mumps, Epstein-Barr virus, herpes zoster, or *Neisseria gonorrhoeae*); palpebral lobe affected more frequently than orbital lobe; most cases associated with systemic infection; typically occurs in children and young adults.

Chronic: Usually due to inflammatory disorders including idiopathic orbital inflammation, sarcoidosis, thyroid ophthalmopathy, Sjögren's syndrome, and benign lymphoepithelial lesions; also seen with syphilis and tuberculosis.

Symptoms

Acute: Temporal upper eyelid redness, swelling, and pain with tearing and discharge.

Chronic: Temporal upper eyelid swelling; occasional redness and discomfort.

Signs

Acute: Edema, tenderness, and erythema of upper eyelid with S-shaped deformity, enlarged and erythematous lacrimal gland (palpebral lobe), preauricular lymphadenopathy, and fever; may have inferonasal globe displacement and proptosis if orbital lobe involved.

Chronic: Tenderness in superotemporal area of upper eyelid, globe displacement, restricted ocular motility, and enlarged lacrimal gland.

Differential Diagnosis

Malignant lacrimal gland neoplasm, preseptal or orbital cellulitis, viral conjunctivitis, chalazion, dermoid tumor, lacrimal gland cyst (dacryops).

Evaluation

Acute:
- Complete ophthalmic history and eye exam with attention to constitutional signs, palpation of parotids, lymph nodes, and upper lid, examination of palpebral lacrimal lobe (lift upper lid) for enlargement, globe retropulsion, and motility
- Check Hertel exophthalmometry
- Lab tests: culture and Gram stain of discharge, CBC with differential; consider blood cultures for suspected systemic involvement
- Orbital CT scan for proptosis, motility restriction, or suspected mass

Chronic:
- Complete ophthalmic history and eye exam with attention to constitutional signs, palpation of parotids, lymph nodes, and upper lid; examination of palpebral lacrimal lobe (lift upper lid) for enlargement, globe retropulsion, motility, and signs of previous anterior or posterior uveitis
- Check Hertel exophthalmometry
- Lab tests: chest radiographs, CBC with differential, angiotensin converting enzyme (ACE), venereal disease research laboratory (VDRL), fluorescent treponemal antibody absorption test (FTA-ABS), purified protein derivative (PPD), anergy panel
- Orbital CT scan
- Consider lacrimal gland biopsy if diagnosis uncertain or malignancy suspected

Management

ACUTE:

- **Mumps/Epstein-Barr virus:** Warm compresses bid to tid
- **Herpes simplex/zoster virus:** Systemic antivirals (acyclovir [Zovirax] 800 mg PO 5 times/day for 10 days or famciclovir [Famvir] 500 mg PO tid for 7 days); in immunocompromised patients use acyclovir 10–12 mg/kg/day IV divided into three doses for 7–10 days

Management Continued

- ■ *Staphylococcus* and *Streptococcus* species: Systemic antibiotic (amoxicillin-clavulanate [Augmentin] 500 mg PO q8h); in severe cases ampicillin-sulbactam [Unasyn] 1.5–3 g IV q6h
- ■ *Neisseria gonorrhoeae*: Systemic antibiotic (ceftriaxone 1 g IV × 1); warm compresses and incision and drainage if suppurative
- ■ *Mycobacterium* species: Surgical excision and systemic treatment with isoniazid (300 mg PO qd) and rifampin (600 mg PO qd) for 6–9 months, follow liver function tests for toxicity; consider adding pyrazinamide (25–35 mg/kg PO qd) for first 2 months
- ■ *Treponema pallidum:* Systemic antibiotic (penicillin G 24 million U/day IV for 10 days)

CHRONIC:

- ■ Treat underlying inflammatory disorder
- ■ Treat infections (rare) as above

Prognosis

Depends on cause; most infections respond well to treatment.

Dacryocystitis

Definition

Acute or chronic infection of the lacrimal sac, often with overlying cellulitis.

Etiology

Streptococcus pneumoniae, Staphylococcus species, and *Pseudomonas* species; *Haemophilus influenzae* in children.

Epidemiology

Conditions that cause lacrimal sac tear stasis and predispose to infection, including strictures, long and narrow nasolacrimal ducts, lacrimal sac diverticulum, trauma, dacryoliths, nasal lacrimal duct obstruction, and inflammatory sinus and nasal problems.

Symptoms

Pain, swelling, and redness over nasal portion of lower eyelid with tearing and crusting; may have fever.

Signs

Edema and erythema below the medial canthal tendon with lacrimal sac swelling; tenderness on palpation of the lacrimal sac, expression of discharge from the punctum; may have fistula formation or lacrimal sac cyst.

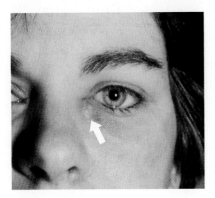

Figure 3–38. Dacryocystitis demonstrating swelling of lacrimal sac of the left eye (arrow).

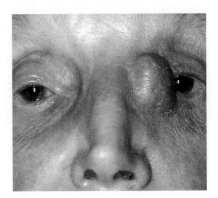

Figure 3–39. Dacryocystitis with massive medial canthal swelling.

Differential Diagnosis

Ethmoid sinusitis, preseptal or orbital cellulitis, lacrimal sac neoplasm, dacryocystocele (infants) and encephalocele (infants, blue mass above medial canthal tendon).

Evaluation

- Complete ophthalmic history with attention to previous history of sinus and/or upper respiratory infection
- Complete eye exam with attention to lids, lacrimal system, expression of discharge from punctum, motility, proptosis, and conjunctiva
- Lab tests: culture and Gram stain any punctal discharge (chocolate agar in children)
- Do not probe nasolacrimal duct during acute infection
- Orbital CT scan for limited motility, proptosis, sinus disease, or atypical cases not responding to antibiotic therapy

Management

- Warm compresses tid

ACUTE:

- Systemic antibiotics (amoxicillin-clavulanate [Augmentin] 500 mg PO tid for 10 days or amoxicillin-sulbactam [Unasyn] 15–30 mg IV q6h); if

Management Continued

penicillin-allergic, use trimethoprim-sulfamethoxazole (Bactrim; one double-strength tablet PO bid for 10 days)
- Topical antibiotic (erythromycin ointment bid) if conjunctivitis exists
- Aspirate lacrimal sac contents with 18 gauge needle for culture and Gram stain
- If pointing abscess, consider incision and drainage
- Consider dacryocystorhinostomy with silicone intubation once infection has resolved; should be performed by an oculoplastic surgeon

CHRONIC:

- Cultures to determine antibiotic therapy (see above)
- Dacryocystorhinostomy usually necessary to relieve obstruction after infection resolved; should be performed by an oculoplastic surgeon

Prognosis

Good; usually responds to therapy, but surgical intervention often required, particularly with chronic dacryocystitis; if untreated, sequelae include mucocele formation, orbital cellulitis, and infectious keratitis.

Nasolacrimal Duct Obstruction (NLDO)

Definition

Obstruction of the nasolacrimal duct; may be congenital or acquired.

Etiology

Congenital: Most frequently due to an imperforate membrane over the valve of Hasner at the nasal end of the duct; occurs clinically in 2–4% of full-term infants at 1–2 weeks of age; bilateral in one third of cases. Spontaneous opening frequently occurs 1–2 months after birth; may be complicated by acute dacryocystitis.

Acquired: Due to chronic sinus disease, involutional stenosis, dacryocystitis, or naso-orbital trauma. Involutional stenosis is the most common cause in older individuals; female predilection (2:1); may be associated with granulomatous diseases such as Wegener's granulomatosis and sarcoidosis; increased risk of dacryocystitis.

Symptoms

Tearing, discharge, crusting, recurrent conjunctivitis.

Signs

Watery eyes, eyelash crusting and debris, mucus reflux from punctum with compression over the lacrimal sac, medial lower eyelid erythema.

Differential Diagnosis

Congenital Tearing: Congenital glaucoma, trichiasis, conjunctivitis, nasal lacrimal duct anomalies (punctal atresia), dacryocystocele, corneal abrasion, corneal trauma from forceps delivery, ocular surface foreign body.

Acquired Tearing: Conjunctivitis, trichiasis, entropion, ectropion, corneal abnormalities, dry eye syndrome, punctal stenosis.

Evaluation

- Complete ophthalmic history and eye exam with attention to lid margins, lashes, puncta, conjunctiva, cornea (diameter, breaks in Descemet's membrane staining with fluorescein), tonometry, palpate over lacrimal sac and observe for reflux of discharge from punctum.

Management

- Warm compresses bid to qid
- Topical antibiotic ointment (erythromycin bid for 1 week) if mucopurulent discharge

CONGENITAL:

- Crigler massage bid to qid (parent places index finger over infant's canaliculi (medial corner of eyelid) and makes several slow downward strokes)
- Nasolacrimal duct probing between age 6 and 13 months if no spontaneous resolution, exact timing for probing is controversial, probing may be repeated; consider silicone intubation of the NLD after one to three unsuccessful attempts

ACQUIRED:

- Treat partial NLDO with antibiotic-steroid preparation (Maxitrol qid)
- Consider silicone intubation of the NLD system for persistent partial obstruction
- Complete NLDO with patent canaliculi and functional lacrimal pump requires dacryocystorhinostomy (anastomosis between lacrimal sac and nasal cavity through a bony ostium); should be performed by an oculoplastic surgeon

Prognosis

Congenital is excellent; acquired is often good, depends on cause of obstruction.

Lacrimal Gland Tumors

Definition

Approximately 50% of all lacrimal gland masses are inflammatory; the other 50% are neoplasms, one half of which are of epithelial origin and the other half of which are primarily lymphoproliferative. Of all epithelial tumors, 50% are benign pleomorphic adenomas, and 50% are malignant. All lesions usually present in the superotemporal quadrant of the orbit.

Benign Mixed Cell Tumor (Pleomorphic Adenoma): Most common epithelial tumor of the lacrimal gland, usually presenting insidiously in the 4th and 5th decade, often with inferior and medial displacement of the globe. A firm, circumscribed mass can be palpated under the superior temporal orbital rim, often with bony cavitation on radiographic images; histologically, these tumors contain a pseudocapsule, a double row of epithelial cells forming lumens, and stroma containing spindle-shaped cells with mucinous, osteoid, or cartilaginous metaplasia.

Malignant Mixed Cell Tumor (Pleomorphic Adenocarcinoma): Occurs in the elderly with pain and rapid progression; contains the same epithelial and mesenchymal features of pleomorphic adenoma, but with malignant components; associated with long-standing or incompletely excised pleomorphic adenomas.

Adenoid Cystic Carcinoma (Cylindroma): Most common malignant tumor of the lacrimal gland, rapid onset with infiltrative capacity; associated with pain due to perineural invasion and bony erosion, often with accompanying proptosis. Histologically, the tumor is composed of densely staining, packed small cells that grow in nests, tubules, or a Swiss-cheese (cribriform) pattern; the basaloid pattern carries the worst prognosis; CT scan shows a poorly-defined mass with adjacent bony destruction.

Symptoms

Upper lid fullness, diplopia, pain.

Signs

Inferior and medial globe displacement, limitation of ocular movements, lid edema and erythema, palpable mass under the superotemporal orbital rim.

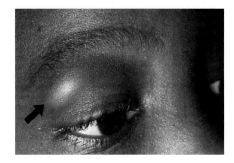

Figure 3–40. Lacrimal gland tumor (arrow).

Differential Diagnosis

Dermoid, sarcoidosis, idiopathic orbital inflammation, lymphoid tumor, dacryops.

Evaluation

- Complete ophthalmic history and eye exam with attention to duration of onset, rate of progression, pain, visual complaints, and constitutional symptoms
- Complete eye exam with attention to lids, lacrimal gland, orbital rim, and motility
- Orbital CT scan demonstrates well-circumscribed mass with lacrimal gland fossa enlargement (pleomorphic adenoma) or an irregular mass with or without adjacent bony erosion (adenoid cystic carcinoma)
- Lacrimal gland biopsy when a malignancy is suspected or the diagnosis is uncertain (do not biopsy suspected pleomorphic adenomas)
- Consider oncology consultation

Management

- **Benign Mixed Tumor (Pleomorphic Adenoma):** En bloc excision via a lateral orbitotomy; rupture of pseudocapsule may lead to recurrence and malignant transformation
- **Pleomorphic Adenocarcinoma:** Same as for adenoid cystic carcinoma
- **Adenoid Cystic Carcinoma (Cylindroma):** Orbital exenteration with adjunctive chemotherapy and radiation after review of biopsy on permanent slide sections; should be performed by an oculoplastic surgeon

Prognosis

- **Benign Mixed Tumor (Pleomorphic Adenoma):** Excellent if tumor is completely excised
- **Pleomorphic Adenocarcinoma:** Similar to adenoid cystic carcinoma
- **Adenoid Cystic Carcinoma (Cylindroma):** Five-year survival rate is 47%, and at 15 years is only 22%; major cause of death is intracranial extension due to perineural spread

Miscellaneous Lesions

Amyloidosis: Localized or systemic disease with deposition of amyloid in various tissues, classified into primary, myeloma-associated, and secondary amyloidosis; the eyelids are a common site of involvement in primary and secondary systemic variants, but the disease can involve all ocular structures including skin, orbit, extraocular muscles, lacrimal gland, orbital nerves, conjunctiva, cornea, anterior chamber, iris, lens, vitreous, retina and retinal vasculature, choroid, optic nerve, and higher visual pathways; may appear as flat or nodular purpuric lesions of the eyelid skin, caruncle, conjunctiva, or lacrimal gland (ruptured, fragile, amyloid-infiltrated blood vessels in abnormal tissue), or may occur without hemorrhage as elevated yellowish waxy papules (often seen in the skin of all four lids); may have dry eye symptoms (with lacrimal and conjunctival involvement); very poor prognosis when associated with multiple myeloma, other forms have variable prognosis depending on underlying disorder and tissues involved.

- Biopsy is gold standard
- Lab tests: serum and urine protein electrophoresis, CBC with differential, serum total protein, albumin and globulin, liver function tests, blood urea nitrogen (BUN) and creatinine, erythrocyte sedimentation rate (ESR), ANA, VDRL, FTA-ABS, urinalysis, PPD, chest radiographs, electrocardiogram (EKG), bone scan
- Surgical excision/debulking, radiotherapy where feasible
- Corticosteroids (multiple myeloma only; contraindicated in primary amyloidosis)

Sarcoidosis: Idiopathic multisystem disease, with abnormalities in cell-mediated and humoral immunity and granulomatous inflammation in many organs; commonly affects the lungs, skin, and eyes including the eyelid skin, lacrimal gland and sac, and nasolacrimal duct; may cause redness, pain, swelling of involved lids or lacrimal glands (usually bilateral), painless subcutaneous nodular masses of eyelids, ptosis, diplopia, severe cicatrizing conjunctival inflammation, conjunctival nodules, keratoconjunctivitis sicca, band keratopathy, granulomatous anterior or posterior uveitis, cataract, chorioretinitis, retinal periphlebitis or neovascularization, optic nerve disease, glaucoma, and orbital involvement; variable prognosis depending on organs involved.

- Biopsy of conjunctival, lacrimal, or eyelid nodule (with stains to rule out acid-fast bacteria)
- Lab tests: ACE, lysozyme, serum calcium, chest radiographs, tuberculin test with anergy panel, upper-body gallium scan, Kveim test (historical), pulmonary function tests
- Topical, peribulbar, and/or systemic steroids, cycloplegics for uveitis (see Chap. 6)
- Panretinal photocoagulation for retinal neovascularization or choroidal neovascular membranes
- May require modified goniotomy, cyclodestructive procedures, or glaucoma drainage implant for uncontrolled glaucoma
- Systemic steroids and chemotherapy for other organ system involvement

Xanthelasma: Xanthomas of the eyelids that appear as flat or slightly elevated creamy yellow plaques; most commonly involving the medial upper lids bilaterally; histologically composed of foamy histiocytes surrounded by localized inflammation; occurs in older patients with hyperlipidemias, or occasionally in normolipidemic patients with lipoprotein abnormalities; may have family history of hypercholesterolemia or hypertriglyceridemia; associated with lipoid granulomatosis (Erdheim-Chester disease, characterized by lipogranulomas containing Touton giant cells in long bones, heart, lungs, kidneys, eyelids, orbit, and optic nerve); excellent prognosis, may recur after excision.

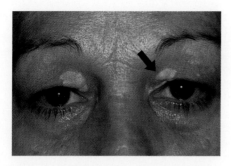

Figure 3–41. Xanthelasma (arrow).

- Lab tests: serum cholesterol and triglycerides
- Full-thickness excision with flaps or grafts as needed
- Carbon dioxide laser treatment

Conjunctiva / Sclera

Trauma

Foreign Body (FB): Exogenous material on, under, or embedded within conjunctiva or sclera; commonly dirt, glass, metal, or cilia; patients usually note foreign body sensation and redness; good prognosis.

- Remove foreign body if present; evert lids to check for foreign body
- Add topical broad-spectrum antibiotic (polymyxin B sulfate–trimethoprim [Polytrim] or bacitracin qid)

Laceration: Partial- or full-thickness cut in conjunctiva and/or partial-thickness cut in the sclera; very important to rule out open globe (see below); good prognosis.

- Complete ophthalmic history and eye exam with attention to evaluating extent of laceration, tonometry, anterior chamber (AC), and ophthalmoscopy
- Perform Seidel test for suspected open globe (see below)
- Conjunctival and partial-thickness scleral lacerations do not require surgical repair; add topical broad-spectrum antibiotic (polymyxin B sulfate–trimethoprim [Polytrim] or bacitracin qid)

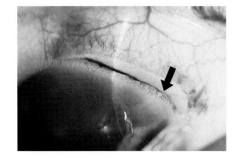

Figure 4–1 Full-thickness corneoscleral limbal laceration (arrow).

Open Globe: Full-thickness defect in eye wall (cornea or sclera) commonly from penetrating or blunt trauma; the latter usually causes rupture at the limbus, just posterior to the rectus muscle insertions, or at previous surgical incision sites; double penetrating injuries are called perforations; an open globe may also be due to corneal or scleral melting. Associated signs include lid and orbital trauma, corneal abrasion or laceration, wound dehiscence, positive Seidel test, low intraocular pressure, flat/shallow anterior chamber, AC cell/flare, hyphema, peaked pupil, iris transillumination defect, sphincter tears, angle recession, iridodialysis, cyclodialysis, iridodonesis, phacodonesis, dislocated lens, cataract, vitreous and retinal hemorrhage, commotio retinae, retinal tear/detachment, choroidal rupture, intraocular foreign body or gas bubbles, and/or extruded intraocular contents. Guarded prognosis.

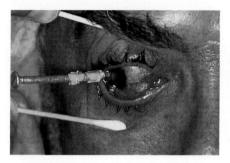

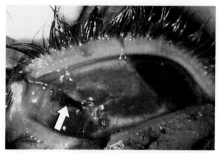

Figure 4–2 Penetrating injury with foreign body (nail) protruding from globe.

Figure 4–3 Open globe demonstrating chemosis, subconjunctival hemorrhage, and uveal prolapse (arrow); also note eyelid lacerations.

OPHTHALMIC EMERGENCY:

- Complete ophthalmic history and eye exam with attention to evaluating extent of laceration, tonometry, Seidel test, anterior chamber lens, and ophthalmoscopy
- Consider B-scan ultrasonography if unable to visualize the fundus
- Consider orbital computed tomography (CT) or orbital radiographs to rule out intraocular foreign body; magnetic resonance imaging (MRI) is contraindicated if foreign body is metallic
- Admit for surgical exploration and repair; protect eye with metal eye shield; minimize ocular manipulations; examine globe only enough to verify the diagnosis of an open globe; remainder of examination and exploration should be performed in the operating room. Postoperatively, start antibiotics and steroids.
  - Subconjunctival antibiotics/steroids:
    Vancomycin (25 mg)
    Ceftazidime (50–100 mg) or gentamicin (20 mg)
    Dexamethasone (12–24 mg)

> **OPHTHALMIC EMERGENCY** *Continued*
> - Broad-spectrum fortified topical antibiotics (alternate every 30 minutes):
>   Vancomycin (25–50 mg/mL q1h)
>   Ceftazidime (50 mg/mL q1h)
> - Topical steroid (prednisolone acetate 1% q1–2h initially) and cycloplegic (scopolamine 0.25% or atropine 1% tid)
> - Systemic IV antibiotics for marked inflammation or severe cases:
>   Vancomycin (1 g IV q12h)
>   Ceftazidime (1 g IV q12h)
> - Small corneal lacerations (<2 mm) that are self-sealing or intermittently Seidel-positive may be treated with a bandage contact lens, topical broad-spectrum antibiotic (ciprofloxacin [Ciloxan] or ofloxacin [Ocuflox] q2h to q6h, cycloplegic (cyclopentolate 1% qd), and an aqueous suppressant (timolol maleate [Timoptic] 0.5% or bromonidine [Alphagan] bid); observe daily for 5–7 days; consider suturing laceration if wound has not sealed after 1 week

Subconjunctival Hemorrhage: Diffuse or focal area of blood under conjunctiva; appears bright red, otherwise asymptomatic; may be idiopathic or associated with trauma, sneezing, coughing, straining, emesis, aspirin or anticoagulant use, or hypertension; excellent prognosis.

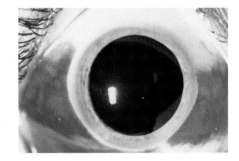

Figure 4–4 Subconjunctival hemorrhage.

- Reassurance if no other ocular findings
- Medical or hematology consultation for recurrent, idiopathic, subconjunctival hemorrhages
- Consider blood pressure measurement and hematology work-up if recurrent

Telangiectasia

Definition

Abnormal, dilated conjunctival capillary formation.

Symptoms

Asymptomatic red spot on eye; patient may have epistaxis and gastrointestinal bleeding depending on etiology.

Signs

Telangiectasia of conjunctival vessels, subconjunctival hemorrhage.

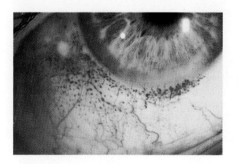

Figure 4–5 Conjunctival telangiectasia.

Differential Diagnosis

Idiopathic, Osler-Weber-Rendu syndrome, ataxia-telangiectasia, Fabry's disease, Sturge-Weber syndrome.

Evaluation

- Complete ophthalmic history and eye exam with attention to conjunctiva, cornea, lens, and ophthalmoscopy
- Consider CT scan for multisystem disorders
- Medical consultation to rule out systemic disease

Management

- No treatment recommended

Prognosis

Usually benign; may bleed; depends on etiology.

Microaneurysm

Definition

Focal dilatation of conjunctival vessel.

Symptoms

Asymptomatic; may notice red spot on eye.

Signs

Microaneurysm; may have associated retinal findings.

Differential Diagnosis

Diabetes mellitus, hypertension, sickle cell anemia (Paton's sign), arteriosclerosis, carotid occlusion, fucosidosis, polycythemia vera.

Evaluation

- Complete ophthalmic history and eye exam with attention to conjunctiva and ophthalmoscopy
- Check blood pressure
- Lab tests: fasting blood glucose (diabetes mellitus), sickle cell prep, hemoglobin electrophoresis (sickle cell)
- Medical consultation

Management

- No treatment recommended
- Treat underlying medical disease

Prognosis

Usually benign.

Dry Eye Syndrome (DES)

Definition

Ocular irritation due to deficiency of one or more tear film components (lipid, aqueous, or mucin).

Etiology

Many conditions may produce a tear film abnormality, including:

Keratoconjunctivitis Sicca: Aqueous tear deficiency; may be associated with Sjögren's syndrome (dry eye, dry mouth, and arthritis), rheumatoid arthritis, and collagen vascular diseases; >95% female.

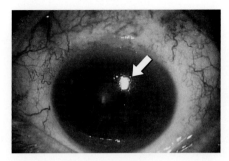

Figure 4–6 Keratoconjunctivitis sicca demonstrating irregular corneal light reflex (arrow).

Acne Rosacea: Inflammatory disease causing meibomian gland dysfunction and blepharoconjunctivitis, corneal vascularization, infiltrates, and ulceration; associated with facial skin changes (erythema, pustules, telangiectasia, rhinophyma); may be exacerbated by foods (eg, alcohol and chocolate) (see Chap. 1).

Vitamin A Deficiency: Conjunctival xerosis and lack of mucin; associated with Bitot's spots (due to gas-producing bacteria *Corynebacterium xerosis*), corneal ulceration, and night blindness (nyctalopia) with progressive retinal degeneration; major cause of worldwide blindness.

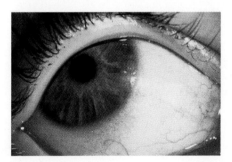

Figure 4–7 Vitamin A deficiency demonstrating diffuse staining of cornea, inferior limbus, and interpalpebral conjunctiva with rose bengal.

Symptoms

Dryness, burning, foreign body sensation, tearing, red eye, discharge, blurred vision, photophobia; symptoms exacerbated by wind, smoke, and reading.

Signs

Blepharitis, conjunctival injection, decreased tear break-up time (TBUT <10 seconds), decreased tear meniscus, tear film debris, filaments, dry corneal surface, irregular/dull corneal light reflex, staining with rose bengal/fluorescein, Bitot's spot (white, foamy patch of keratinized bulbar conjunctiva [pathognomonic for vitamin A deficiency]). In vitamin A deficiency, severe cases may cause corneal ulceration, descemetocele and/or perforation.

Differential Diagnosis

See above; also deficiency in lipid (blepharitis), aqueous (lacrimal gland tumor, Riley-Day syndrome, radiation), mucin (Stevens-Johnson syndrome, ocular cicatricial pemphigoid, radiation, chemical burn, trachoma), or other (ectropion, entropion, lagophthalmos, Bell's palsy, thyroid ophthalmopathy, conjunctivitis, medicamentosa).

Evaluation

- Complete ophthalmic history and eye exam with attention to lids, conjunctiva, cornea, tear film, and rose bengal/flourescein staining
- **Schirmer's test:** Two tests exist, but they are usually not performed as originally described. One is done without and one is done with topical anesthesia. The inferior fornix is dried with a cotton-tipped applicator, and a strip of standardized filter paper (Whatman #41, 5 mm width) is placed over each lower lid at the junction of the lateral and middle thirds. After 5 minutes, the strips are removed and the amount of wetting is measured. Normal results are ≥15 mm without anesthesia (basal + reflex tearing), and ≥10 mm with anesthesia (basal tearing)
- Consider lab tests: tear lactoferrin and lysozyme (decreased), and tear osmolarity (>310 mOsm/L)
- Electroretinogram (ERG; reduced), electro-oculogram (EOG; abnormal), and dark adaptation (prolonged) in vitamin A deficiency
- Consider medical consultation for systemic diseases

Management

- Topical lubrication with nonpreserved artificial tears (see Appendix) up to q1h and ointment (Refresh P.M.) at bedtime
- Consider acetylcysteine 10% (Mucomyst qd to qid), punctal occlusion (temporary first, then permanent if successful), lacriserts, bandage contact lens, moist chamber goggles, lid taping at bedtime, and/or tarsorrhaphy for more severe cases
- **Acne rosacea:** Oral doxycycline (50–100 mg PO qd to bid for 1 month, may require long-term treatment) and topical metronidazole (Metrogel) to facial skin
- **Vitamin A deficiency:** Vitamin A replacement (vitamin A 15,000 IU PO qd)

Prognosis

Depends on underlying condition; severe cases may be difficult to manage.

Inflammation

Definition

Chemosis: Edema of conjunctiva; may be mild with boggy appearance or massive with tense ballooning.

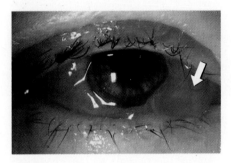

Figure 4–8 Chemosis with extensive ballooning of conjunctiva (arrow) and prolapse over lower lid nasally.

Follicles: Small, translucent, avascular mounds of plasma cells and lymphocytes seen in epidemic keratoconjunctivitis (EKC), herpes simplex virus (HSV) blepharoconjunctivitis, chlamydia keratoconjunctivitis, molluscum contagiosum blepharoconjunctivitis, or drug reactions.

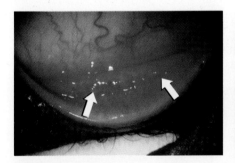

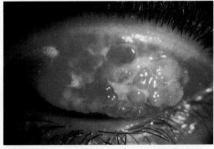

Figure 4–9 Follicular conjunctivitis demonstrating inferior palpebral follicles (arrows).

Figure 4–10 Large, gelatinous, tarsal follicles in a patient with acute trachoma.

Granuloma: Collection of giant multinucleated cells seen in chronic inflammation from sarcoid, foreign body, or chalazion.

Hyperemia: Redness/injection of conjunctiva.

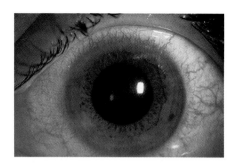

Figure 4–11 Hyperemia.

Membranes: A true membrane is a firmly adherent, fibrinous exudate that bleeds and scars when removed; seen in bacterial conjunctivitis (*Streptococcus* species, *Neisseria gonorrhoeae* (GC), *Corynebacterium diphtheriae*), Stevens-Johnson syndrome, and burns; a pseudomembrane is a loosely attached, avascular, fibrinous exudate seen in epidemic keratoconjunctivitis (EKC) and mild allergic or bacterial conjunctivitis.

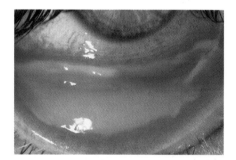

Figure 4–12 Pseudomembrane in a patient with epidemic keratoconjunctivitis.

Papillae: Vascular reaction consisting of fibrovascular mounds with central vascular tuft; nonspecific finding seen with any conjunctival irritation or conjunctivitis; can be large ("cobblestones" or giant papillae).

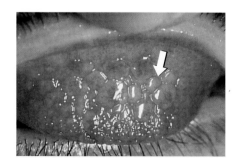

Figure 4–13 Large papillae (arrow) in a patient with vernal keratoconjunctivitis.

Phlyctenule ("Blister"): Focal, nodular, vascularized, infiltrate of polymorphonuclear leukocytes (PMN) and lymphocytes with central necrosis due to hypersensitivity to *Staphylococcus* species, *Mycobacterium* species, *Candida* species, *Coccidioides, Chlamydia,* or nematodes; located on the bulbar conjunctiva or at the limbus; can march across cornea, causing vascularization and scarring behind the leading edge.

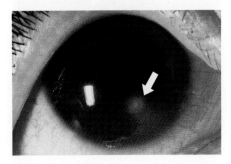

Figure 4–14 Phlyctenule (arrow) creeping across the cornea with trailing vascularization.

Symptoms

Red eye, swelling, itching, foreign body sensation; may have discharge, photophobia, and tearing.

Signs

See above; depends on type of inflammation.

Differential Diagnosis

Any irritation of conjunctiva (allergic, infectious, autoimmune, chemical, foreign body, idiopathic).

Evaluation

- Complete ophthalmic history and eye exam with attention to preauricular lymphadenopathy, everting lids, conjunctiva, cornea, and characteristics of discharge if present
- Lab tests: cultures/smears of conjunctiva, cornea, and discharge for infectious causes

Management

- Treatment depends on etiology; usually supportive
- Topical vasoconstrictor, nonsteroidal anti-inflammatory drug (NSAID) antihistamine, and/or mast cell stabilizer (naphazoline–pheniramine maleate [Naphcon-A], ketorolac tromethamine [Acular], levocabastine [Livostin], lodoxamide tromethamine 0.1% [Alomide], olopatadine [Patanol] or cromolyn sodium 4% [Crolom] bid to qid); severe cases

Management *Continued*

may require topical steroid (prednisolone acetate 1% qid) and/or topical antibiotic (polysporin or erythromycin qid)
- Membranes and pseudomembranes may require debridement
- Discontinue offending agent if patient is allergic

Prognosis

Depends on etiology; most are benign and self-limited (see Conjunctivitis section).

Conjunctivitis

Definition

Infectious or noninfectious inflammation of the conjunctiva.

ALLERGIC:

Atopic (AKC): Occurs in adults; not seasonal; associated with atopy (rhinitis, asthma, dermatitis); similar features as vernal keratoconjunctivitis but papillae usually smaller and conjunctiva has milky edema; also thickened and erythematous lids, corneal neovascularization, cataracts (10%), and keratoconus.

Giant Papillary Conjunctivitis (GPC): Occurs in contact-lens wearers (>95% of GPC cases); also secondary to prosthesis, foreign body, or exposed suture; signs include itching, ropy discharge, blurry vision, and pain with contact lens use.

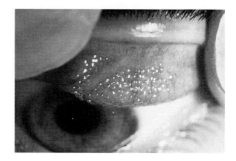

Figure 4–15 Giant papillary conjunctivitis.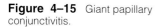

Seasonal: Seen in all ages; associated with hayfever, airborne allergens.

Superior Limbic Keratoconjunctivitis (SLK): Occurs in middle-aged females; 50% have thyroid disease; usually bilateral and asymmetric; may be secondary to contact lens use (see Chap. 5); signs include boggy edema, redundancy and injection of superior conjunctiva, superficial punctate keratitis, filaments, and no discharge; symptoms are worse than signs.

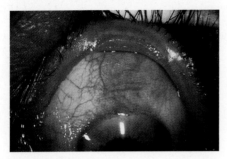

Figure 4–16 Superior limbic keratoconjunctivitis demonstrating staining of the superior conjunctiva with rose bengal.

Vernal Keratoconjunctivitis (VKC): Occurs in children; seasonal (warm months); male predilection; lasts 5–10 years, then resolves; associated with family history of atopy; signs include intense itching, ropy discharge, giant papillae (cobblestones), Horner-Trantas dots (collections of eosinophils at limbus), shield ulcer, and keratitis in 50%; more than two eosinophils per high-power field is pathognomonic.

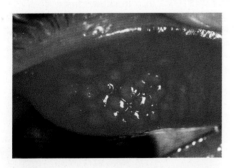

Figure 4–17 Vernal keratoconjunctivitis demonstrating "cobblestones" (giant papillae).

BACTERIAL:

Usually caused by *Staphylococcus aureus, Streptococcus pneumoniae, Haemophilus* species, *Moraxella catarrhalis,* and *Neisseria gonorrhoeae;* spectrum of presentations ranging from mild (signs include minimal lid edema, scant purulent discharge, moderate conjunctival injection, and no corneal involvement) to severe (signs include marked lid swelling, copious purulent discharge, extensive conjunctival injection, subconjunctival hemorrhage, chemosis, and membranes); *N. gonorrhoeae* can invade intact corneal epithelium and cause infectious keratitis (see Chap. 5).

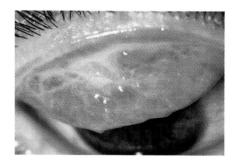

Figure 4–18 Bacterial conjunctivitis with mucopurulent discharge.

CHLAMYDIAL:

Trachoma: Leading cause of blindness worldwide; caused by serotypes A–C; signs include follicles, Herbert's pits (scarred limbal follicles), superior pannus, superficial punctate keratitis (SPK), upper tarsal scarring (Arlt's line).

Inclusion Conjunctivitis (TRIC): Caused by serotypes D–K; signs include chronic, follicular conjunctivitis, subepithelial infiltrates, and no membrane; associated with urethritis in 5%.

Lymphogranuloma Venereum: Caused by serotype L; associated with Parinaud's oculoglandular syndrome (see below), conjunctival granulomas, and interstitial keratitis.

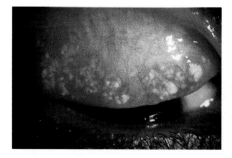

Figure 4–19 Trachoma demonstrating upper tarsal scarring.

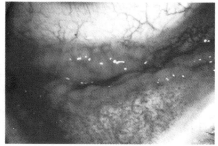

Figure 4–20 Chlamydial conjunctivitis with follicles.

KAWASAKI'S DISEASE:

Mucocutaneous lymph node syndrome of unknown etiology; seen in children <5 years old; more common in Japanese; diagnosis based on 5 of 6 criteria: (1) fever (≥ 5 days), (2) bilateral conjunctivitis, (3) oral mucosal changes (erythema, fissures, "strawberry tongue"), (4) rash, (5) cervical lymphadenopathy, and (6) peripheral extremity changes (edema, erythema, desquamation); associated with polyarteritis especially of coronary arteries; may be fatal (1–2%).

LIGNEOUS:

Rare, idiopathic, bilateral, membranous conjunctivitis seen in children; develop a thick, white, woody infiltrate/plaque located on the upper tarsal conjunctiva.

PARINAUD'S OCULOGLANDULAR SYNDROME:

Unilateral conjunctivitis with conjunctival granulomas and preauricular/ submandibular lymphadenopathy; may have fever, malaise, and/or rash; due to cat-scratch fever, tularemia, sporotrichosis, tuberculosis, syphilis, lymphogranuloma venereum, Epstein-Barr virus, mumps, fungi, malignancy, and sarcoidosis.

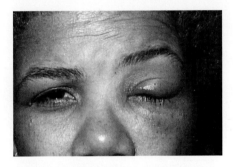

Figure 4–21 Parinaud's oculoglandular syndrome.

OPHTHALMIA NEONATORUM:

Occurs in newborns; may be toxic (silver nitrate) or infectious (bacteria [especially *Neisseria gonorrhoeae*], herpes simplex virus, chlamydia [may have otitis and/or pneumonitis]).

VIRAL:

Adenovirus: Most common cause of viral conjunctivitis ("pink eye"); signs include lid edema, serous discharge, pseudomembranes; may have preauricular node (PAN) and corneal subepithelial infiltrates; transmitted by contact and contagious for 12–14 days; several different types:

■ **Epidemic keratoconjunctivitis (EKC):** Types 8 and 19
■ **Pharyngoconjunctival fever:** Types 3 and 7

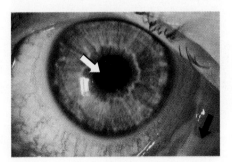

Figure 4–22 Adenoviral conjunctivitis due to EKC demonstrating subepithelial infiltrates (white arrow) and pseudomembrane (black arrow).

Herpes Simplex Virus (HSV): Primary disease in children causes bilateral lid vesicles; may also have fever, preauricular lymphadenopathy, and an upper respiratory infection.

Symptoms

Red eye, swelling, itching, burning, foreign body sensation, tearing, discharge, crusting of lashes; may have photophobia and decreased vision.

Signs

Normal or decreased visual acuity, lid edema, conjunctival injection, chemosis, papillae, follicles, membranes, petechial hemorrhages, concretions, discharge; may have preauricular lymphadenopathy, subepithelial infiltrates, punctate staining, corneal ulcers, and/or cataract.

Differential Diagnosis

See above; also medicamentosa (toxic reaction commonly associated with preservatives in medications, as well as antivirals, antibiotics, miotics, dipivefrin [Propine], apraclonidine [Iopidine], and atropine), dacryocystitis, nasolacrimal duct obstruction.

Evaluation

- Complete ophthalmic history and eye exam with attention to preauricular lymphadenopathy, everting lids, characteristics of discharge, conjunctiva, cornea, and anterior chamber
- Lab tests: consider cultures/smears of conjunctiva and cornea (mandatory for suspected bacterial cases)
- Consider pediatric consultation

Management

- Treatment depends on etiology; usually supportive with medications, compresses, and debridement of membranes for symptomatic relief

ALLERGIC:

- Topical vasoconstrictor, NSAID, antihistamine, and/or mast cell stabilizer (naphazoline–pheniramine maleate [Naphcon-A], ketorolac tromethamine [Acular], olopatadine [Patanol], levocabastine [Livostin], lodoxamide tromethamine 0.1% [Alomide], or cromolyn sodium 4% [Crolom] bid to qid)
- Consider mild topical steroid (start with fluorometholone qid, change to prednisolone acetate 1% qid to q1h in severe cases), especially for vernal keratoconjunctivitis
- Consider systemic antihistamine (Benadryl 25–50 mg PO q6h prn)

Management Continued

- **Giant Papillary Conjunctivitis:** Clean, change, or discontinue use of contact lenses; change contact lens cleaning solution to preservative-free (see Chap. 5)
- **Superior Limbic Keratoconjunctivitis:** Silver nitrate solution, bandage contact lens, conjunctival cautery, or conjunctival recession (see Chap. 5)
- **Vernal Keratoconjunctivitis:** Consider topical cyclosporine (1–2%) qid

BACTERIAL:

- Topical broad-spectrum antibiotic (ciprofloxacin [Ciloxan] or ofloxacin [Ocuflox] qid)
  - May require systemic antibiotics especially in children
  - Remove discharge with irrigation and membranes with sterile cotton-tipped applicator

KAWASAKI'S DISEASE:

- Pediatric consultation and hospital admission; systemic steroids are contraindicated

LIGNEOUS:

- May respond to topical steroids, mucolytics, or cyclosporine

OTHER INFECTIONS:

- *Neisseria gonorrhoeae,* chlamydia, and Parinaud's oculoglandular syndrome (eg, cat-scratch disease, tularemia, syphilis, tuberculosis, etc) require systemic antibiotics based on causative organism

VIRAL:

- Topical lubrication with artificial tears (see Appendix) and topical vasoconstrictor, NSAID, antihistamine, and/or mast cell stabilizer (naphazoline–pheniramine maleate [Naphcon-A], ketorolac tromethamine [Acular], levocabastine [Livostin], lodoxamide tromethamine 0.1% [Alomide], olopatadine [Patanol], or cromolyn sodium 4% [Crolom] bid to qid)
- Add topical antibiotic (polymyxin B sulfate–trimethoprim [Polytrim] qid, erythromycin or bacitracin ointment qd to tid) for corneal epithelial defects
- Add topical steroid (fluorometholone qid) for subepithelial infiltrates in epidemic keratoconjunctivitis
- Add topical antiviral (trifluridine [Viroptic] 5 times/day) for herpes simplex

Prognosis

Usually good; subepithelial infiltrates in adenoviral conjunctivitis cause variable decreased vision for months.

Conjunctival Degenerations

Definition

Secondary degenerative changes of the conjunctiva.

Amyloidosis: Yellow-white or salmon-colored, avascular deposits; may be due to primary (localized) or secondary (systemic) amyloidosis.

Concretions: Yellow-white inclusion cysts filled with keratin and epithelial debris in fornix or palpebral conjunctiva; associated with aging and chronic conjunctivitis; can erode overlying conjunctiva, causing foreign body sensation; easily excised.

Pingueculae: Yellow-white, subepithelial deposits of abnormal collagen at the nasal and/or temporal limbus; due to actinic changes; elastotic degeneration seen histologically; may calcify over time.

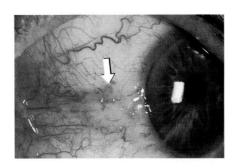

Figure 4–23 Pinguecula (arrow).

Pterygium: Triangular fibrovascular tissue in interpalpebral space involving cornea; often preceded by pinguecula; destroys Bowman's membrane; may have iron line at leading edge (Stocker's line); induces astigmatism and may cause decreased vision.

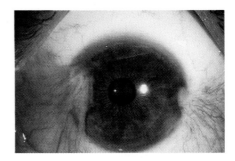

Figure 4–24 Large nasal and smaller temporal pterygia.

Symptoms

Asymptomatic; may have red eye, foreign body sensation, decreased vision; may notice bump or growth; may have contact lens intolerance.

Signs

See above.

Differential Diagnosis

Cyst, squamous cell carcinoma, conjunctival intra-epithelial neoplasia, episcleritis, scleritis, phlyctenule.

Evaluation

■ Complete ophthalmic history and eye exam with attention to conjunctiva and cornea.

Management

- No treatment recommended
- Topical lubrication with artificial tears (see Appendix) up to q1h
- Consider limited use of vasoconstrictor (naphazoline [Naphcon] qid) for inflamed pterygium, and/or excision of pterygium for chronic inflammation, cosmesis, contact lens intolerance, or involvement of visual axis

Prognosis

Good; about one third of pterygia recur after simple excision, recurrences are reduced by conjunctival autograft, beta irradiation, thiotepa, or mitomycin C.

Ocular Cicatricial Pemphigoid (OCP)

Definition

Systemic vesiculobullous disease of mucous membranes resulting in bilateral, chronic, cicatrizing conjunctivitis; other mucous membranes frequently involved, including oral (up to 90%), esophageal, tracheal, and genital; skin involved in up to 30% of cases.

Etiology

Usually idiopathic (probably autoimmune mechanism) or drug-induced (may occur with epinephrine, timolol, pilocarpine, echothiophate iodide [Phospholine Iodide], or idoxuridine).

Epidemiology

Incidence of 1 in 20,000; usually occurs in females (2:1) >60 years old; associated with HLA-DR4, DQw3.

Symptoms

Red eye, dryness, foreign body sensation, tearing, decreased vision; may have dysphagia or difficulty breathing.

Signs

Normal or decreased visual acuity, conjunctival injection and scarring, dry eye, symblepharon (fusion/attachment of eyelid to bulbar conjunctiva), ankyloblepharon (fusion/attachment of upper and lower eyelids), foreshortened fornices, trichiasis, entropion, keratitis, corneal ulcer/scarring/vascularization, conjunctival and corneal keratinization, and oral lesions; corneal perforation and endophthalmitis can occur.

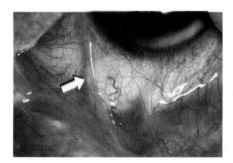 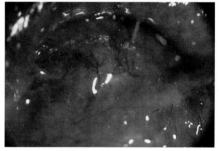

Figure 4–25 Ocular cicatricial pemphigoid demonstrating symblepharon (arrow) and foreshortening of the inferior fornix.

Figure 4–26 Ocular cicatricial pemphigoid demonstrating advanced stage with corneal vascularization, symblepharon, and ankyloblepharon formation.

Differential Diagnosis

Stevens-Johnson syndrome, chemical burn, squamous cell carcinoma, scleroderma, infectious or allergic conjunctivitis, trachoma, sarcoidosis, ocular rosacea, radiation, linear immunoglobulin A dermatosis, practolol-induced conjunctivitis.

Evaluation

- Complete ophthalmic history and eye exam with attention to conjunctiva and cornea
- Conjunctival biopsy (immunoglobulin and complement deposition in basement membrane)

Management

- Topical lubrication with nonpreserved artificial tears (see Appendix) up to q1h and ointment (Refresh P.M.) at bedtime
- Add topical antibiotic (polymyxin B sulfate-trimethoprim [Polytrim] qid or erythromycin tid) for corneal epithelial defects
- Consider punctal occlusion, tarsorrhaphy
- Often requires treatment with systemic steroids and/or immunosuppressives (dapsone contraindicated in patients with G6PD deficiency); should be performed by a cornea or uveitis specialist
- Consider surgery for entropion and trichiasis, release of symblepharon, and mucous membrane grafting; keratoprosthesis used in advanced cases

Prognosis

Poor; chronic progressive disease with remissions and exacerbations, surgery often initiates exacerbations.

Stevens-Johnson Syndrome (SJS, Erythema Multiforme Major)

Definition

Acute, usually self-limited (up to 6 weeks), cutaneous, bullous disease with mucosal ulceration resulting in acute membranous conjunctivitis.

Etiology

Usually drug-induced (may occur with sulfonamides, penicillin, aspirin, barbiturates, isoniazid, or phenytoin [Dilantin]) or infectious (herpes simplex virus, *Mycoplasma* species, adenovirus, *Streptococcus* species).

Symptoms

Fever, upper respiratory infection, headache, malaise, skin eruption, decreased vision, pain, red eye, swelling, and oral mucosal ulceration.

Signs

Fever, skin eruption (target lesions), mucous membrane ulceration and crusting, decreased visual acuity, conjunctival injection, discharge, membranes, dry eye, symblepharon (fusion/attachment of eyelid to bulbar conjunctiva), trichiasis, keratitis, corneal ulcer/scarring/vascularization/keratinization.

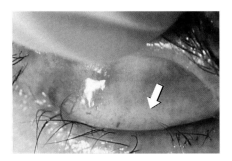

Figure 4–27 Stevens-Johnson syndrome demonstrating tarsal scarring (arrow).

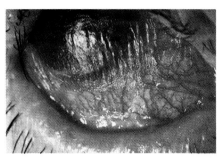

Figure 4–28 Stevens-Johnson syndrome demonstrating keratinization of the ocular surface.

Differential Diagnosis

Ocular cicatricial pemphigoid, chemical burn, squamous cell carcinoma, scleroderma, infectious or allergic conjunctivitis, trachoma, sarcoidosis, ocular rosacea, radiation.

Evaluation

- Complete ophthalmic history and eye exam with attention to systemic mucous membranes, conjunctiva, and cornea
- Medical consultation

Management

- Supportive, topical lubrication with nonpreserved artificial tears (see Appendix) up to q1h and ointment (Refresh P.M.) at bedtime
- Add topical antibiotic (polymyxin B sulfate–trimethoprim [Polytrim] qid or erythromycin tid) for corneal epithelial defects
- Consider topical steroid (prednisolone acetate 1% up to q2h) depending on severity of inflammation
- Consider systemic steroids (prednisone 60–100 mg PO qd) in very severe cases
- Check purified protein derivative (PPD), blood glucose, and chest radiographs before starting systemic steroids
- Add H_2-blocker (ranitidine [Zantac] 150 mg PO bid) when taking steroids
- May require punctal occlusion, tarsorrhaphy for more severe cases
- Consider surgery for trichiasis, symblepharon, or corneal scarring

Prognosis

Fair; not progressive (in contrast to ocular cicatricial pemphigoid), recurrences are rare, but up to 30% mortality.

Conjunctival Tumors

Definition

CONGENITAL:

Hamartoma: Derived from abnormal rest of cells, composed of tissues normally found at same location (eg, telangiectasia, lymphangioma).

Choristoma: Derived from abnormal rest of cells, composed of tissues not normally found at that location:

- **Dermoid:** White-yellow, solid, round, elevated nodule often with visible hairs on surface and lipid deposition anterior to its corneal edge; composed of dense connective tissue with pilosebaceous units and stratified squamous epithelium; usually located at inferotemporal limbus; may be part of Goldenhar's syndrome with dermoids, preauricular skin tags, and vertebral anomalies.
- **Dermolipoma:** Similar appearance to dermoid, but composed of adipose tissue with keratinized surface; usually located superotemporally extending into orbit.
- **Epibulbar Osseous Choristoma:** Solitary, white nodule composed of compact bone that develops from episclera; freely moveable; usually located superotemporally.

CYST:

Fluid-filled cavity within the conjunctiva, defined by its lining (ductal or inclusion); often due to trauma or inflammation, can be congenital.

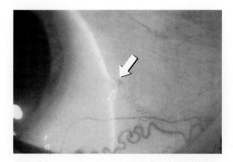

Figure 4–29 Conjunctival inclusion cyst (arrow).

EPITHELIAL:

Papilloma: Red, gelatinous lesions composed of proliferative epithelium with fibrovascular cores; may be pedunculated or sessile, solitary or multiple; often associated with human papillomavirus.

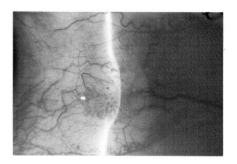

Figure 4–30 Papilloma.

Conjunctival Intraepithelial Neoplasia (CIN): White, gelatinous, conjunctival dysplasia confined to the epithelium; usually begins at limbus and is a precursor of squamous cell carcinoma.

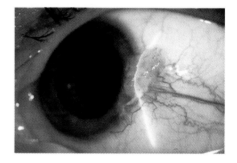

Figure 4–31 Conjunctival intraepithelial neoplasia demonstrating pink, gelatinous, vascularized appearance at the limbus.

Squamous Cell Carcinoma (SCC): Interpalpebral, exophytic, gelatinous, papillary appearance with loops of vessels; may have superficial invasion and extend onto cornea; deep invasion and metastasis are rare.

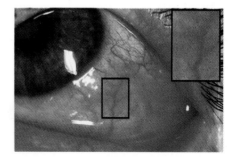

Figure 4–32 Squamous cell carcinoma appearing as a pink, gelatinous growth.

MELANOCYTIC:

Nevus: Mobile, discrete, elevated, variably pigmented lesion that contains cysts; may be junctional, subepithelial, or compound; may enlarge during puberty; rarely becomes malignant.

Ocular Melanocytosis: Unilateral, increased uveal, scleral, and episcleral pigmentation appearing as blue-gray patches; more common in Caucasians.

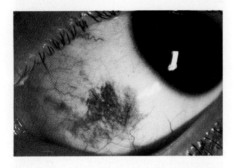

Figure 4–33 Ocular melanocytosis.

Oculodermal Melanocytosis (Nevus of Ota): Increased uveal, scleral, episcleral, and periorbital skin pigmentation; more common in Asians and African Americans; uveal melanoma may rarely develop in Caucasians (see Chap. 10).

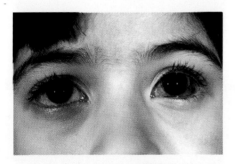

Figure 4–34 Oculodermal melanocytosis (nevus of Ota) of the left eye.

Primary Acquired Melanosis (PAM): Mobile, patchy, diffuse, flat, brown lesions without cysts; indistinct margins and may grow; occurs in middle-aged adults; histologically may have atypia; malignant potential (30%).

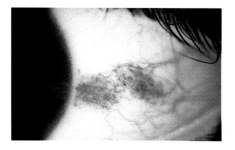

Figure 4–35 Primary acquired melanosis.

Secondary Acquired Melanosis: Hyperpigmentation due to racial variations, actinic stimulation, radiation, pregnancy, Addison's disease, or inflammation; usually perilimbal.

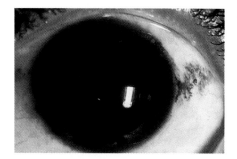

Figure 4–36 Secondary acquired melanosis (racial pigmentation).

Malignant Melanoma: Nodular, pigmented lesion containing vessels, but no cysts; may arise from PAM, nevi, or de novo; 20–40% mortality.

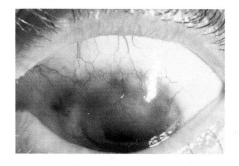

Figure 4–37 Malignant melanoma.

STROMAL:

Cavernous Hemangioma: Red patch on conjunctiva; may bleed and be associated with other ocular hemangiomas or systemic disease.

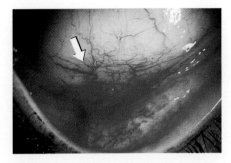

Figure 4–38 Cavernous hemangioma (arrow).

Juvenile Xanthogranuloma (JXG): Yellow-orange conjunctival nodules composed of vascularized, lipid-containing histiocytes; can also involve iris and skin; often regresses spontaneously.

Kaposi's Sarcoma (KS): Single or multiple, flat or elevated, deep red to purple plaques (malignant granulation tissue) on palpebral conjunctiva; may involve orbit; occurs in immunocompromised individuals, especially HIV-positive patients.

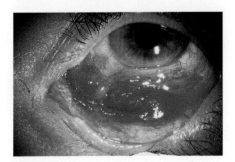

Figure 4–39 Kaposi's sarcoma.

Lymphangiectasis: Cluster of elevated clear cysts that represent dilated lymphatics; may have areas of hemorrhage.

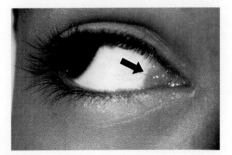

Figure 4–40 Lymphangiectasis (arrow).

Lymphoid: Single or multiple, smooth, flat, salmon-colored patches; usually occurs in middle-aged adults; spectrum of disease from benign reactive lymphoid hyperplasia to malignant lymphoma (non-Hodgkin's); may develop systemic lymphoma.

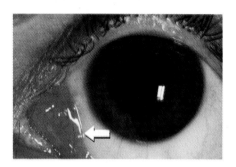

Figure 4–41   Lymphoid tumor with salmon-patch appearance (arrow).

Pyogenic Granuloma: Red, fleshy, polypoid mass at the site of chronic inflammation; often follows surgical or accidental trauma; misnomer, as it is neither pyogenic nor a granuloma, but rather granulation tissue.

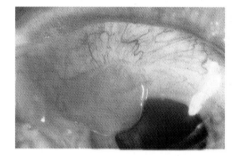

Figure 4–42   Pyogenic granuloma.

CARUNCLE:

Tumors that affect the conjunctiva may also occur in the caruncle, including (in order of frequency): papilloma, nevus, inclusion cyst, malignant melanoma, also sebaceous cell carcinoma, and oncocytoma (oxyphilic adenoma; fleshy, yellow-tan cystic mass from transformation of epithelial cells of accessory lacrimal glands; slowly progressive).

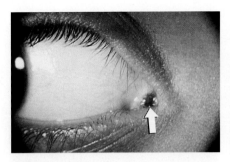

Figure 4–43 Nevus of the caruncle (arrow).

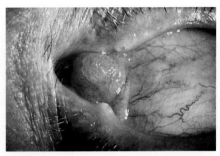

Figure 4–44 Papilloma of the caruncle.

Symptoms

Asymptomatic; may notice discoloration or growth of the lesion.

Signs

Conjunctival lesion (see above), may have involvement of lids, cornea, rarely intraocular or intraorbital extension.

Differential Diagnosis

See above.

Evaluation

- Complete ophthalmic history and eye exam with attention to skin, everting lids, conjunctiva, cornea, and ophthalmoscopy
- Consider biopsy
- Medical consultation and systemic work-up for malignant and lymphoproliferative processes

Management

- Depends on etiology; options include observation, radiation, cryotherapy, chemotherapy, excision, and enucleation; should be performed by a cornea or tumor specialist

Prognosis

Depends on etiology; good except malignant and lymphoid tumors.

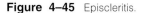 **Episcleritis**

Definition

Sectoral (70%) or diffuse (30%) inflammation of episclera.

Epidemiology

80% simple; 20% nodular; 33% bilateral.

Etiology

Idiopathic, tuberculosis, syphilis, herpes zoster, rheumatoid arthritis, other collagen vascular diseases.

Symptoms

Asymptomatic; may have mild pain and/or red eye.

Signs

Subconjunctival and conjunctival injection, usually sectoral; may have chemosis, episcleral nodules, anterior chamber cell/flare.

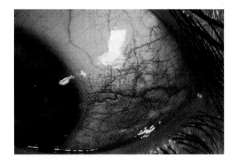

Figure 4–45 Episcleritis.

Differential Diagnosis

Scleritis, iritis, phlyctenule, myositis.

Evaluation

- Complete ophthalmic history and eye exam with attention to pattern of conjunctival and scleral injection and blanching with topical phenylephrine (scleritis is painful, has violaceous hue, and does not blanch with topical vasoconstrictor [phenylephrine 2.5%]), and anterior chamber
- Consider scleritis work-up in recurrent or bilateral cases (see Scleritis section)

Management

- No treatment recommended
- Consider limited use of vasoconstrictor (naphazoline–pheniramine maleate [Naphcon] qid), mild topical steroid (fluorometholone qid), or oral NSAID (indomethacin 50 mg PO qd to bid) if severe

Prognosis

Good; usually self-limited; may be recurrent in 67% of cases.

Scleritis

Definition

Inflammation of sclera, can be anterior (98%) or posterior (2%).

Epidemiology

Anterior form may be diffuse (40%), nodular (44%), or necrotizing (14%) with or without (scleromalacia perforans) inflammation; >50% bilateral; associated systemic disease in 50% of cases.

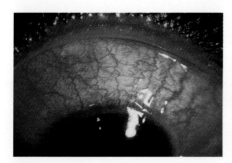

Figure 4–46 Scleritis.

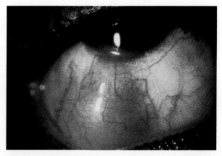

Figure 4–47 Nodular scleritis.

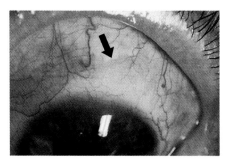 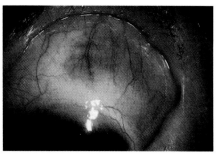

Figure 4–48 Necrotizing scleritis with thinning of sclera superiorly (arrow).

Figure 4–49 Scleromalacia perforans.

Etiology

Collagen vascular disease in 30% of cases (most commonly rheumatoid arthritis, ankylosing spondylitis, lupus erythematosus, polyarteritis nodosa, Wegener's granulomatosis, and relapsing polychondritis); also herpes zoster, syphilis, tuberculosis, leprosy, gout, porphyria, post-surgical, and idiopathic.

Symptoms

Pain, photophobia, swelling, red eye, decreased vision (except scleromalacia).

Signs

Normal or decreased visual acuity, subconjunctival and conjunctival injection with violaceous hue, chemosis, scleral edema, scleral nodule(s), globe tenderness to palpation; may have anterior chamber cell/flare (30%), corneal infiltrate or thinning, scleral thinning (30%); posterior type may have chorioretinal folds and/or focal serous retinal detachment.

Differential Diagnosis

Episcleritis, iritis, phlyctenule, retrobulbar mass, myositis, scleral ectasia/staphyloma.

Evaluation

- Complete ophthalmic history and eye exam with attention to pattern of conjunctival and scleral injection and failure of area to blanch with topical vasoconstrictor (phenylephrine 2.5%), cornea, anterior chamber, and ophthalmoscopy
- B-scan ultrasonography: thickened sclera and "T-sign" in posterior scleritis
- Lab tests: complete blood count (CBC), rheumatoid factor (RF), antinuclear antibody (ANA), antineutrophil cytoplasmic antibody (ANCA), Venereal Disease Research Laboratory (VDRL), fluorescent treponemal antibody absorption test (FTA-ABS), purified protein derivative (PPD) and controls, and chest radiographs
- Medical consultation

Management

- Depending on severity, consider using one or a combination of the following:
- Systemic NSAID (indomethacin 50 mg PO bid to tid)
- Systemic steroids (prednisone 60–100 mg PO qd); *Note:* topical steroids and NSAIDs are ineffective
- Check PPD, blood glucose, and chest radiographs before starting systemic steroids
- Add H_2-blocker (ranitidine [Zantac] 150 mg PO bid) when taking oral NSAIDs or steroids
- Consider immunosuppressive agents (see Anterior Uveitis section in Chap. 6) in severe cases; should be administered by a uveitis specialist
- Sub-Tenon's steroid injection is contraindicated
- May require surgery (patch graft) for globe perforation

Prognosis

Depends on etiology; poor for necrotizing form, which may perforate; scleromalacia perforans rarely perforates; recurrences common.

Scleral Discoloration

Definition

Alkaptonuria/Ochronosis: Recessive inborn error of metabolism (accumulation of homogentisic acid) causing brown pigment deposits in eyes, ears, nose, joints, and heart; triangular patches in interpalpebral space near limbus, pigmentation of tarsus and lids.

Ectasia/Staphyloma: Congenital, focal area of scleral thinning usually near limbus; underlying uvea is visible and may bulge through defect; perforation is uncommon.

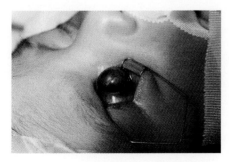

Figure 4–50 Scleral and corneal staphyloma with bulging blue appearance.

Osteogenesis Imperfecta: Congenital disorder of collagen; sclera is thin and appears blue due to underlying uvea (also seen in Ehlers-Danlos syndrome).

Scleral Icterus: Yellow sclera seen in hyperbilirubinemia.

Senile Scleral Plaque: Blue-gray discoloration of sclera located near horizontal rectus muscle insertions due to hyalinization; seen in elderly patients.

Symptoms

Asymptomatic; may notice scleral discoloration.

Signs

Focal or diffuse discoloration of sclera in one or both eyes.

Differential Diagnosis

See above; also foreign body, melanoma, mascara, intrascleral nerve loop, adrenochrome deposits (epinephrine), scleromalacia perforans.

Evaluation

- Complete ophthalmic history and eye exam with attention to conjunctiva, sclera, and ophthalmoscopy
- B-scan ultrasonography and gonioscopy to rule out suspected extension of uveal melanoma
- Medical consultation for systemic diseases

Management

- No treatment recommended
- Treat underlying disorder

Prognosis

Good; discoloration itself is benign.

Cornea

Trauma

Birth Trauma: Vertical or oblique breaks in Descemet's membrane due to forceps injury at birth; acute corneal edema and breaks/scars in Descemet's membrane that usually resolve; associated with astigmatism and amblyopia in later life.

- No treatment required

Chemical/Thermal Burn: Corneal tissue destruction (epithelium and stroma) due to chemical (acid or base) or thermal (eg., welding, intense sunlight, tanning lamp) injury; alkali causes most severe injury and may cause perforation; patients note pain, foreign-body sensation, photophobia, tearing, and red eye; may have normal or decreased visual acuity, conjunctival injection, ciliary injection, epithelial defects that stain with fluorescein, and scleral/limbal blanching due to ischemia in severe chemical burns; prognosis variable, worst for severe alkali burns.

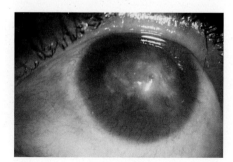

Figure 5–1 Corneal scarring and vascularization due to a chemical injury.

OPHTHALMIC EMERGENCY:

- Immediate copious irrigation with sterile water, saline, or Ringer's solution
- Measure pH before and after irrigation, continue irrigation until pH is neutralized
- Remove any chemical particulate matter from surface of eye and evert lids to sweep fornices with sterile cotton swab
- Topical lubrication with nonpreserved artificial tears (see Appendix) up to q1h and ointment (Refresh P.M.) at bedtime, broad-spectrum topical antibiotic (ciprofloxacin [Ciloxan] or ofloxacin [Ocuflox] qid), and cycloplegic (cyclopentolate 1% tid, scopolamine 0.25% or atropine 1% bid to qid depending on severity)
- For more severe damage, consider topical steroids (prednisolone acetate 1% up to q2h then taper; only use during first week, then if steroids are still necessary, change to medroxyprogesterone [Provera 1%]), topical citrate (10% qid) or sodium ascorbate (10% qid and 2 g PO qid), collagenase inhibitor (acetylcysteine [Mucomyst] up to q4h)
- May require treatment of increased intraocular pressure (see Chap. 11)
- In severe cases, surgery may be required, including symblepharon lysis, conjunctival/mucous membrane transplantation, and tarsorrhaphy; later consider penetrating keratoplasty or keratoprosthesis

Corneal Abrasion: Corneal epithelial defect usually due to trauma; patients note pain, foreign-body sensation, photophobia, tearing, and red eye; may have normal or decreased visual acuity, conjunctival injection, and an epithelial defect that stains with fluorescein.

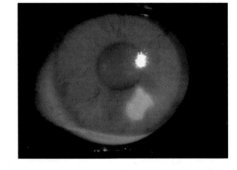

Figure 5–2 Corneal abrasion demonstrating fluorescein staining.

- Topical antibiotic drop (polymyxin B sulfate–trimethoprim [Polytrim] or tobramycin [Tobrex] qid) or ointment (polymyxin B sulfate–bacitracin zinc [Polysporin] qid)
- Consider topical nonsteroidal anti-inflammatory drugs (NSAIDs; [Acular or Voltaren] tid × 48–72h) for pain

- Consider topical cycloplegic (cyclopentolate 1% qd) for pain and photophobia
- Pressure patch or bandage contact lens if area >10 mm² (***Note:*** Do not patch if patient is contact lens wearer; or there is corneal infiltrate or injury caused by plant material, as these scenarios represent high risk for infectious keratitis if patched; no patching necessary if area of abrasion is <10 mm²)

Foreign Body (FB): Foreign material on or in cornea; usually metal, glass, or organic material; may have associated rust ring if metallic; patients note pain, foreign-body sensation, photophobia, tearing, and red eye; may have normal or decreased visual acuity, conjunctival injection, ciliary injection, foreign body, rust ring, epithelial defect that stains with fluorescein, corneal edema, anterior chamber (AC) cell/flare; may be asymptomatic if deep and chronic; good prognosis unless rust ring or scarring involves visual axis.

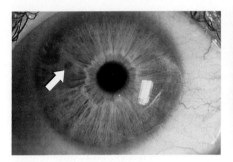 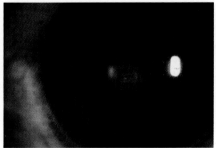

Figure 5–3 Metallic foreign body (arrow).   **Figure 5–4** Rust ring from iron foreign body.

- Removal of foreign material with needle or foreign body removal instruments unless it is deep, nonpenetrating, unexposed, and inert material (may be observed).
- Remove rust ring with Alger brush or automated burr
- Seidel test if deep foreign body to rule out open globe (see below)
- Topical antibiotic (polymyxin B sulfate–trimethoprim [Polytrim] or tobramycin [Tobrex] qid) and cycloplegic (cyclopentolate 1% qd)
- Pressure patch or bandage contact lens as needed (same indications as for corneal abrasion; see above)

Laceration: Partial or full-thickness cut in cornea (see Open Globe section in Chap. 4) due to trauma; patients note pain, foreign-body sensation, photophobia, tearing, and red eye; may have normal or decreased visual acuity, conjunctival injection, ciliary injection, intraocular foreign body, corneal laceration, corneal edema, breaks/scars in Descemet's membrane, anterior chamber cell/flare, low intraocular pressure; good prognosis unless laceration crosses visual axis.

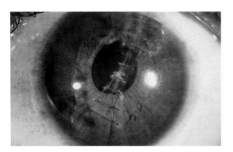

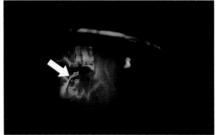

Figure 5–5 Corneal laceration after surgical repair; note nylon sutures.

Figure 5–6 Corneal laceration demonstrating positive Seidel test (bright stream of fluorescein around the central suture [arrow]).

- **Seidel test** (to rule out open globe): Concentrated fluorescein is used to cover the suspected leakage site by placing a drop of sterile 2% fluorescein in the eye or wetting a sterile fluorescein strip and painting the area of the wound. Slit lamp examination is then performed looking for a stream of diluted fluorescein emanating from the wound. This will appear as a fluorescent yellow area on a dark blue background with the cobalt blue light, or a light yellow-green area on a dark orange background with the white light.
- Partial-thickness lacerations require topical broad spectrum antibiotic (ciprofloxacin [Ciloxan] or ofloxacin [Ocuflox] qid) and cycloplegic (cyclopentolate 1% or scopolamine 0.25% tid)
- Daily follow-up until wound has healed
- Pressure patch or bandage contact lens as needed; if wound gape exists, consider surgical repair
- Full-thickness lacerations usually require surgical repair (see Open Globe section in Chap. 4)
- Consider orbital radiographs or computed tomography (CT) to rule out intraocular foreign body when full-thickness laceration exists; magnetic resonance imaging (MRI) contraindicated

Recurrent Erosion: Recurrent bouts of pain, foreign-body sensation, photophobia, tearing, red eye, and spontaneous corneal epithelial defect usually upon awakening; associated with anterior basement membrane dystrophy in 50% of cases, or previous traumatic corneal abrasion (usually from fingernail, paper, or brush); also seen in Meesmann's, Reis-Bücklers, lattice, granular, Fuchs', and posterior polymorphous dystrophies.

- Same treatment as for corneal abrasion until re-epithelialization occurs, then add hypertonic saline ointment (Adsorbonac or Muro 128 5% at bedtime for 3 months)
- Topical lubrication with nonpreserved artificial tears (see Appendix) up to q1h
- Consider debridement, bandage contact lens, anterior stromal puncture/reinforcement, or phototherapeutic keratectomy (PTK) for multiple recurrences

Peripheral Ulcerative Keratitis

Definition

Marginal Keratolysis: Acute corneal ulceration/melting due to autoimmune or collagen vascular disease (lupus erythematosus, rheumatoid arthritis, polyarteritis nodosa, and Wegener's granulomatosis); rapid progression, usually in one sector; corneal epithelium absent; may perforate; melting resolves after healing of overlying epithelium.

Mooren's Ulcer: Idiopathic, inflammatory, painful, progressive, peripheral thinning and ulceration that spreads circumferentially and then centrally with undermining of the leading edge; neovascularization may occur; two types:

(1) More common (75%), benign, and unilateral; seen in older patients; responds to conservative management
(2) Progressive and bilateral; seen in younger patients; more common in African-American males; may perforate; may be associated with coexistent parasitemia

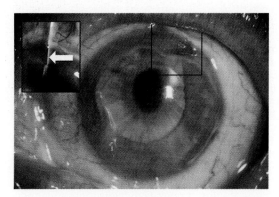

Figure 5–7 Mooren's ulcer; inset demonstrates undermining of the ulcer's leading edge seen with fine slit beam (arrow).

Staphylococcal Marginal Keratitis: Peripheral, white, corneal infiltrate(s) and ulceration 1–2 mm from limbus with intervening clear zone; often stains with fluorescein; due to immune response (hypersensitivity) to *Staphylococcus aureus;* associated with staphylococcal blepharitis, phlyctenule, and vascularization; may progress to ring ulcer or become superinfected; more common in patients with ocular rosacea.

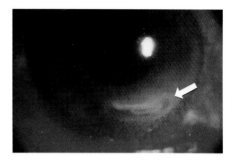

Figure 5–8 Staphylococcal marginal keratitis (arrow).

Terrien's Marginal Degeneration: Noninflammatory, slowly progressive, peripheral thinning of cornea with pannus; starts superiorly and spreads circumferentially; epithelium intact; slight male predilection; causes progressive against-the-rule astigmatism; rarely perforates.

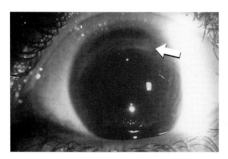

Figure 5–9 Terrien's marginal degeneration (arrow).

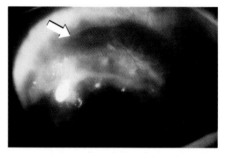

Figure 5–10 Same patient as shown in Figure 5–9, demonstrating peripheral thinning (arrow) with vascularization.

Symptoms

Asymptomatic; may have pain, discharge, photophobia, red eye, and decreased vision.

Signs

Normal or decreased visual acuity, blepharitis, conjunctival injection, ciliary injection, corneal infiltrate with or without overlying epithelial defect, corneal thinning, corneal edema, anterior chamber cell/flare, hypopyon; may have associated scleritis in marginal keratolysis

Differential Diagnosis

Infectious ulcer, sterile ulcer (diagnosis of exclusion), ocular rosacea, pellucid marginal degeneration.

Evaluation

- Complete ophthalmic history and eye exam with attention to lids, keratometry, cornea, fluorescein staining, anterior chamber, and ophthalmoscopy
- Consider corneal topography (computerized videokeratography)
- Lab tests: complete blood count (CBC), erythrocyte sedimentation rate (ESR), rheumatoid factor (RF), antinuclear antibody (ANA), antineutrophil cytoplasmic antibody (ANCA); consider hepatitis C antigen (Mooren's)
- Consider cultures/smears to rule out infectious etiology
- Medical or rheumatology consultation for systemic disorders or when treatment with immunosuppressives is anticipated

Management

- Lid hygiene with warm compresses and lid scrubs for blepharitis
- Consider oral doxycycline (50–100 mg PO qd) for recurrent blepharitis
- Consider protective eye wear to prevent perforation
- Topical lubrication with nonpreserved artificial tears (see Appendix) up to q1h and ointment (Refresh P.M.) at bedtime
- Topical steroid (prednisolone acetate 1% or fluorometholone qid, adjust and taper as necessary)
- Add cycloplegic (cyclopentolate 1% bid) if AC cell/flare exists
- Add antibiotic (polymyxin B sulfate–trimethoprim [Polytrim] or tobramycin [Tobrex] qid) if epithelial defect exists
- Consider collagenase inhibitor (acetylcysteine [Mucomyst] qd to qid)
- Consider oral steroids (prednisone 60–100 mg PO qd) for significant, progressive thinning; check purified protein derivative (PPD), blood glucose, and chest radiographs before starting systemic steroids
- Add H_2-blocker (ranitidine [Zantac] 150 mg PO bid) when taking systemic steroids
- May require immunosuppressive agents, lamellar keratectomy with conjunctival resection, or penetrating keratoplasty if significant thinning exists; should be managed by a cornea specialist

Prognosis

Depends on etiology; poor for marginal keratolysis and Mooren's ulcer.

Contact Lens–Related Problems

Definition

A variety of abnormalities induced by contact lenses (CL). Several types of lenses exist: hard (polymethylmethacrylate [PMMA]), rigid gas permeable (RGP), and soft (SCL). These lenses can be either daily-wear (DWCL) or extended-wear

(EWCL) and are used primarily to correct refractive errors (myopia, hyperopia, astigmatism, and presbyopia), but can also serve as a therapeutic bandage lens for unhealthy corneal surfaces or even for cosmetic use (to apparently change iris color or create a pseudo-pupil).

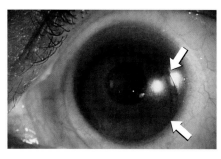
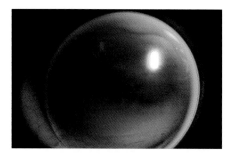

Figure 5–11 Hard contact lens (arrows).

Figure 5–12 Rigid gas permeable contact lens demonstrating fluorescein staining pattern.

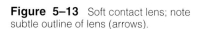

Figure 5–13 Soft contact lens; note subtle outline of lens (arrows).

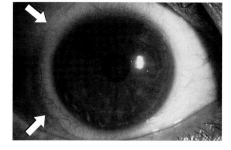

Symptoms

Foreign-body sensation, decreased vision, red eye, tearing, itching, burning, pain, lens awareness, and reduced contact lens wear time.

Signs

Corneal Abrasion: Corneal fluorescein staining due to epithelial defect (see Trauma: Corneal Abrasion section); contact lens–related etiologies include foreign bodies, poor fit, corneal hypoxia, poor contact lens insertion/removal technique.

Corneal Hypoxia: *Acute:* conjunctival injection and epithelial defect (polymethyl-methacrylate [PMMA] contact lens). *Chronic:* punctate staining, corneal epithelial microcysts, stromal edema, and corneal neovascularization.

Contact Lens–Related Dendritic Keratitis: Conjunctivitis, pseudodendritic lesions.

Contact Lens Solution Hypersensitivity/Toxicity: Conjunctival injection, diffuse corneal punctate staining and/or erosion; seen with solutions that contain preservatives (eg, thimerosal).

Corneal Neovascularization: 1–2 mm superior corneal pannus in soft contact lens wearer; >2 mm is serious; may develop scarring, lipid deposits, stromal hemorrhage.

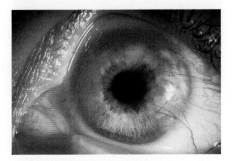

Figure 5–14 Contact lens–induced corneal neovascularization.

Damaged Contact Lens: Pain with lens insertion and prompt relief with removal, look for chips in rigid lenses and fissures in soft lenses.

Deposits on Contact Lens: Significant contact lens deposits (film or bumps), conjunctival injection, corneal erosion, excess contact lens movement, giant papillary conjunctivitis; old contact lens.

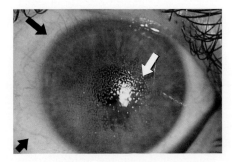

Figure 5–15 Calcium phosphate deposits (white arrow) on soft contact lens (black arrows).

Giant Papillary Conjunctivitis (GPC): Due to contact lens protein deposits, conjunctival contact lens–related mechanical irritation, or soft contact lens material sensitivity reaction. Signs include large upper lid tarsal conjunctival papillae

(>0.33 mm), ropy mucous discharge, contact lens coating, and possible contact lens decentration secondary to papillae; also seen with exposed sutures and ocular prosthesis (see Fig. 4–15).

Infectious Keratitis: Pain, red eye, infiltrate with epithelial defect, and anterior chamber cell/flare; contact lens–related corneal infiltrates should be treated as an infection, suspect *Pseudomonas* or *Acanthamoeba*; seen more often in extended-wear and soft contact lens wearers.

Sterile Corneal Infiltrates: Small (1 mm), peripheral, often multifocal, whitish, nummular, corneal lesions; corneal epithelium usually intact.

Poor Fit (Loose): Upper eyelid irritation, limbal injection, excess contact lens movement with blinking, poor contact lens centration, lens edge bubbles, lens edge stand-off, variable keratometry mires with blinking, and lower portion of retinoscopy reflex darker and faster.

Poor Fit (Tight): Injection or indentation around limbus, minimal contact lens movement with blinking, blurred retinoscopic reflex, corneal edema, and distorted keratometry mires clear with blinking.

Superior Limbic Keratoconjunctivitis (SLK): Contact lens–related etiologies include contact lens hypersensitivity reaction and poor contact lens fit. Upper tarsal micropapillae, superior limbal injection, fluorescein staining of superior bulbar conjunctiva, and 12 o'clock micropannus are seen (see Fig. 4–16).

Superficial Punctate Keratitis (SPK): Contact lens–related etiologies include poor lens fit, dry eye, and contact lens solution reaction; punctate fluorescein staining of corneal surface

Evaluation

- Complete ophthalmic history with attention to contact lens wear and care habits
- Complete eye exam with attention to contact lens fit, contact lens surface, everting upper lids, conjunctiva, keratometry, cornea, and fluorescein staining
- Consider corneal topography (computerized videokeratography)
- Consider dry eye evaluation: tear meniscus, tear break-up time (TBUT), rose bengal staining, and Schirmer's testing (see Chap. 4)
- Lab tests: cultures/smears of cornea, contact lens, contact lens case, and contact lens solutions if infiltrate exists to rule out infection

Management

- **Corneal Abrasion:** Treat as for traumatic corneal abrasion *except* do *not* patch any size abrasion (see Trauma: Corneal Abrasion section).
- **Corneal Hypoxia:**
  - *Acute:* Suspend contact lens use; topical antibiotic ointment (polymyxin B sulfate–bacitracin zinc [Polysporin] tid for 3 days); when acute hypoxia has resolved, re-fit with higher Dk/L (oxygen transmissibility) contact lens
  - *Chronic:* Suspend contact lens use or decrease contact lens wear time; re-fit with higher Dk/L contact lens
- **Corneal Neovascularization:** If neovascularization >2 mm, suspend contact lens use and re-fit with higher Dk/L contact lens
- **Contact Lens–Related Dendritic Keratitis:** Suspend contact lens use until resolved
- **Contact Lens Solution Hypersensitivity/Toxicity:** Identify and discontinue toxic source; suspend contact lens use until corneal surface has healed; thoroughly clean, rinse, and disinfect contact lenses; educate patient on proper contact lens care or change system of care; replace soft contact lenses or polish rigid contact lens; topical antibiotic ointment (erthyromycin or bacitracin tid for 3 days); do *not* patch
- **Damaged Contact Lens:** Replace defective contact lens
- **Deposits on Contact Lens:** Review contact lens cleaning procedures; institute regular enzyme cleaning (SCL or RGP), frequent replacement schedule, or use of disposable contact lenses; polish rigid contact lens.
- **Giant Papillary Conjunctivitis:**
  - *Mild:* Replace contact lenses and reinstruct patient in thorough contact lens cleaning; decrease contact lens wear time; increase frequency of enzyme cleanings; change to frequent or disposable contact lenses, or change lens material from SCL to RGP; topical lodoxamide tromethamine 0.1% (Alomide qid) or cromolyn sodium 4% (Crolom qid)
  - *Severe:* Suspend contact lens use; short course of mild topical steroid (prednisolone acetate 1% or fluorometholone qid)
- **Multiple Sterile Corneal Infiltrates:** Suspend contact lens use until condition resolves; use nonpreserved solutions; must treat as corneal infection (see Infectious Keratitis section)
- **Poor Fit (Loose):** Increase sagittal vault; choose steeper base curve and/or larger diameter contact lens
- **Poor Fit (Tight):** Decrease sagittal vault; choose flatter base curve and/or smaller diameter contact lens
- **Superior Limbic Keratoconjunctivitis:** Suspend contact lens use; replace and/or clean contact lenses; use nonpreserved contact lens solutions (no thimerosal); for persistent cases, consider topical steroid (prednisolone acetate 1% or fluorometholone qid) or silver nitrate 0.5–1% solution

Management Continued

- **Superficial Punctate Keratitis:** Suspend contact lens use until corneal surface has healed; topical lubrication with artificial tears (see Appendix) up to q1h; re-fit contact lens; consider punctal plugs for dry eyes
- **Infectious Keratitis:** (see Infectious Keratitis section)
  - Suspend contact lens use
  - Lab tests: cultures of cornea and contact lens solution
  - Topical broad-spectrum antibiotics (fluoroquinolone [Ocuflox or Ciloxan] or a fortified antibiotic q1h) (see Infectious Keratitis section for specific treatment); be alert for *Pseudomonas* and *Acanthamoeba;* do ***not*** patch any epithelial defects if infectious etiology is suspected

Prognosis

Usually good except for corneal infections.

Miscellaneous

Definitions

Dellen: Areas of corneal thinning secondary to corneal drying from an adjacent area of tissue elevation; appears as focal thinning with overlying pooling of fluorescein dye; usually seen near pterygium or filtering bleb.

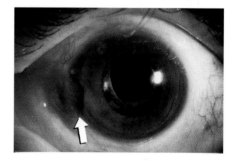

Figure 5–16 Dellen appears as depression/thinning of cornea nasally (arrow).

Exposure Keratopathy: Drying of cornea with subsequent epithelial breakdown; due to neurotrophic (cranial nerve V palsy, cerebrovascular accident, aneurysm, multiple sclerosis, tumor, herpes simplex, herpes zoster), neuroparalytic (cranial nerve VII palsy), lid malposition, nocturnal lagophthalmos, or any cause of proptosis with lagophthalmos; sequelae include filamentary keratitis, corneal ulcer, and corneal vascularization.

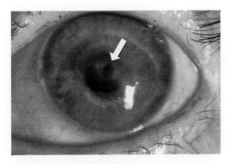

Figure 5–17 Exposure keratopathy with rose bengal staining and a neurotrophic ulcer (arrow).

Filamentary Keratitis: Strands of mucus and desquamated epithelial cells adherent to corneal epithelium due to many conditions including any cause of dry eye, patching, recurrent erosion, bullous keratopathy, superior limbic keratoconjunctivitis, herpes simplex, medicamentosa, or ptosis; blinking causes pain as filaments pull on intact epithelium.

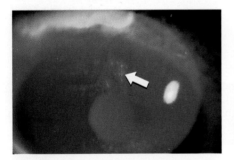

Figure 5–18 Filamentary keratitis demonstrating diffuse fluorescein staining of cornea and brighter staining of corneal filaments (arrow).

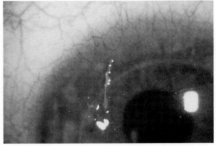

Figure 5–19 Corneal filament.

Keratic Precipitates (KP): Fine, medium, or large deposits of inflammatory cells on the corneal endothelium due to a prior episode of inflammation; usually round white spots, but can be translucent or pigmented; may have mutton-fat (in granulomatous uveitis) or stellate (in Fuchs' heterochromic iridocyclitis) appearance; often melt/disappear or become pigmented with time.

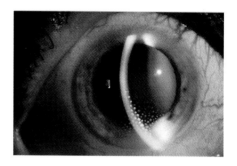

Figure 5–20 White, mutton-fat, granulomatous, keratic precipitates in a patient with toxoplasmosis.

Superficial Punctate Keratitis (SPK): Nonspecific, pinpoint, epithelial defects; punctate staining with fluorescein; associated with blepharitis, any cause of dry eye, trauma, foreign body, trichiasis, ultraviolet or chemical burn, medicamentosa, contact lens–related, exposure, and conjunctivitis.

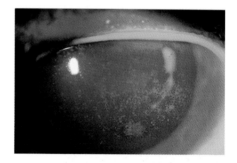

Figure 5–21 Superficial punctate keratitis.

Thygeson's Superficial Punctate Keratitis: Bilateral, recurrent, gray-white, slightly elevated lesions (similar to subepithelial infiltrates in adenoviral keratoconjunctivitis) in a white and quiet eye, minimal or no staining with fluorescein; unknown etiology; usually occurs in 2nd–3rd decade.

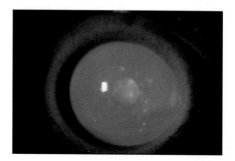

Figure 5–22 Thygeson's superficial punctate keratitis demonstrating white, stellate, corneal opacities with cobalt blue light.

Symptoms

Asymptomatic; may have dryness, foreign-body sensation, discharge, tearing, photophobia, red eye, and decreased vision.

Signs

Normal or decreased visual acuity, lagophthalmos, conjunctival injection, decreased corneal sensation, corneal staining, superficial punctate keratitis (inferiorly or in a central band in exposure keratopathy), filaments (stain with fluorescein), subepithelial infiltrates, keratic precipitates, anterior chamber cell/flare.

Differential Diagnosis

See above.

Evaluation

- Complete ophthalmic history and eye exam with attention to lids, conjunctiva, cornea, anterior chamber, and cranial nerve testing

Management

- Topical lubrication with nonpreserved artificial tears (see Appendix) up to q1h and ointment (Refresh P.M.) at bedtime
- Add antibiotic ointment (erythromycin or bacitracin tid) for moderate SPK and exposure keratitis; consider cycloplegic (cyclopentolate 1% or scopolamine 0.25% bid) and pressure patch (except in contact lens wearer) if severe
- Consider punctal occlusion, lid-taping at bedtime, moist chamber goggles, bandage contact lens, or tarsorrhaphy for moderate to severe dry eye symptoms and exposure keratitis
- Clean, change, or discontinue contact lenses
- Debridement of filaments with sterile cotton-tipped applicator, consider collagenase inhibitor (acetylcysteine [Mucomyst] qd to qid) or bandage contact lens for prolonged episodes of filamentary keratitis
- Add mild topical steroid (fluorometholone qid for 1–2 weeks then taper slowly) for Thygeson's SPK
- Consider bandage contact lens for comfort

Prognosis

Usually good.

Corneal Edema

Definition

Focal or diffuse hydration and swelling of corneal stroma (stromal edema due to endothelial dysfunction) and/or corneal epithelium (intercellular/microcystic edema due to increased intraocular pressure or epithelial hypoxia).

Symptoms

Asymptomatic; may have photophobia, foreign-body sensation, tearing, pain, halos around lights, decreased vision.

Signs

Normal or decreased visual acuity, poor corneal light reflex, thickened cornea, epithelial microcysts and bullae, nonhealing epithelial defects, superficial punctate keratitis, stromal haze, Descemet's folds, guttata, anterior chamber cell/flare, decreased or increased intraocular pressure, iridocorneal touch, aphakia, pseudophakia, vitreous in anterior chamber.

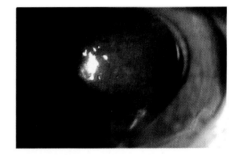

Figure 5–23 Pseudophakic bullous keratopathy demonstrating corneal edema with central corneal folds, hazy stroma, and distorted light reflex.

Differential Diagnosis

Inflammation, infection, Fuchs' dystrophy, posterior polymorphous dystrophy (PPMD), congenital hereditary endothelial dystrophy (CHED), hydrops (keratoconus or pellucid marginal degeneration), acute angle-closure glaucoma, congenital glaucoma, previous ocular surgery (aphakic/pseudophakic bullous keratopathy [ABK/PBK] or graft failure), contact lens overwear, hypotony, birth trauma, iridocorneal endothelial (ICE) syndrome, Brown-McLean syndrome (peripheral edema in aphakic patients possibly from endothelial contact with floppy iris), anterior segment ischemia.

Evaluation

■ Complete ophthalmic history and eye exam with attention to cornea, pachymetry (central thickness >0.610 mm indicates edema), tonometry, anterior chamber, gonioscopy, iris, and specular microscopy

Management

- Symptomatic relief with hypertonic saline ointment (Adsorbonac or Muro 128 5% tid); consider topical steroid (prednisolone acetate 1% up to qid) and cycloplegic (scopolamine 0.25% bid to qid)
- Add broad-spectrum topical antibiotic (polymyxin B sulfate–trimethoprim [Polytrim] or tobramycin [Tobrex] qid) for epithelial defects; consider bandage contact lens or tarsorrhaphy for persistent epithelial defects
- Treat underlying cause (eg, penetrating keratoplasty for ABK, PBK, Fuchs' dystrophy, and CHED; intraocular pressure control and iridotomy for angle-closure glaucoma; observation for hydrops and birth trauma)

Prognosis

Depends on etiology.

Graft Failure

Definition

Failure (edema and opacification) of corneal graft due to primary donor failure (early), allograft rejection (late; usually from endothelial rejection, epithelial rejection rarely causes graft failure), or a variety of other insults including increased intraocular pressure, neovascularization, and recurrence of primary disease.

Symptoms

Pain, photophobia, red eye, and decreased vision.

Signs

Decreased visual acuity, conjunctival injection, ciliary injection, corneal edema, vascularization, subepithelial infiltrates, epithelial rejection line, endothelial rejection line (Khodadoust line), keratic precipitates, anterior chamber cell/flare; may have increased intraocular pressure.

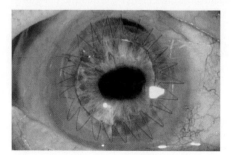

Figure 5–24 Clear corneal graft with running suture; note anterior chamber intraocular lens implant.

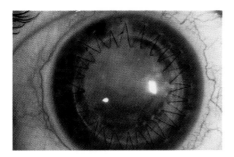 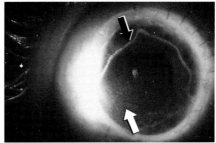

Figure 5–25 Graft failure with opaque cornea.

Figure 5–26 Graft failure with rejection line (black arrow) and keratic precipitates (white arrow).

Differential Diagnosis

Endophthalmitis, herpes simplex keratitis, adenoviral keratoconjunctivitis, anterior uveitis.

Evaluation

■ Complete ophthalmic history and eye exam with attention to conjunctiva, cornea, pachymetry, suture integrity, tonometry, and anterior chamber

Management

■ Topical steroid (prednisolone acetate 1% up to q1h initially, taper slowly), cycloplegic (cyclopentolate 1% or scopolamine 0.25% tid); consider systemic steroids (prednisone 60–80 mg PO qd initially, then taper rapidly over 5–7 days), or sub-Tenon steroid injection (triamcinolone acetonide 40 mg/mL); check purified protein derivative (PPD), blood glucose, and chest radiographs before starting systemic steroids

■ Add H_2-blocker (ranitidine [Zantac] 150 mg PO bid) when taking systemic steroids

■ Topical cyclosporine is controversial

■ Treat recurrent herpes simplex virus keratitis if this is the inciting event with systemic antivirals (acyclovir 400 mg PO tid for 10–21 days, then bid for 12–18 months)

■ May require treatment of increased intraocular pressure (see Chap. 11)

Prognosis

Often good if treated early and aggressively; poorer prognosis for a penetrating keratoplasty secondary to prior graft failure, herpes simplex keratitis, acute corneal ulcer, chemical burn, and eyes with other ocular disease (dry eye syndrome, exposure keratopathy, ocular cicatricial pemphigoid, Stevens-Johnson syndrome, uveitis, and glaucoma); better prognosis for a penetrating keratoplasty secondary to corneal edema (aphakic/pseudophakic bullous keratopathy, Fuchs' dystrophy), keratoconus, corneal scar/opacity, and dystrophy.

Infectious Keratitis (Corneal Ulcer)

Definition

Destruction of corneal tissue (epithelium and stroma) due to inflammation from an infectious organism. Risks include contact lens wear, trauma, dry eyes, exposure keratopathy, bullous keratopathy, neurotrophic cornea, and lid abnormalities.

Etiology

BACTERIAL:

Most common infectious source; usually due to *Pseudomonas aeruginosa, Staphylococcus aureus, Staphylococcus epidermidis, Streptococcus pneumoniae, Haemophilus influenzae, Moraxella catarrhalis;* beware of *Neisseria* species, *Corynebacterium diphtheriae, Haemophilus aegyptius,* and *Listeria* because they can penetrate intact epithelium; *Streptococcus viridans* causes crystalline keratopathy (central branching cracked-glass appearance without epithelial defect; associated with chronic topical steroid use).

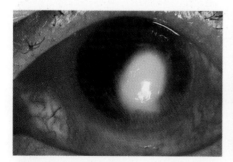 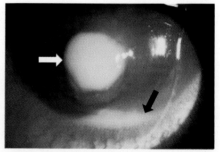

Figure 5–27 Bacterial keratitis demonstrating *Streptococcus pneumoniae* corneal ulcer.

Figure 5–28 Bacterial keratitis demonstrating *Pseudomonas aeruginosa* corneal ulcer (white arrow) with surrounding corneal edema and hypopyon (black arrow).

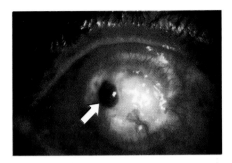

Figure 5–29 Perforated corneal ulcer with iris plugging wound (arrow).

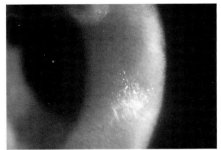

Figure 5–30 Crystalline keratopathy due to *Streptococcus viridans*.

FUNGAL:

Usually *Aspergillus, Candida,* or *Fusarium* species; often have satellite infiltrates, feathery edges, endothelial plaques; can penetrate Descemet's membrane; associated with trauma, especially involving vegetable matter.

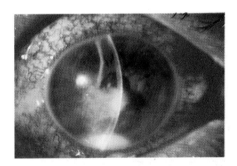

Figure 5–31 Fungal keratitis demonstrating feathery borders and hypopyon.

PARASITIC:

Acanthamoeba:

Resembles herpes simplex virus epithelial keratitis early, perineural and ring infiltrates later; usually seen in contact lens wearers who use nonsterile water or have poor contact lens cleaning habits. Patients usually have pain out of proportion to signs.

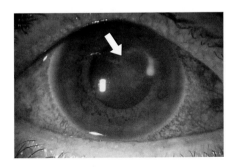

Figure 5–32 Acanthamoeba keratitis demonstrating ring infiltrate (arrow).

Microsporidia: Causes diffuse epithelial keratitis with small, white, intraepithe-lial infiltrates (organisms); seen in patients with AIDS.

VIRAL:

Herpes Simplex Virus (HSV):

Recurrent HSV is the most common cause of central infectious keratitis; associated with sun exposure, fever, stress, menses, trauma, illness, and immunosuppression; recurrence rate = 25% in 1st year, 50% in 2nd year; several types of HSV infection exist:

- *Epithelial keratitis:* Can present as a superficial punctate keratitis, dendrite (ulcerated, classically with terminal bulbs), or geographic ulcer; associated with scarring and decreased corneal sensation
- *Disciform keratitis:* Self-limited (2–6 months), cell-mediated, immune reaction with focal disc-like area of stromal edema, folds, fine keratic precipitates, and scarring
- *Necrotizing interstitial keratitis:* Antigen-antibody-complement mediated; dense stromal inflammation and ulceration with severe iritis
- *Endotheliitis:* Corneal edema, keratic precipitates, increased intraocular pressure, anterior chamber cell/flare

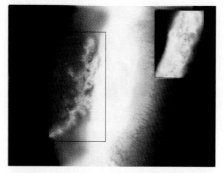

Figure 5–33 Herpes simplex epithelial keratitis demonstrating dendrite with terminal bulbs; inset shows staining of dendrite with rose bengal.

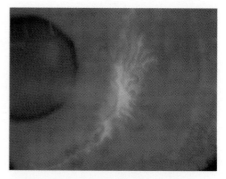

Figure 5–34 Same patient as shown in Figure 5–33 demonstrating staining of dendrite with fluorescein.

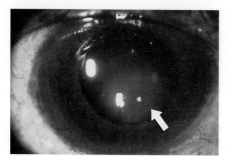

Figure 5–35 Herpes simplex disciform keratitis (arrow).

Herpes Zoster Virus (HZV): Causes a pseudodendrite (coarser, heaped-up epithelial plaque without terminal bulbs) or superficial punctate keratitis with iritis and increased intraocular pressure; may develop sector iris atrophy.

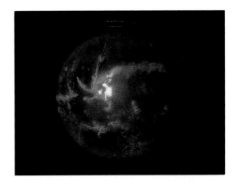

Figure 5–36 Herpes zoster ophthalmicus demonstrating staining of coarse, dendriform, corneal lesion with fluorescein.

Symptoms

Pain, discharge, tearing, photophobia, red eye, decreased vision; may notice white spot on cornea.

Signs

Normal or decreased visual acuity, conjunctival injection, ciliary injection, white corneal infiltrate with overlying epithelial defect that stains with fluorescein, satellite lesions (fungal), corneal edema, Descemet's folds, dendrite (HSV), pseudodendrite (HZV), cutaneous herpes vesicles, perineural and ring infiltrates *(Acanthamoeba),* corneal thinning, descemetocele, anterior chamber cell/flare, hypopyon, mucopurulent discharge, increased intraocular pressure.

Differential Diagnosis

Sterile ulcer, shield ulcer (vernal keratoconjunctivitis), staphylococcal marginal keratitis, epidemic keratoconjunctivitis (EKC) subepithelial infiltrates, ocular rosacea, marginal keratolysis, Mooren's ulcer, Terrien's marginal degeneration, corneal abrasion, recurrent erosion, stromal scar, Thygeson's superficial punctate keratitis, metaherpetic/trophic ulcer (noninfectious, nonhealing epithelial defect with heaped-up gray edges due to HSV basement membrane disease with possible neurotrophic component), tyrosinemia (pseudodendrite).

Evaluation

- Complete ophthalmic history with attention to contact lens use and care regimen
- Complete eye exam with attention to cornea (sensation, size and depth of ulcer, character of infiltrate, fluorescein and rose bengal staining, amount of thinning), tonometry, and anterior chamber

- Lab tests: Scrape corneal ulcer with sterile spatula or blade and smear on microbiology slides; send for routine cultures (bacteria), Sabouraud's media (fungi), chocolate agar *(H. influenzae, N. gonorrhoeae),* Gram stain (bacteria), Giemsa stain (fungi, *Acanthamoeba*); consider calcofluor white *(Acanthamoeba)* and acid fast *(Mycobacteria)* if these entities are suspected
- Consider biopsy for progressive disease, culture-negative ulcer, or deep abscess (usually fungal, *Acanthamoeba,* crystalline)

Management

- Suspend contact lens use
- May require treatment of increased intraocular pressure (see Chap. 11), especially HZV
- Consider bandage contact lens or tarsorrhaphy to heal persistent epithelial defects; glue and contact lens to seal small perforations; and penetrating keratoplasty; *never patch* corneal ulcer
- Ulcers require daily follow-up initially, and severe ones require hospital admission
- If organism is in doubt, treat as a bacterial ulcer until culture results return

BACTERIAL:

- **Small Infiltrates** (<2 mm): Broad-spectrum topical antibiotic (ciprofloxacin [Ciloxan] or ofloxacin [Ocuflox] q1h initially, then taper slowly)
- **Larger Ulcers:** Broad-spectrum *fortified* topical antibiotics (tobramycin 13.6 mg/mL and cefazolin 50 mg/mL or vancomycin 50 mg/mL [in penicillin- and cephalosporin-allergic patients] alternating q1h [which means taking a drop every 30 minutes] for 24–72 hours, then taper slowly); consider subconjunctival antibiotic injections in noncompliant patients
- Tailor antibiotic choices as culture and Gram stain results return
- Topical cycloplegic (scopolamine 0.25% or atropine 1% bid to qid)
- Topical steroid (prednisolone acetate 1% with lower frequency than topical antibiotics) should be avoided until improvement is noted (usually after 48–72 hours)
- Systemic antibiotics for corneal perforation or scleral involvement

FUNGAL:

- Topical antifungal (natamycin 50 mg/mL q1h, amphotericin B 1–2.5 mg/mL q1h, or miconazole 10 mg/mL q1h for 24–72 hours, then taper slowly)
- For severe infection, add systemic antifungal (ketoconazole 200–400 mg PO qd or amphotericin B 1 mg/kg IV over 6 hours)
- Topical cycloplegic (scopolamine 0.25% or atropine 1% bid to qid)
- Topical steroids are **contraindicated**

Management Continued

PARASITIC:

- *Acanthamoeba:* Topical agents (combination of propamidine isethionate [Brolene] 0.1% or hexamidine 0.1%, and miconazole 1% or clotrimazole 1%, and polyhexamethylene biguanide (PHBG) [Baquacil] 0.02% or chlorhexidine 0.02%, q1h [for 1 week], then taper very slowly over 2–3 months), topical broad-spectrum antibiotic (neomycin or paromomycin q2h), and oral antifungal (ketoconazole 200 mg or itraconazole 100 mg PO bid)
- Topical steroids are controversial, consider for severe necrotizing keratitis (prednisolone phosphate 1% qid)
- Topical cycloplegic (scopolamine 0.25% or atropine 1% bid to qid)
- *Microsporidia:* Topical fumagillin up to q2h initially, then taper slowly

VIRAL:

- **HSV Epithelial Keratitis:** Topical antiviral (trifluridine [Viroptic] 9 times/day or vidarabine monohydrate [Vira-A] 5 times/day for 10–14 days); consider oral antiviral (acyclovir 400 mg PO tid for 10–21 days, then prophylaxis with 400 mg bid for up to 1 year [or longer after penetrating keratoplasty]), débride dendrite
- **HSV Disciform or Endotheliitis:** Topical steroid (prednisolone phosphate 0.12–1.0% qd to qid depending on severity of inflammation, adjust and then taper slowly over months depending on response); consider cycloplegic (scopolamine 0.25% bid to qid); add topical antiviral (trifluridine [Viroptic] qid) if epithelium is involved or prophylactically when using steroid doses greater than prednisolone phosphate 0.12% bid (alternatively, can use acyclovir 400 mg PO bid)
- **HSV Metaherpetic/Trophic Ulcer:** Topical lubrication with nonpreserved artificial tears (see Appendix) up to q1h and ointment (Refresh P.M.) at bedtime; broad-spectrum topical antibiotic (polymyxin B sulfate–trimethoprim [Polytrim], tobramycin [Tobrex], ciprofloxacin [Ciloxan], or ofloxacin [Ocuflox] qid), bandage contact lens; add mild topical steroid (fluorometholone qd to bid) if stromal inflammation exists
- **HZV:** Systemic antivirals (acyclovir 800 mg PO 5 times a day for 10 days), topical steroids (prednisolone acetate 1% qid to q4h, then taper slowly over months), cycloplegic (scopolamine 0.25% bid to qid); add topical antibiotic ointment (erythromycin or bacitracin tid) if conjunctival or corneal involvement

Prognosis

Depends on organism, size, location, and response to treatment; sequelae may range from a small corneal scar without alteration of vision to corneal perforation requiring emergent grafting; poor prognosis for fungal and *Acanthamoeba* keratitis; herpes simplex and *Acanthamoeba* commonly recur in corneal graft.

Interstitial Keratitis (IK)

Definition

Diffuse or sectoral vascularization and scarring of corneal stroma due to non-necrotizing inflammation and edema; may be acute or chronic.

Etiology

Most commonly congenital syphilis (90% of cases), tuberculosis, and herpes simplex; also herpes zoster, leprosy, onchocerciasis, mumps, lymphogranuloma venereum, sarcoidosis, and Cogan's syndrome (triad of interstitial keratitis, vertigo, and deafness).

Symptoms

Acute: Decreased vision, pain, photophobia, red eye.

Chronic: Usually asymptomatic.

Signs

Normal or decreased visual acuity.

Acute: Conjunctival injection, salmon patch (stromal vascularization), stromal edema, anterior chamber cell/flare, keratic precipitates.

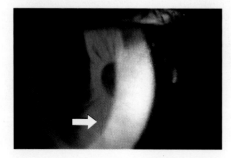

Figure 5–37 Interstitial keratitis demonstrating central scarring and extensive corneal neovascularization (arrow).

Chronic: Deep corneal haze, scarring, thinning, vascularization, ghost vessels; other stigmata of congenital syphilis (optic nerve atrophy, salt-and-pepper fundus, deafness, notched teeth, saddle nose, sabre shins).

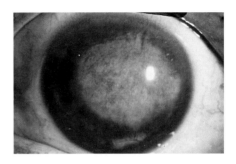

Figure 5–38 Interstitial keratitis demonstrating ghost vessels.

Evaluation

- Complete ophthalmic history and eye exam with attention to lids, conjunctiva, cornea, anterior chamber, and ophthalmoscopy
- Lab tests: Venereal Disease Research Laboratory (VDRL), fluorescent treponemal antibody absorption test (FTA-ABS), purified protein derivative (PPD), and chest radiographs; consider angiotensin converting enzyme (ACE)
- Consider medical and otolaryngology (Cogan's syndrome) consultation

Management

ACUTE:

- Topical steroid (prednisolone acetate 1% qid to q4h, then taper) and cycloplegic (scopolamine 0.25% bid to qid)

CHRONIC:

- Treat underlying cause (eg, syphilis, tuberculosis)
- May require penetrating keratoplasty if vision is affected by corneal scarring
- Early oral steroids in Cogan's syndrome may prevent permanent hearing loss

Prognosis

Good; corneal opacity is nonprogressive.

Pannus

Definition

Superficial vascularization and scarring of peripheral cornea due to inflammation; histologically, fibrovascular tissue between epithelium and Bowman's layer; two types:

- **Inflammatory:** Bowman's layer destruction, with inflammatory cells
- **Degenerative:** Bowman's layer intact, with areas of calcification

Symptoms

Asymptomatic; may have decreased vision if visual axis is involved.

Signs

Vascularization and opacification of cornea past the normal peripheral vascular arcade; micropannus (1–2 mm), gross pannus (>2 mm).

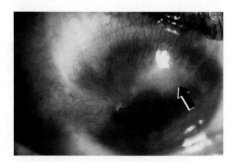

Figure 5–39 Large pannus in a patient with a chemical burn (arrow).

Differential Diagnosis

Trachoma, contact lens–related neovascularization, vernal keratoconjunctivitis, superior limbic keratoconjunctivitis, atopic keratoconjunctivitis, staphylococcal blepharitis, ocular rosacea, herpes simplex, chemical injury, phlyctenulosis, ocular cicatricial pemphigoid, Stevens-Johnson syndrome, aniridia, or idiopathic.

Evaluation

- Complete ophthalmic history and eye exam with attention to everting lids, conjunctiva, and cornea

Prognosis

Good; may progress.

Degenerations

Definition

Acquired lesions secondary to aging or previous corneal insult.

Arcus Senilis: Bilateral, white ring in peripheral cornea; seen in elderly individuals due to lipid deposition at level of Bowman's and Descemet's membrane; clear zone exists between arcus and limbus; check lipid profile if patient is <40 years old; unilateral is due to contralateral carotid occlusive disease; congenital form is called arcus juvenilis.

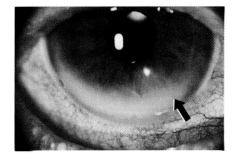

Figure 5–40   Arcus senilis (arrow).

Band Keratopathy: Interpalpebral, subepithelial, patchy calcific changes in Bowman's membrane; swiss-cheese pattern; seen in chronic ocular inflammation (edema, uveitis, glaucoma, interstitial keratitis, phthisis, dry eye syndrome), hypercalcemia, gout, mercury vapors, or hereditary.

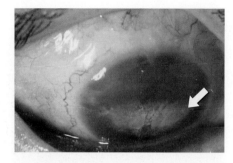

Figure 5–41 Band keratopathy (arrow).

Crocodile Shagreen: Bilateral, gray-white opacification at level of Bowman's layer (anterior) or the deep stroma (posterior); mosaic/cracked-ice pattern.

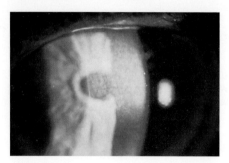

Figure 5–42 Posterior crocodile shagreen with hazy, cracked-ice appearance.

Furrow Degeneration: Corneal thinning in the clear zone between arcus senilis and limbus (more apparent than real); perforation is rare; nonprogressive.

Lipid Keratopathy: Yellow-white, subepithelial and stromal infiltrate with feathery edges due to lipid deposition from chronic inflammation and vascularization.

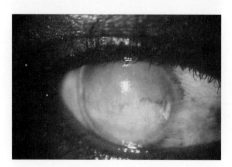

Figure 5–43 Lipid keratopathy.

Spheroidal Degeneration (Actinic/Labrador Keratopathy/Bietti's Nodular Dystrophy): Bilateral, elevated, interpalpebral, yellow, stromal droplets due to sun exposure; male predilection; associated with band keratopathy.

Salzmann's Nodular Degeneration: Elevated, smooth, opaque, blue-white, subepithelial, hyaline nodules due to chronic keratitis; female predilection.

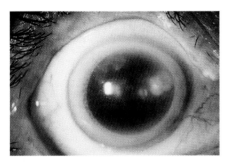

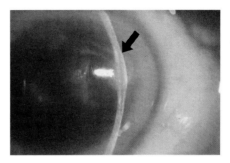

Figure 5–44 Salzmann's nodular degeneration.

Figure 5–45 Same patient as shown in Figure 5–44, demonstrating elevation of nodule with fine slit beam (arrow).

White Limbal Girdle of Vogt: Bilateral, white, needle-like opacities in interpalpebral peripheral cornea; seen in elderly patients; two types:

- **Type I:** calcific (lucid interval at limbus)
- **Type II:** elastotic (no lucid interval)

Symptoms

Asymptomatic; may have tearing, photophobia, decreased vision, and foreign-body sensation.

Signs

Normal or decreased visual acuity, corneal opacity.

Differential Diagnosis

See above, corneal dystrophy, metabolic disease, corneal deposition.

Evaluation

- Complete ophthalmic history and eye exam with attention to cornea

Management

- No treatment recommended
- Consider 3% topical sodium ethylene diaminetetraacetic acid (EDTA) chelation, superficial keratectomy, phototherapeutic keratectomy, or penetrating keratoplasty for band keratopathy
- Salzmann's nodules often respond to superficial keratectomy

Prognosis

Good, most are benign incidental findings; poor for band and lipid keratopathy as these are secondary to chronic processes.

Ectasias

Definition

Keratoconus (KC): Bilateral, asymmetric, cone-shaped deformity of the cornea due to progressive paracentral corneal thinning; patients develop irregular astigmatism, corneal striae, superficial scarring from breaks in Bowman's membrane, acute painful stromal edema from breaks in Descemet's membrane (hydrops); usually sporadic, but may have positive family history (10% of cases); associated with atopy and vernal keratoconjunctivitis (eye-rubbing), Down's syndrome, Marfan's syndrome, and contact lens wear (polymethylmethacrylate [PMMA]).

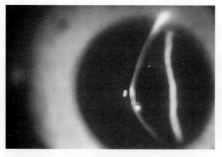

Figure 5–46 Keratoconus demonstrating central "nipple" cone with fine slit beam.

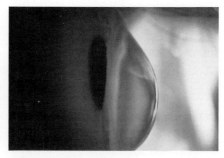

Figure 5–47 Keratoconus demonstrating inferior "sagging" cone.

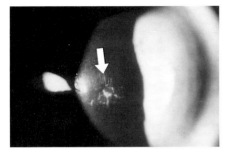

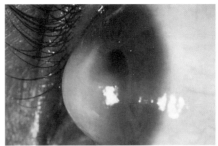

Figure 5–48 Keratoconus demonstrating central scarring and Vogt's striae (arrow).

Figure 5–49 Hydrops in a patient with keratoconus.

Keratoglobus: Rare, globular deformity of the cornea due to diffuse thinning that is maximal at the base of the protrusion; sporadic; associated with Ehlers-Danlos syndrome.

Pellucid Marginal Degeneration: Bilateral, inferior, peripheral corneal thinning (2 mm from limbus) with protrusion above thinned area; patients develop irregular astigmatism; no scarring, cone, or striae seen.

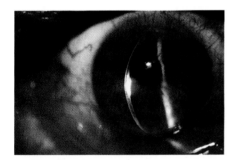

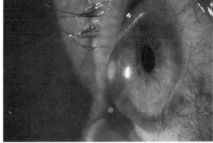

Figure 5–50 Pellucid marginal degeneration demonstrating inferior thinning.

Figure 5–51 Side view of same patient as shown in Figure 5–50.

Symptoms

Decreased vision; may have sudden loss of vision, pain, photophobia, tearing, and red eye in hydrops.

Signs

Decreased visual acuity, abnormally shaped cornea, astigmatism, irregular keratometer mires; in keratoconus may have central thinning, scarring, Fleischer's ring (epithelial iron deposition around base of cone, best seen with blue light), Vogt's striae (deep, stromal, vertical stress lines at apex of cone), Munson's sign (protrusion of lower lid with downgaze), and Rizzuti's sign (triangle of light on iris from penlight beam focused by cone); in keratoconus and pellucid marginal degeneration may have hydrops (opaque edematous cornea, ciliary injection, and anterior chamber cell/flare).

Differential Diagnosis

See above; Terrien's marginal degeneration.

Evaluation

- Complete ophthalmic history and eye exam with attention to cornea, keratometry, retinoscopy reflex, and anterior chamber
- Corneal topography (computerized videokeratography)

Management

- Correct refractive errors with spectacles or rigid gas permeable contact lens (RGP)
- Consider penetrating keratoplasty when acuity declines or if patient is intolerant of contact lenses
- Supportive treatment for acute hydrops with hypertonic saline ointment (Adsorbonac or Muro 128 5% qid); add topical broad-spectrum antibiotic (polymyxin B sulfate–trimethoprim [Polytrim] or tobramycin [Tobrex] qid) for epithelial defect; consider topical steroid (prednisolone acetate 1% qid) and cycloplegic (cyclopentolate 1% tid) for severe pain
- Corneal refractive surgery contraindicated in these unstable corneas

---

Prognosis

Good; penetrating keratoplasty has high success rate for keratoconus and keratoglobus.

Congenital Anomalies

Definition

Cornea Plana (autosomal dominant/autosomal recessive [AD/AR]): Flat cornea (curvature often as low as 20–30 diopters); corneal curvature equal to scleral curvature is pathognomonic; associated with sclerocornea and microcornea; increased incidence of angle-closure glaucoma; mapped to chromosome 12q.

Dermoid: Choristoma composed of dense connective tissue with pilosebaceous units and stratified squamous epithelium; usually located at inferotemporal limbus, can involve entire cornea; may cause astigmatism and amblyopia; may be associated with preauricular skin tags and vertebral anomalies (Goldenhar's syndrome).

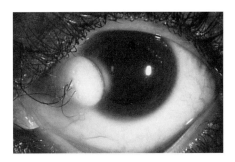

Figure 5–52 Limbal dermoid with corneal lipid deposition along anterior edge.

Haab's Striae: Horizontal breaks in Descemet's membrane due to increased intraocular pressure in children with congenital glaucoma.

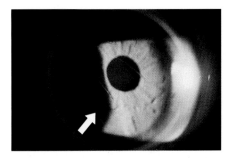

Figure 5–53 Haab's striae (arrow).

Megalocornea (X-Linked): Enlarged cornea (horizontal diameter ≥13 mm); male predilection (90%); usually isolated, nonprogressive, and bilateral; associated with weak zonules and lens subluxation.

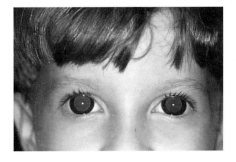

Figure 5–54 Megalocornea.

Microcornea (AD/AR): Small cornea (diameter <10 mm); increased incidence of hyperopia and angle-closure glaucoma.

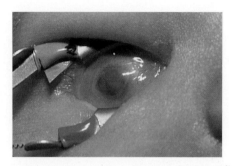

Figure 5–55 Microcornea.

Posterior Keratoconus: Focal, central indentation of posterior cornea with scarring; rare, usually unilateral, and nonprogressive; female predilection; no change in anterior corneal surface.

Sclerocornea: Scleralized peripheral or entire cornea; nonprogressive, 50% sporadic, 50% hereditary (AR more severe); 90% bilateral; associated with cornea plana (80%).

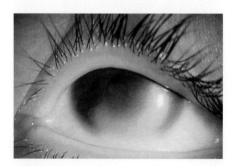

Figure 5–56 Sclerocornea.

Symptoms

Asymptomatic; may have decreased vision.

Signs

Normal or decreased visual acuity, abnormal corneal size or shape, corneal opacity, edema, or scarring; may have other anterior segment abnormalities (angle, iris, or lens) and increased intraocular pressure.

Differential Diagnosis

Microphthalmos, nanophthalmos, congenital glaucoma (buphthalmos), interstitial keratitis, anterior keratoconus, birth trauma.

Evaluation

- Complete ophthalmic history and eye exam with attention to refraction, cornea, keratometry, tonometry, gonioscopy, iris, lens, and ophthalmoscopy
- May require examination under anesthesia in a child

Management

- Correct any refractive error
- May require patching/occlusion therapy for amblyopia (see Chap. 12), treatment of increased intraocular pressure (see Congenital Glaucoma section in Chap. 11), or even penetrating keratoplasty in severe cases
- Consider surgical excision of dermoid

Prognosis

Depends on etiology.

Dystrophies

Definition

Primary, inherited, corneal diseases without prior corneal pathology or systemic disease; usually bilateral, symmetric, and progressive with early onset.

ANTERIOR (EPITHELIAL AND BOWMAN'S MEMBRANE):

Anterior Basement Membrane (ABM/Epithelial Basement Membrane [EBM]/ Map-Dot-Fingerprint [MDF]/Cogan's Microcystic) (AD):

Most common anterior corneal dystrophy; intra- and subepithelial basement membrane reduplication causing abnormal epithelial adhesion and recurrent erosions; intraepithelial microcysts (dots) and subepithelial ridges and lines (map-like and fingerprint-like) are also seen; 10% with ABM dystrophy develop recurrent erosions, whereas 50% of patients with recurrent erosions have ABM dystrophy; may develop scarring and decreased vision starting after age 30 years; slight female predilection.

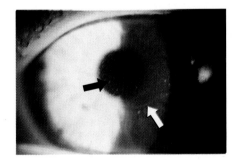

Figure 5–57 Anterior basement membrane dystrophy demonstrating central dots (black arrow) and lines (white arrow).

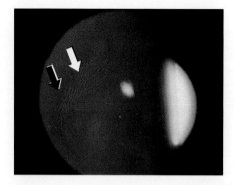

Figure 5–58 Anterior basement membrane dystrophy demonstrating dots (black arrow) and lines (white arrow) as viewed with retroillumination.

Gelatinous Drop-Like (AR): Rare, subepithelial, central, mulberry-like, protuberant opacity; composed of amyloid; lack Bowman's membrane; decreased vision, photophobia, and tearing occur in 1st decade.

Meesmann's (AD): Intraepithelial microcystic blebs concentrated in the interpalpebral zone extending to the limbus; surrounded by clear epithelium; blebs contain PAS positive material ("peculiar substance") and appear as numerous dots with retroillumination; rare and bilateral; develop recurrent erosions, but retain good vision.

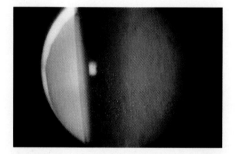

Figure 5–59 Meesmann's dystrophy as viewed with retroillumination.

Reis-Bücklers (AD): Progressive subepithelial opacification and scarring of Bowman's membrane with honeycomb appearance; recurrent erosions early, often in the 1st or 2nd decade; often recurs after penetrating keratoplasty; mapped to chromosome 5q.

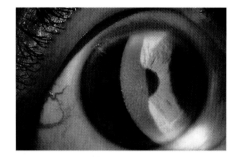

Figure 5–60 Reis-Bücklers dystrophy.

STROMAL:

Avellino (AD):

Combination of granular and lattice (see below) with discrete granular-like opacities; intervening stroma contains lattice-like branching lines and dots (not clear like granular); composed of a combination of hyaline and amyloid that stains with Congo red and Masson's trichrome; mapped to chromosome 5q.

Central Cloudy (AD): Small, indistinct, cloudy gray areas in central posterior stroma with intervening clear cracks (like crocodile shagreen, but does not extend to periphery); nonprogressive; usually asymptomatic.

Central Crystalline (Schnyder's) (AD): Central, yellow-white ring of fine, needle-like, polychromatic crystals with stromal haze; also have dense arcus and limbal girdle; composed of cholesterol and neutral fats that stain with Oil-red-O; very rare and nonprogressive; associated with hyperlipidemia, genu valgum, and xanthelasma; usually asymptomatic; mapped to chromosome 1p.

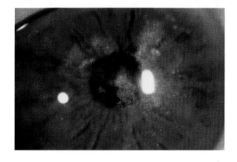

Figure 5–61 Central crystalline dystrophy.

Congenital Hereditary Stromal (CHSD) (AD): Superficial, central, feathery, diffuse opacity; alternating layers of abnormal collagen lamellae; nonprogressive; associated with amblyopia, esotropia, and nystagmus.

Fleck (François-Neetans') (AD): Subtle, gray-white, dandruff-like specks that extend to the limbus; composed of abnormal glycosaminoglycans that stain with alcian blue; can be unilateral and asymmetric; nonprogressive and usually asymptomatic.

Granular (AD): Most common stromal dystrophy; central, discrete, white, bread-crumb or snowflake-like opacities; intervening stroma usually clear, but may become hazy late; corneal periphery spared; composed of hyaline that stains with Masson's trichrome; decreased vision late, erosions rare; mapped to chromosome 5q.

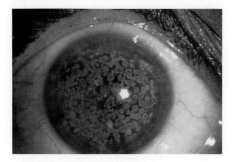

Figure 5–62 Granular dystrophy.

Lattice (AD): Refractile branching lines, white dots, and central haze; intervening stroma becomes cloudy, with ground-glass appearance; composed of amyloid that stains with Congo red; recurrent erosions common, decreased vision in 3rd decade; often recurs after penetrating keratoplasty; mapped to chromosome 5q.

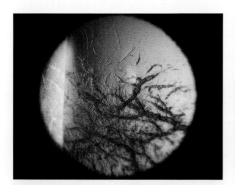

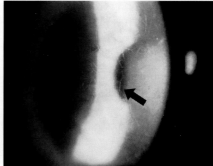

Figure 5–63 Lattice dystrophy demonstrating branching lines as viewed with retroillumination.

Figure 5–64 Lattice dystrophy demonstrating branching lines (arrow).

Macular (AR): Diffuse haze with focal, irregular, gray-white spots that have a sugar-frosted appearance; extends to limbus; composed of abnormal glycosaminoglycans that stain with alcian blue; rare; decreased vision early, recurrent erosions occasionally; mapped to chromosome 16q.

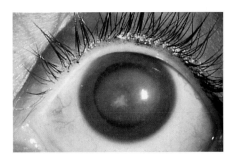

Figure 5–65 Macular dystrophy.

Pre-Descemet's (Deep Filiform) (?AD): Fine, gray, posterior opacities; various morphologies; composed of lipid; onset in 4th to 7th decade; four types: pre-Descemet's, polymorphic stromal, cornea farinata, and pre-Descemet's associated with ichthyosis and pseudoxanthoma elasticum; usually asymptomatic.

POSTERIOR (ENDOTHELIAL):

Congenital Hereditary Endothelial (CHED) (AR>AD):

Opacified, edematous corneas at birth due to endothelial dysfunction; rare; mapped to chromosome 20p; two types:

(1) More common, autosomal recessive, no pain or tearing, nonprogressive
(2) Autosomal dominant, delayed onset (age 1–2 years old); painful with tearing; progressive; may require penetrating keratoplasty

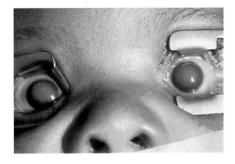

Figure 5–66 Congenital hereditary endothelial dystrophy.

Fuchs' Endothelial (AD): Cornea guttata (thickened Descemet's membrane with PAS-positive excrescences [orange-peel appearance]) and endothelial dysfunction; decreased endothelial cell density, increased pleomorphism, and increased polymegathism; early stromal edema, late epithelial edema, bullae, and fibrosis; female predilection; may have decreased vision (worse in the morning), pain with ruptured bullae, and subepithelial scarring.

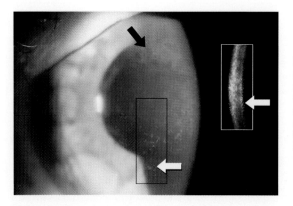

Figure 5–67 Fuchs' endothelial dystrophy demonstrating guttata (white arrow) and endothelial scarring (black arrow); inset demonstrates guttata (white arrow) and corneal edema when viewed with fine slit beam.

Posterior Polymorphous (PPMD) (AD): Asymmetric patches of grouped vesicles, scalloped bands, and geographic, gray, hazy areas; epithelial-like endothelium (loss of contact inhibition with proliferation and growth over angle and iris); may develop stromal edema, iris and pupil changes similar to those in iridocorneal endothelial (ICE) syndrome (see Chap. 7), broad peripheral anterior synechiae, and glaucoma; usually asymptomatic; mapped to chromosome 20q.

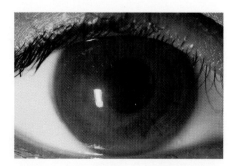

Figure 5–68 Posterior polymorphous dystrophy demonstrating diffuse, hazy, endothelial opacities.

Symptoms

Asymptomatic; may have pain, foreign-body sensation, tearing, photophobia, decreased vision.

Signs

Normal or decreased visual acuity, corneal opacities.

Differential Diagnosis

See above, corneal degeneration, corneal deposition, metabolic diseases.

Evaluation

- Complete ophthalmic history and eye exam with attention to refraction, cornea, tonometry, gonioscopy, iris, and ophthalmoscopy
- B-scan ultrasonography if unable to visualize the fundus
- Consider pachymetry and specular microscopy for Fuchs' dystrophy
- Lab tests: lipid profile for Schnyder's central crystalline

Management

- No treatment recommended
- Topical lubrication with nonpreserved artificial tears (see Appendix) up to q1h, hypertonic saline ointment (Adsorbonac or Muro 128 5% at bedtime)
- May require treatment of recurrent erosions (see Trauma: Recurrent Erosion section)
- May require superficial keratectomy, phototherapeutic keratectomy, lamellar keratoplasty, or penetrating keratoplasty if scarring across the visual axis exists

Prognosis

Usually good; may recur in graft (Reis-Bücklers' > macular > granular > lattice); may develop glaucoma in posterior polymorphous.

Metabolic Diseases

Definition

Hereditary (AR) enzymatic deficiencies that result in accumulation of substances in various tissues as well as bilateral corneal opacities.

Etiology

Mucopolysaccharidoses, mucolipidoses, sphingolipidoses, gangliosidosis type 1; corneal clouding not seen in Hunter's or Sanfilippo's syndromes.

Symptoms

Decreased vision, white cornea.

Signs

Decreased visual acuity; may have nystagmus, cataracts, retinal pigment epithelial changes, macular cherry red spot, optic nerve atrophy, and other systemic abnormalities.

Differential Diagnosis

See above; congenital glaucoma, congenital hereditary endothelial dystrophy, birth trauma, Peter's anomaly, sclerocornea, dermoid.

Evaluation

- Complete ophthalmic history and eye exam with attention to cornea, tonometry, lens, and ophthalmoscopy
- Pediatric consultation

Management

- Treat underlying disease
- May require penetrating keratoplasty

Prognosis

Poor.

Depositions

Definition

Pigment or crystal deposition at various levels of the cornea.

Calcium: Yellow-white deposits in Bowman's membrane (see Degeneration: Band Keratopathy section).

Copper:

- **Chalcosis:** Green-yellow pigmentation of Descemet's membrane and iris; causes sunflower cataract; seen with intraocular foreign body composed of <85% copper; pure copper causes suppurative endophthalmitis.

- **Wilson's Disease:** 95% have Kayser-Fleischer ring at Descemet's membrane (brown-yellow-green peripheral pigmentation that starts inferiorly, no clear interval at limbus).

Figure 5–69 Copper deposition in a patient with Wilson's disease, demonstrating peripheral, brown, Kayser-Fleischer ring (arrows).

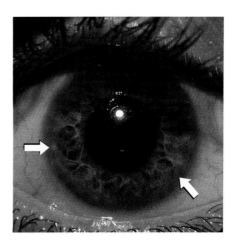

Cysteine (Cystinosis): Stromal, polychromatic crystals.

Drugs:

- **Epinephrine:** Black, conjunctival and corneal adrenochrome deposits

- **Ciprofloxacin:** White, corneal precipitate over epithelial defect

- **Gold (Chrysiasis):** Deposits in conjunctival and stromal periphery; dose-related

- **Mercury:** Preservative in drops causes orange-brown band in Bowman's membrane

- **Silver (Argyrosis):** Conjunctival and deep stromal deposits

- **Thorazine/Stelazine:** Brown, stromal deposits; also anterior subcapsular lens deposits

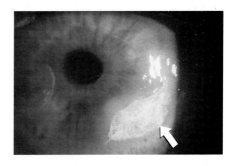

Figure 5–70 Drug deposition demonstrating chalky, white, ciprofloxacin (Ciloxan) precipitates (arrow).

- **Immunoglobulin (Multiple Myeloma):** Stromal deposits (also seen in Waldenström's macroglobulinemia and benign monoclonal gammopathy)

Iron:

- **Blood Staining:** Stromal deposits, after hyphema

- **Ferry Line:** Epithelial deposits, under filtering bleb

- **Fleischer Ring:** Epithelial deposits, at base of cone in keratoconus

- **Hudson-Stahli Line:** Epithelial deposits, across inferior one third of cornea

- **Siderosis:** Stromal deposits, from intraocular metallic foreign body

- **Stocker Line:** Epithelial deposits, at head of pterygium

Lipid/Cholesterol (Dyslipoproteinemias):

- **Hyperlipoproteinemia:** Arcus in types 2, 3, and 4

- **Fish Eye Disease:** Diffuse corneal clouding, denser in periphery

- **Lecithin-Cholesterol Acyltransferase (LCAT) Deficiency:** Dense arcus and diffuse, fine, gray, stromal dots

- **Tangier's Disease:** Familial high-density lipoprotein deficiency; diffuse or focal, small, deep, stromal opacities

Melanin:

- **Krukenberg Spindle:** Endothelial deposits, central vertical patch seen in pigment dispersion syndrome

- **Scattered Endothelial Pigment:** Ingested by abnormal endothelial cells (Fuchs' dystrophy)

Tyrosine (Tyrosinemia): Epithelial and subepithelial pseudo-dendritic opacities; may ulcerate and lead to vascularization and scarring.

Urate (Gout): Epithelial, subepithelial, and stromal, fine, yellow crystals; may form brown, band keratopathy with ulceration and vascularization.

Symptoms
Asymptomatic; may have photophobia, and rarely decreased vision.

Signs
Normal or decreased visual acuity, corneal deposits, may have iris heterochromia (siderosis and chalcosis), cataract (Wilson's disease, intraocular metallic foreign body, tyrosinemia).

Differential Diagnosis

See above; cornea verticillata (brown, epithelial, whorl pattern involving inferior and paracentral cornea; seen in Fabry's disease or from chloroquine, amiodarone, indomethacin, chlorpromazine, tamoxifen toxicity), dieffenbachia plant sap, ichthyosis (may have fine, white, deep, stromal opacities), hyperbilirubinemia.

Evaluation

■ Complete ophthalmic history and eye exam with attention to conjunctiva, cornea, anterior chamber, iris, and lens
■ Electroretinogram (ERG) for intraocular metallic foreign body
■ Medical consultation for systemic diseases

Management

■ Treat underlying disease, remove offending agent
■ May require surgical removal of intraocular metallic foreign body

Prognosis

Good except for siderosis, chalcosis, Wilson's disease, and multiple myeloma.

Enlarged Corneal Nerves

Definition

Prominent, enlarged corneal nerves.

Etiology

Multiple endocrine neoplasia type IIb (MEN-IIb), leprosy, Fuchs' dystrophy, amyloidosis, keratoconus, ichthyosis, Refsum's syndrome, neurofibromatosis, congenital glaucoma, trauma, posterior polymorphous dystrophy, and idiopathic.

Symptoms

Asymptomatic.

Signs

Prominent, white, branching, linear opacities in cornea.

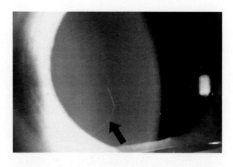

Figure 5–71   Enlarged corneal nerves (arrow).

Differential Diagnosis

See above; lattice dystrophy.

Evaluation

- Complete ophthalmic history and eye exam with attention to cornea, tonometry, lens, and ophthalmoscopy
- Medical consultation for systemic diseases

Management

- No treatment recommended
- Treat underlying medical disorder

Prognosis

Enlarged nerves are benign; underlying cause may have poor prognosis (MEN-IIb).

Tumors

Definition

Corneal intraepithelial neoplasia (CIN) or squamous cell carcinoma (SCC) involving the cornea; usually arises from conjunctiva near limbus.

Epidemiology

Usually unilateral; male predilection (95%); associated with ultraviolet radiation, human papilloma virus, and heavy smoking.

Symptoms

Asymptomatic; may have foreign-body sensation, red eye, decreased vision, or notice growth (white spot) on cornea.

Signs

Gelatinous, thickened, white, nodular or smooth, limbal/corneal mass; may also have vascularization, conjunctival injection, and abnormal vessels.

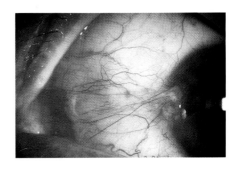

Figure 5–72 Corneal intraepithelial neoplasia.

Differential Diagnosis

Pinguecula, pterygium, pannus, dermoid, Bitot's spot, papilloma, pyogenic granuloma, pseudoepitheliomatous hyperplasia (PEH), benign hereditary intraepithelial dyskeratosis (BHID).

Evaluation

■ Complete ophthalmic history and eye exam with attention to conjunctiva and cornea

Management

■ Excision with cryotherapy, radiation, or mitomycin C by a cornea or tumor specialist

Prognosis

Good if completely excised; 50% recur; rarely invasive or metastatic.

Anterior Chamber

Anterior Chamber Cell/Flare

Definition

Cells and increased protein (flare) in the anterior chamber due to breakdown of the blood-aqueous barrier by inflammation.

Cells: Appear as small particles floating in the aqueous; usually white blood cells; sometimes red blood cells (hyphema) or pigment cells (from iris after dilation and in pigment dispersion syndrome).

Flare: Appears as hazy/cloudy aqueous; severe fibrinous exudate has jelly-like/plasmoid appearance (4^+ flare [see under Signs]).

Etiology

Exudation from blood vessels due to anterior segment inflammation; usually uveitis, trauma, postoperative, and keratitis.

Symptoms

Variable pain, photophobia, tearing, red eye, decreased vision; may be asymptomatic.

Signs

Normal or decreased visual acuity, ciliary injection, miosis, anterior chamber cell/flare (best seen when viewed with a short narrow slit lamp beam directed at an angle through the pupil (see Fig. 6–1) producing an effect similar to shining a flashlight through a dark room; cells demonstrate brownian motion and flare looks like smoke in the light beam; graded on a 1 to 4 scale [ie, 1^+ = 0–10 cells; 2^+ = 11–20 cells; 3^+ = 21–50 cells; 4^+ = >50 cells]); may have keratic precipitates (KP), keratitis, iris nodules, posterior synechiae, increased or decreased intraocular pressure (IOP), hypopyon, hyphema, pseudohypopyon, cataract, vitritis, or retinal/choroidal lesions.

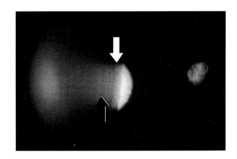

Figure 6–1 Grade 4+ anterior chamber cell/flare (black arrow) visible with fine slit beam between the cornea (white arrow) and iris.

Differential Diagnosis

See above.

Evaluation

- Complete ophthalmic history and eye exam with attention to cornea, tonometry, anterior chamber, gonioscopy, iris, lens, and ophthalmoscopy
- Consider uveitis work-up (see Anterior Uveitis section)

> ### Management
>
> - Treat underlying cause
> - Topical steroid (prednisolone acetate 1% up to q1h initially, then taper slowly) and cycloplegic (cyclopentolate 1%, scopolamine 0.25%, or atropine 1% bid to tid)
> - May require intraocular pressure control (see Chap. 11; do not use miotics), sub-Tenon steroid injection (triamcinolone acetonide 40 mg/mL), systemic steroids (prednisone 60–100 mg PO qd), or cytotoxic agents (see Anterior Uveitis section)

Prognosis

Depends on etiology.

Hypotony

Definition

Low intraocular pressure (IOP <10 mm Hg); functional and structural changes usually occur with pressures ≤5 mm Hg.

Symptoms

Asymptomatic; may have pain and decreased vision.

Signs

Normal or decreased visual acuity, low intraocular pressure; may have corneal folds, anterior chamber cell/flare, shallow anterior chamber, chorioretinal folds, choroidal effusion, cystoid macular edema (CME), positive Seidel test, filtering bleb, optic disc edema, squared-off globe.

Differential Diagnosis

Trauma (blunt, penetrating, or surgical), wound leak, bleb overfiltration, ciliary body shut down, cyclodialysis, choroidal effusion, retinal detachment, pharmacologic, systemic disorder (bilateral hypotony), uveitis, phthisis.

Evaluation

- Complete ophthalmic history and eye exam with attention to cornea, tonometry, anterior chamber, gonioscopy, and ophthalmoscopy
- Check Seidel test (see Chap. 5, Trauma: Laceration section) to rule out open globe or wound leak in traumatic or postsurgical cases

Management

- Treat underlying problem
- Topical cycloplegic (cyclopentolate 1% or scopolamine 0.25% bid to tid)
- Add topical antibiotic for wound leak (ciprofloxacin [Ciloxan] or ofloxacin [Ocuflox] qid)
- May require surgical repair of wound leak, retinal detachment, ciliary body detachment, or drainage of choroidals
- Bandage contact lens or pressure patch may work with small leaks
- Consider Simmons' shell for bleb overfiltration

Prognosis

Depends on etiology.

Hyphema

Definition

Blood in the anterior chamber. Hyphema forms a layer of blood, whereas a microhyphema cannot be visualized with the naked eye (can only see red blood cells floating in anterior chamber with slit lamp examination).

Etiology

Usually a result of trauma (60% also have angle recession); may be spontaneous when associated with neovascularization of the iris and/or angle, iris lesions, or malpositioned/loose intraocular lens (IOL).

Symptoms

Decreased vision; may have pain, photophobia, red eye.

Signs

Normal or decreased visual acuity, red blood cells in the anterior chamber (layer or clot); may have subconjunctival hemorrhage, increased intraocular pressure, rubeosis, iris sphincter tears, iris lesion, unusually deep anterior chamber, angle recession, iridodonesis, iridodialysis, cyclodialysis, and other signs of ocular trauma; may have IOL implant.

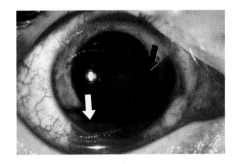

Figure 6–2 Hyphema demonstrating layered blood inferiorly (white arrow) and suspended red blood cells and clot (black arrow).

Differential Diagnosis

Trauma, uveitis-glaucoma-hyphema (UGH) syndrome, juvenile xanthogranu-loma, leukemia, child abuse, postoperative, Fuchs' heterochromic iridocyclitis, rubeosis iridis, malpositioned or loose IOL.

Evaluation

- Complete ophthalmic history and eye exam with attention to cornea, tonome-try, anterior chamber, iris, and ophthalmoscopy; wait 2–4 weeks to perform go-nioscopy and scleral depression in traumatic cases
- Lab tests: sickle cell prep and hemoglobin electrophoresis to rule out sickle cell disease
- B-scan ultrasonography if unable to visualize the fundus to rule out open globe; consider ultrasound biomicroscopy (UBM) to evaluate angle structures

Management

- Topical steroid (prednisolone acetate 1% up to q1h initially, then taper over 3–4 weeks as hyphema and inflammation resolve)
- Topical cycloplegic (scopolamine 0.25% or atropine 1% bid to tid)
- Consider aminocaproic acid (Amicar; 50–100 mg/kg q4h)

Management Continued

- Intraocular pressure control as needed (see Chap. 11; do not use carbonic anhydrase inhibitors in patients with sickle cell disease; do not use miotics)
- Counsel patient to avoid aspirin-containing products, sleep with head of bed elevated at 30-degree angle, metal eye shield over injured eye at all times, and bedrest
- Follow closely every day for first 5 days (when rebleed risk is highest) then slowly space out visits
- May require anterior chamber washout for corneal blood staining, uncontrolled elevated intraocular pressure, persistent clot, rebleed (8-ball hyphema); intraocular lens (IOL) removal or exchange for UGH syndrome and malpositioned IOLs

Prognosis

Good in traumatic cases if intraocular pressure is controlled and there is no rebleed; may be at risk for angle recession glaucoma in the future.

Hypopyon

Definition

Layer of white blood cells in anterior chamber.

Etiology

Sterile (HLA-B27 associated uveitis and Behçet's), infectious, and pseudohypopyon (pigment cells, ghost cells, tumor cells, macrophages).

Symptoms

Pain, red eye, and decreased vision.

Signs

Normal or decreased visual acuity, conjunctival injection, hypopyon, and anterior chamber cell/flare; may have corneal infiltrate, keratic precipitates, iris nodules, cataract, vitritis, vitreous hemorrhage, tumor, retinal/choroidal lesions.

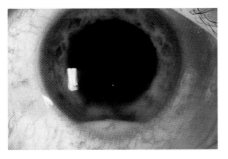

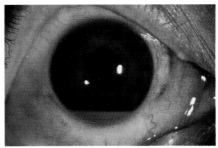

Figure 6–3 Hypopyon.

Figure 6–4 Pseudohypopyon composed of khaki-colored ghost cells.

Differential Diagnosis

Corneal ulcer, uveitis, endophthalmitis, pseudohypopyon.

Evaluation

- Complete ophthalmic history and eye exam with attention to cornea, tonometry, anterior chamber, iris, lens, and ophthalmoscopy
- B-scan ultrasonography if unable to visualize the fundus
- Lab tests: cultures/smears for infectious keratitis or endophthalmitis (see Endophthalmitis section)
- Consider uveitis work-up (see Anterior Uveitis section)

Management

- Antimicrobials if infectious (see Infectious Keratitis and Endophthalmitis sections)
- Topical cycloplegic (cyclopentolate 1% or scopolamine 0.25% bid to tid)
- Topical steroid (prednisolone acetate 1% up to q1h then taper over weeks; use caution if infectious etiology is suspected)
- Monitor treatment response by hypopyon resorption
- Rarely requires surgery, except in cases of endophthalmitis

Prognosis

Depends on etiology and treatment response.

Endophthalmitis

Definition

Intraocular infection; may be acute, subacute, or chronic; localized or involving anterior and posterior segments.

Etiology

Postoperative (70%):

■ **Acute Postoperative (<6 weeks after surgery):** 94% gram-positive bacteria including coagulase-negative staphylococci (70%), *Staphylococcus aureus* (10%), *Streptococcus* species (11%); only 6% gram-negative organisms.

■ **Delayed Postoperative (>6 weeks after surgery):** *Propionibacterium acnes*, coagulase-negative staphylococci, and fungi (*Candida* species).

■ **Conjunctival Filtering Bleb Associated:** *Streptococcus* species (47%), coagulase-negative staphylococci (22%), *Haemophilus influenzae* (16%).

Post-Traumatic (20%):

Bacillus (*B. cereus)* species (24%), *Staphylococcus* species (39%), and gram-negative organisms (7%).

Endogenous (8%):

Rare, usually fungal (*Candida* species); bacterial endogenous is very rare and due to *Staphylococcus aureus* and gram-negative bacteria; seen in debilitated, septicemic, or immunocompromised patients.

Epidemiology

Incidence of endophthalmitis following penetrating trauma is 3–7%, may be as high as 30% after injuries in rural settings; risk factors include retained intraocular foreign body, delayed surgery (>24 hours), rural setting (soil contamination), disrupted crystalline lens. Incidence of endophthalmitis following cataract surgery is <0.1%; risk factors include loss of vitreous, disrupted posterior capsule, poor wound closure, and prolonged surgery.

Symptoms

Pain, photophobia, discharge, red eye, decreased vision; may be asymptomatic or have chronic uveitis appearance in delayed onset and endogenous cases.

Signs

Decreased visual acuity (usually severe; only 14% of patients in the Endophthalmitis Vitrectomy Study (EVS) had better than 5/200 vision), lid edema, proptosis, conjunctival injection, chemosis, wound abscess, corneal edema, keratic precipitates, anterior chamber cell/flare, hypopyon, vitritis, poor red reflex; may have positive Seidel test and other signs of an open globe (see Chap. 4).

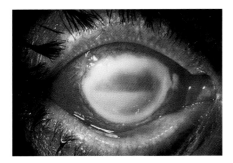

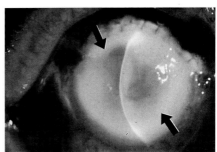

Figure 6–5 Endophthalmitis with hypopyon.

Figure 6–6 *Staphylococcus* endophthalmitis with ring infiltrate (arrows).

Differential Diagnosis

Uveitis, sterile inflammation (usually from prolonged intraoperative manipulations, especially involving vitreous, contaminants on intraocular lens implant or surgical instruments, retained lens material, or rebound inflammation after sudden decrease in postoperative medications), intraocular foreign body, intraocular tumor, sympathetic ophthalmia, anterior segment ischemia (from carotid artery disease [ocular ischemic syndrome] or following muscle surgery [usually on three or more rectus muscles in same eye at the same surgery]).

Evaluation

- Complete ophthalmic history and eye exam with attention to visual acuity, surgical incision integrity, conjunctiva, cornea, tonometry, anterior chamber, vitreous cells, red reflex, and ophthalmoscopy
- B-scan ultrasonography if unable to visualize the fundus
- Lab tests: **STAT** evaluation of intraocular fluid cultures and smears; conjunctival and nasal swabs can also be collected for culture, but have low yield
- Medical consultation for endogenous endophthalmitis

Management

OPHTHALMIC EMERGENCY

ACUTE POSTOPERATIVE ENDOPHTHALMITIS:

- If vision is better than light perception (>LP), then anterior chamber and vitreous tap for collection of specimens for culture, and injection of intravitreal antibiotics (see below)
- If vision is LP only, then anterior chamber tap, pars plana vitrectomy, and injection of intravitreal antibiotics (EVS conclusions); should be managed by a vitreoretinal specialist

Management Continued

- Intravitreal antibiotics/steroids:
  Vancomycin (1 mg/0.1 mL)
  Ceftazidime (2.25 mg/0.1 mL) or amikacin (0.4 mg/0.1 mL)
  Dexamethasone (0.4 mg/0.1 mL); controversial, since intravitreal steroids were not evaluated in the EVS
- Subconjunctival antibiotics/steroids:
  Vancomycin (25 mg)
  Ceftazidime (100 mg) or gentamicin (20 mg)
  Dexamethasone (12–24 mg)
- Broad-spectrum fortified topical antibiotics (alternate every 30 minutes):
  Vancomycin (50 mg/mL q1h)
  Ceftazidime (50 mg/mL q1h)
- Topical steroid (prednisolone acetate 1% q1–2h initially) and cycloplegic (atropine 1% tid or scopolamine 0.25% qid)
- Systemic IV antibiotics for marked inflammation, severe cases, or rapid onset (controversial, since EVS found no benefit with systemic antibiotics):
  Vancomycin (1 g IV q12h)
  Ceftazidime (1 g IV q12h)

SUB-ACUTE, DELAYED, ENDOGENOUS, FILTERING BLEB ASSOCIATED, AND POST-TRAUMATIC:

- EVS study guidelines do not apply and treatment should be based on clinical situation:
  - Intravitreal antibiotics/steroids similar to acute postoperative guidelines (see above); add amphotericin B (0.005 mg/0.1 mL) if endogenous fungal or delayed onset
  - Subconjunctival antibiotics/steroids similar to acute postoperative guidelines
  - Broad-spectrum fortified topical antibiotics similar to acute postoperative guidelines; add amphotericin B 1–2.5 mg/mL q1h or natamycin 50 mg/mL q1h if fungal (poor penetration)
  - Topical steroid (prednisolone acetate 1% q1–2h initially) and cycloplegic (atropine 1% tid)
  - Systemic IV antibiotics for marked inflammation similar to acute postoperative guidelines
  - Systemic antifungals (amphotericin B 0.25–1.0 mg/kg IV divided equally q6h) if disseminated disease exists
  - Delayed postoperative may require capsulectomy and IOL exchange

- Consider repeat tap (or pars plana vitrectomy) and intravitreal injections if clinical picture is worse after 48–72 hours
- Tailor antibiotic choices based on culture results

Prognosis

Depends on etiology, duration, and organism; usually poor, especially for traumatic cases.

Angle-Closure Glaucoma (ACG)

Definition

Glaucoma due to obstruction of trabecular meshwork by peripheral iris; may be primary or secondary, with and without pupillary block; may be acute, subacute, intermittent, or chronic.

Etiology

Primary Angle-Closure With Pupillary Block: Lens-iris apposition, which interferes with aqueous flow and causes iris to bow forward and occlude the trabecular meshwork

Primary Angle-Closure Without Pupillary Block: Plateau iris syndrome.

Secondary Angle-Closure With Pupillary Block: Lens-induced (eg, phacomorphic, dislocated lens, microspherophakia), seclusio pupillae, aphakic/pseudophakic pupillary block, silicone oil nanophthalmos.

Secondary Angle-Closure Without Pupillary Block: Due to posterior pushing mechanism from tumors, choroidal hemorrhage or effusion, scleral buckle, swelling after panretinal photocoagulation, ciliary block/malignant glaucoma, persistent hyperplastic primary vitreous, retinopathy of prematurity; or anterior pulling mechanism in neovascular glaucoma, postinflammatory peripheral anterior synechiae, iridocorneal endothelial syndrome, epithelial downgrowth, fibrous ingrowth, posterior polymorphous dystrophy.

Epidemiology

Female predilection (4:1); higher incidence in Asians and Eskimos; approximately 5% of the general population >60 years old have occludable angles, 0.5% of these develop angle-closure; usually bilateral (develops in 50% of untreated fellow eyes within 5 years); associated with hyperopia, nanophthalmos, anterior chamber depth <2.5 mm, thicker lens, and lens subluxation.

Symptoms

Acute Angle-Closure: Pain, red eye, photophobia, decreased/blurred vision, halos around lights, headache, nausea, emesis.

Chronic Angle-Closure: Asymptomatic; may have decreased vision or constricted visual fields in late stages.

Signs

Acute Angle-Closure: Decreased visual acuity, increased intraocular pressure, ciliary injection, corneal edema, anterior chamber cell/flare, shallow anterior chamber, narrow angles on gonioscopy, mid-dilated, nonreactive pupil, iris bombé (deep centrally, shallow peripherally), retinal vascular occlusions; may have signs of previous attacks including sector iris atrophy (especially superiorly), anterior subcapsular lens opacities (glaukomflecken), dilated irregular pupil, and peripheral anterior synechiae (PAS).

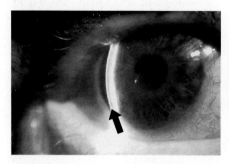
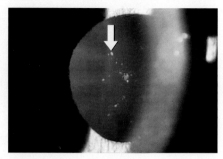

Figure 6–7   Primary angle-closure glaucoma with very shallow anterior chamber and iridocorneal touch (no space between slit beam view of cornea and iris; arrow).

Figure 6–8   Glaukomflecken (arrow).

Chronic Angle-Closure: Narrow angles, increased intraocular pressure, peripheral anterior synechiae, cupping of optic nerve.

Evaluation

- Complete ophthalmic history and eye exam with attention to pupils, cornea, tonometry, anterior chamber, iris, indentation gonioscopy, lens, and ophthalmoscopy
- Check visual fields
- Consider provocative testing (prone test, dark-room test, prone dark-room test, and pharmacologic dilation; intraocular pressure increase of >8 mm Hg is considered positive)

Management

PRIMARY ACUTE ANGLE-CLOSURE:

- Topical β-blocker (timolol [Timoptic] 0.5% q15 minutes × 2, then bid), alpha-agonist (apraclonidine [Iopidine] 1% q15 minutes × 2), and topical steroid (prednisolone acetate 1% q15 minutes × 4, then q1h)
- Topical miotic (pilocarpine 1–2% × 1 initially, then qid if effective; usually not effective if IOP > 40 mm Hg due to iris sphincter ischemia; in 20% of patients pilocarpine will exacerbate the situation due to forward displacement of the lens-iris diaphragm); can also consider topical alpha-antagonist (thymoxamine 0.5% q15 minutes for 2–3h)
- Systemic acetazolamide (Diamox 500 mg PO **STAT,** then bid) and hyperosmotic (isosorbide up to 2 g/kg PO of 45% solution)

Management Continued

- Laser peripheral iridotomy (LPI) ± iridoplasty is definitive treatment after acute attack is broken medically; may require application of topical glycerin (Ophthalgan) to clear corneal edema for adequate visualization for laser
- Prophylactic LPI in fellow eye with narrow angle to prevent an acute attack in the future
- If unable to perform LPI, consider surgical iridectomy
- Consider goniosynechiolysis for recent peripheral anterior synechiae (<12 months)
- Plateau iris syndrome may require long-term miotic therapy and peripheral iridectomy to reduce risk of pupillary block; consider laser iridoplasty

SECONDARY ACUTE ANGLE-CLOSURE:

- Treat underlying problem:
  - Laser peripheral iridotomy for pupillary block
  - Topical cycloplegic (scopolamine 0.25% qid or atropine 1% bid) for malignant glaucoma, microsphcrophakia, post-scleral buckle or after panretinal photocoagulation (do not use miotics); may require pars plana vitrectomy and lens extraction in refractory cases of malignant glaucoma or Nd: YAG laser disruption of the anterior hyaloid face in pseudophakic and aphakic patients
  - Topical cycloplegic (scopolamine 0.25% qid), steroid (prednisolone acetate 1% qid), and panretinal photocoagulation for neovascular glaucoma
  - Cataract extraction may be necessary in some cases of lens-induced angle-closure glaucoma

CHRONIC ANGLE-CLOSURE:

- Laser peripheral iridotomy even without evidence of pupillary block

Prognosis

Primary Acute Angle-Closure: Good if prompt treatment is initiated.

Secondary Angle-Closure: Poorer since usually due to chronic process; depends on extent of optic nerve damage and subsequent intraocular pressure control.

Anterior Uveitis (Iritis, Iridocyclitis)

Definition

Inflammation of the anterior uvea (iris and ciliary body) with exudation of blood cells and proteins into the anterior chamber secondary to breakdown of the blood-aqueous barrier and increased vascular permeability from a variety of disorders.

Etiology

May be nongranulomatous (lymphocyte and plasma cell infiltrates) or granulomatous (epithelioid and giant cell infiltrates).

ACUTE NONGRANULOMATOUS:

Ankylosing Spondylitis: Patients develop lower back pain and stiffness after in-
activity; also associated with aortitis and pulmonary apical fibrosis; arthritis less
severe in women, but eye disease can still be severe; 88% are HLA-B27 positive;
sacroiliac radiographs often show sclerosis and narrowing of joint spaces

Behçet's Disease: Triad of recurrent hypopyon iritis, aphthous stomatitis, and genital ulcers; iritis usually bilateral with posterior involvement (see Chap. 10); more
common in Asians; associated with HLA-B5 (subtypes Bw51 and B52) and HLA-B12

Idiopathic: Responsible for most cases of anterior uveitis

Inflammatory Bowel Disease: Rare in Crohn's disease (2.4%), 5–10% in ulcerative colitis; associated with sacroiliitis; 60% of patients with sacroiliitis are HLA-
B27 positive

Glaucomatocyclitic Crisis (Posner-Schlossman Syndrome): Unilateral, mild,
recurrent iritis with markedly elevated intraocular pressure, corneal edema, fine
keratic precipitates, and a mid-dilated pupil; crisis episodes can last hours to
days; associated with HLA-Bw54

Herpes Simplex and Herpes Zoster Ophthalmicus (HZO): Patients often exhibit
keratic precipitates in a diffuse distribution; elevated intraocular pressure common;
also associated with iris atrophy (simplex at pupillary border; zoster is segmental)

Kawasaki's Disease: Acute exanthematous disease seen in children (see Chap. 4)

Lyme Disease: Patients have classic cutaneous erythema chronicum migrans at
the site of a tick bite; due to *Borrelia burgdorferi* transmitted by *Ixodes dammini*
or *pacificus* tick; 1–3 months later can develop neurologic symptoms including encephalitis, meningitis; also iritis, vitritis, and optic neuritis; late stages have
chronic skin changes and chronic arthritis; may develop cardiac manifestations

Postoperative: Ocular surgery produces variable anterior chamber inflammation

Psoriatic Arthritis: Patients have sausage digits from terminal phalangeal joint
arthritic involvement, subungual hyperkeratosis, erythematous rash, nail pitting, and onycholysis; associated with sacroiliitis; no iritis seen when psoriasis
appears without arthritis; associated with HLA-B27

Reiter's Syndrome: Triad of nonspecific urethritis, polyarthritis (80%), and mucopurulent, papillary conjunctivitis with iritis; arthritis starts within 30 days of
infection; also associated with keratoderma blennorrhagicum, circinate balanitis,
plantar fasciitis, Achilles tendinitis, sacroiliitis, palate/tongue ulcers, and nail
pitting; seen in young males (90%); may be triggered by diarrhea or infectious
dysentery; 85–95% are HLA-B27 positive

Also, Systemic Lupus Erythematosus, Traumatic, and Wegener's Granulomatosis

CHRONIC NONGRANULOMATOUS:

Juvenile Rheumatoid Arthritis (JRA): Leading cause of uveitis in children; type I is pauciarticular (90%), rheumatoid factor (RF) negative, antinuclear antibody (ANA) positive, female predilection (4:1), no sacroiliitis, and earlier onset (by age 4 years); type II is pauciarticular, RF negative, ANA negative, HLA-B27 positive, slight male predilection, sacroiliitis common, and later onset (by age 8 years); both have chronic course with poor prognosis

Fuchs' Heterochromic Iridocyclitis: Unilateral problem with diffuse iris stromal atrophy, diffuse, white, stellate keratic precipitates, fine neovascularization of the angle, fine vitreous opacities, and minimal inflammation; predilection for blue-eyed patients; iris of affected eye may be lighter; good prognosis; topical steroids not indicated

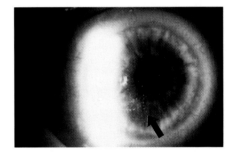

Figure 6–9 Fuchs' heterochromic iridocyclitis with fine, white, stellate keratic precipitates (arrow).

GRANULOMATOUS:

Sarcoidosis, tuberculosis, syphilis, brucellosis, toxoplasmosis, leprosy, lens-induced (phacoanaphylactic endophthalmitis is an immune-mediated reaction to lens particles after surgery or rarely spontaneously), Vogt-Koyanagi-Harada syndrome (VKH), and sympathetic ophthalmia (see Chap. 10).

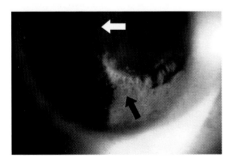

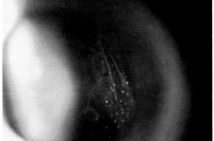

Figure 6–10 Granulomatous uveitis demonstrating inflammatory iris nodules, keratic precipitates (black arrow), and posterior synechiae (white arrow).

Figure 6–11 Anterior vitreous cells visible with fine slit beam behind the lens.

HLA Associations (Located on Chromosome 6):

A11	Sympathetic ophthalmia
A29	Birdshot retinochoroidopathy
B5	Behçet's disease
B7	Presumed ocular histoplasmosis syndrome, serpiginous choroidopathy, ankylosing spondylitis
B8	Sjögren's syndrome
B12	Ocular cicatricial pemphigoid
B27	Ankylosing spondylitis (88%), Reiter's syndrome (85–95%), inflammatory bowel disease (60%), psoriatic arthritis (also B17)
B54	Posner-Schlossman syndrome
DR4	Vogt-Koyanagi-Harada syndrome, ocular cicatricial pemphigoid

Symptoms

Pain, photophobia, tearing, red eye; may have decreased vision.

Signs

Normal or decreased visual acuity, ciliary injection, miosis, anterior chamber cell/flare; may have fine (nongranulomatous) or mutton-fat (granulomatous) keratic precipitates (KP), keratitis, iris nodules (Koeppe, Busacca), increased or decreased intraocular pressure, peripheral anterior synechiae (PAS), posterior synechiae, hypopyon (especially HLA-B27 associated and Behçet's), cataract, vitritis, retinal/choroidal lesions, cystoid macular edema (CME).

Differential Diagnosis

Masquerade Syndromes: Retinal detachment, retinoblastoma, malignant melanoma, leukemia, large cell lymphoma (reticulum cell sarcoma), juvenile xanthogranuloma (JXG), intraocular foreign body, spill-over syndromes from any posterior uveitis (most commonly toxoplasmosis).

Evaluation

- Complete ophthalmic history and eye exam with attention to corneal sensation, character of keratic precipitates, tonometry, anterior chamber, iris, vitreous cells, and ophthalmoscopy
- Unilateral, nongranulomatous iritis is often idiopathic and treated without extensive work-up
- If uveitis is recurrent, bilateral, granulomatous, or involving the posterior segment, consider work-up as clinical examination and history dictate
- Lab tests: complete blood count (CBC), erythrocyte sedimentation rate (ESR), ANA, RF (juvenile rheumatoid arthritis), serum lysozyme, angiotensin converting enzyme (ACE; sarcoidosis), Venereal Disease Research Laboratory (VDRL), fluorescent treponemal antibody absorption test (FTA-ABS; syphilis), serum haplotyping (see above), Lyme titer, purified protein derivative (PPD) and controls (tuberculosis), herpes simplex and herpes zoster titers, enzyme-linked immunosorbent assay (ELISA) for Lyme immunoglobulin M (IgM) and immunoglobulin

G (IgG), chest radiographs (sarcoidosis, ankylosing spondylitis), sacroiliac radiographs (ankylosing spondylitis), knee radiographs (juvenile rheumatoid arthritis), gallium scan (sarcoidosis), and urethral cultures (Reiter's syndrome)
- Medical or rheumatology consultation

Management

- Topical steroid (prednisolone acetate 1% up to q2h initially, then taper very slowly over weeks to months depending on etiology and response)
- Topical cycloplegic (cyclopentolate 1%, scopolamine 0.25%, or atropine 1% bid to tid)
- Consider aspirin (325–500 mg PO qd) or nonsteroidal anti-inflammatory drugs (indomethacin 25 mg PO tid) for ankylosing spondylitis, juvenile rheumatoid arthritis, and psoriatic arthritis
- Colchicine (0.6 mg PO bid) for Behçet's disease (see Chap. 10) is controversial
- Treat elevations in intraocular pressure as needed, especially glaucomatocyclitic crisis (see Chap. 11; do not use miotics)
- Systemic antibiotics for Lyme disease, tuberculosis, syphilis, toxoplasmosis (see Chap. 10)
- Topical antivirals (trifluridine [Viroptic] 9 times/day) for herpes simplex infections with concomitant corneal epithelial involvement
- Systemic antivirals (acyclovir 800 mg 5 times/day for 10 days) for herpes zoster
- Consider oral steroids (prednisone 60–100 mg PO qd); check PPD, blood glucose, and chest radiographs before starting systemic steroids
- Add H_2-blocker (ranitidine [Zantac] 150 mg PO bid) when taking systemic steroids
- Consider sub-Tenon steroid injection (triamcinolone acetonide 40 mg/mL)
- Consider immunomodulating agents including alkylating agents (cyclophosphamide 1–2 mg/kg/day, chlorambucil 2–8 mg/day), antimetabolites (azathioprine 50–150 mg/day, methotrexate 7.5–15.0 mg/day), or T-cell suppressors (cyclosporine 5 mg/kg/day) for vision threatening inflammation and/or lack of response to steroids, especially in Behçet's, juvenile rheumatoid arthritis, sympathetic ophthalmia, Vogt-Koyanagi-Harada syndrome, and serpiginous choroidopathy; should be managed by a uveitis specialist

Prognosis

Depends on etiology; most are benign. Poor if sequelae of chronic inflammation exist including cataract, glaucoma, posterior synechiae, band keratopathy, iris atrophy, cystoid macular edema, retinal detachment, optic neuritis, neovascularization, hypotony, phthisis.

Uveitis-Glaucoma-Hyphema (UGH) Syndrome

Definition

Triad of findings found in patients with closed-loop and rigid anterior chamber, iris-supported, or loose sulcus intraocular lenses secondary to trauma to angle structures, iris, or ciliary body.

Symptoms

Pain, photophobia, red eye, and decreased vision.

Signs

Decreased visual acuity, increased intraocular pressure, anterior chamber cell/flare, hyphema, intraocular lens implant; may have corneal edema.

Differential Diagnosis

Neovascular glaucoma, trauma.

Evaluation

- Complete ophthalmic history and eye exam with attention to cornea, tonometry, anterior chamber, gonioscopy, iris, and ophthalmoscopy

Management

- Intraocular pressure control as needed (see Chap. 11; do not use miotics)
- Topical steroid (prednisolone acetate 1% up to q1h then taper slowly over weeks to months) and cycloplegic (scopolamine 0.25% tid or atropine 1% bid)
- Usually requires surgery for intraocular lens removal or exchange, and possibly subsequent glaucoma surgery

Prognosis

Poor.

Iris / Pupils

Trauma

Angle Recession: Tear in ciliary body between longitudinal and circular muscle fibers; associated with hyphema; 10% develop glaucoma if >2/3 angle involved.

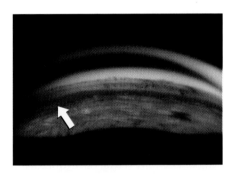

Figure 7–1 Gonioscopy view of angle recession demonstrating deepened angle and blue-gray face of the ciliary body (arrow).

Cyclodialysis: Disinsertion of ciliary body from scleral spur.

Iridodialysis: Disinsertion of iris root from ciliary body; appears as peripheral iris hole; usually related to trauma and associated with hyphema at time of injury.

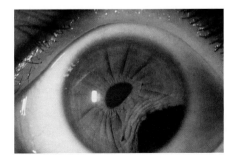

Figure 7–2 Iridodialysis.

Sphincter Tears: Small radial iris tears at pupillary margin; usually due to blunt trauma; associated with hyphema at time of injury; may result in permanent pupil dilation.

Symptoms

Pain, photophobia, red eye, and decreased vision.

Signs

Normal or decreased visual acuity, conjunctival injection, subconjunctival hemorrhage, anterior chamber (AC) cell/flare, hyphema, unusually deep anterior chamber, iris tears, abnormal pupil, angle tears, iridodonesis; may have other signs of ocular trauma including lid or orbital trauma, dislocated lens, phacodonesis, cataract, vitreous hemorrhage, commotio retinae, retinal tear/detachment, choroidal rupture, and/or traumatic optic neuropathy; may have signs of glaucoma with increased intraocular pressure, optic nerve cupping, and visual field defects.

Differential Diagnosis

See above, distinguish by careful gonioscopy; also, surgical iridectomy or iridotomy, essential iris atrophy, Reiger's anomaly

Evaluation

- Complete ophthalmic history and eye exam with attention to cornea, tonometry, iris, lens, and ophthalmoscopy
- Check gonioscopy and scleral depression if globe is intact and there is no hyphema
- B-scan ultrasonography if unable to visualize the fundus; consider ultrasound biomicroscopy (UBM) to evaluate angle structures and localize the injury
- Rule out open globe and intraocular foreign body (see Chap. 4)

Management

- No treatment required for sphincter tears or angle recession
- May require treatment of increased intraocular pressure (see Chap. 11)
- Observe patients for signs of angle recession glaucoma
- Consider cosmetic contact lens or surgical repair of dilated nonreactive pupil
- Consider surgical or laser reattachment if persistent hypotony accompanies a cyclodialysis
- Consider a cosmetic contact lens or surgical repair if disabling glare or diplopia accompanies an iridodialysis
- Treat other traumatic injuries as indicated

Prognosis

Depends on amount of damage; poor when associated with angle recession glaucoma or chronic hypotony

Pigment Dispersion Syndrome

Definition

Liberation of pigment from the iris with subsequent accumulation on anterior segment structures.

Etiology

Chafing of posterior iris surface on zonules produces pigment dispersion.

Epidemiology

More common in 20- to 50-year-old Caucasian males and in patients with myopia; affected females are usually older; associated with lattice degeneration in 20% of cases and retinal detachment in up to 5% of cases.

Symptoms

Asymptomatic.

Signs

Radial, mid-peripheral, iris transillumination defects, pigment on corneal endothelium (Krukenberg spindle), posterior bowing of midperipheral iris, dark pigment band overlying trabecular meshwork, pigment in iris furrows and on anterior lens capsule; may have signs of glaucoma with increased intraocular pressure, optic nerve cupping, and visual field defects (see below); may have pigmented anterior chamber cells, especially following pupillary dilation.

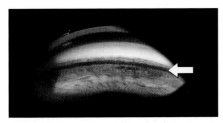

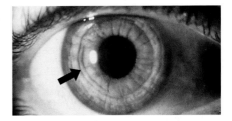

Figure 7–3 Pigment dispersion syndrome demonstrating pigment deposition on the trabecular meshwork that appears as a dark brown band (arrow) when viewed with gonioscopy.

Figure 7–4 Pigment dispersion syndrome demonstrating pigment deposition in concentric rings on the iris surface (arrow).

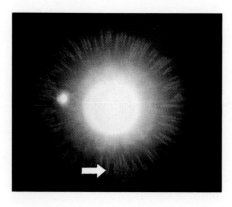

Figure 7–5 Pigment dispersion syndrome demonstrating radial, midperipheral, slit-like iris transillumination defects (arrow).

Differential Diagnosis

Uveitis, albinism, pseudoexfoliation syndrome, iris atrophy.

Evaluation

- Complete ophthalmic history and eye exam, with attention to cornea, tonometry, anterior chamber, the pattern of iris transillumination, gonioscopy, lens, and ophthalmoscopy
- Check visual fields in patients with elevated intraocular pressure or optic nerve cupping to rule out glaucoma

Management

- No treatment recommended
- Observe patients for signs of pigmentary glaucoma (see below)
- May require treatment of increased intraocular pressure (see Chap. 11)

Prognosis

Usually good; poor if pigmentary glaucoma develops.

Pigmentary Glaucoma (PG)

Definition

A form of secondary open-angle glaucoma caused by pigment liberated from the posterior iris surface (eg, a sequela of uncontrolled, increased, intraocular pressure in pigment dispersion syndrome).

Epidemiology

25 to 50% of patients with pigment dispersion syndrome develop glaucoma; same associations as in pigment dispersion syndrome (see above).

Mechanism

Obstruction of the trabecular meshwork by dispersed pigment and pigment-laden macrophages. Pigment overwhelms trabecular meshwork endothelial cells' phagocytic activity.

Symptoms

Asymptomatic; may have decreased vision or constricted visual fields in late stages; exercise or pupillary dilation can cause pigment release with acute elevation of intraocular pressure and symptoms including halos around lights and blurred vision.

Signs

Normal or decreased visual acuity, large fluctuations in intraocular pressure (especially with exercise); similar ocular signs as in pigment dispersion syndrome (see above), optic nerve cupping, nerve fiber layer defects, and visual field defects.

Differential Diagnosis

Primary open-angle glaucoma, other secondary open-angle glaucomas

Evaluation

- Complete ophthalmic history and eye exam with attention to cornea, tonometry, anterior chamber, gonioscopy, iris, lens, and ophthalmoscopy
- Check visual fields
- Stereo optic nerve photos are useful for comparison at subsequent evaluations

Management

- Choice and order of topical glaucoma medications depend on many factors, including patient's age, intraocular pressure level and control, and amount and progression of optic nerve cupping and visual field defects. Treatment options are presented in the Primary Open-Angle Glaucoma (POAG) section (see Chap. 11)
- Consider initial treatment with pilocarpine 1–4% qid to minimize iris contact with lens zonules
- Laser trabeculoplasty is effective, but action may be short-lived
- If posterior bowing of the iris exists, then consider laser peripheral iridotomy (LPI) to alter iris configuration and minimize pigment liberation
- May require glaucoma filtering surgery if medical treatment fails

Prognosis

Poorer than primary open-angle glaucoma.

Corectopia

Definition

Displaced or ectopic pupil.

Symptoms

Asymptomatic; may have decreased vision.

Signs

Normal or decreased visual acuity, distorted pupil.

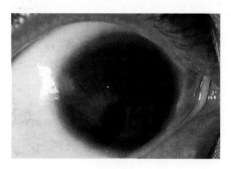

Figure 7–6 Corectopia.

Differential Diagnosis

Mesodermal dysgenesis syndromes, iridocorneal endothelial (ICE) syndromes, chronic uveitis, trauma, postoperative, ectopia lentis et pupillae.

Evaluation

- Complete ophthalmic history and eye exam with attention to cornea, tonometry, anterior chamber, iris, and lens
- Rule out open globe (peaked pupil after trauma, see Chap. 4)

Management

- No treatment recommended
- May require treatment of increased intraocular pressure or iritis (see Chaps. 6, 11)

Prognosis

Usually benign; depends on etiology

Seclusio Pupillae

Definition

Posterior synechiae (iris adhesions to the lens) at the pupillary border for 360 degrees. *Note:* different from occlusio pupillae, which is a fibrotic membrane across the pupil.

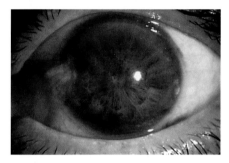

Figure 7–7 Seclusio pupillae.

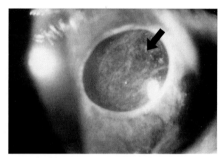

Figure 7–8 Occlusio pupillae with thin, white, fibrotic membrane (arrow) and neovascularization covering the pupil.

Symptoms

Asymptomatic; may have pain, red eye, and decreased vision.

Signs

Normal or decreased visual acuity, posterior synechiae, poor or irregular pupil dilation, increased intraocular pressure, acute or chronic signs of iritis, including anterior chamber cell/flare, keratic precipitates (KP), iris atrophy, iris nodules, cataract, and cystoid macular edema.

Differential Diagnosis

As for anterior uveitis (see Chap. 6).

Evaluation

- Complete ophthalmic history and eye exam with attention to cornea, tonometry, anterior chamber, gonioscopy, iris, and ophthalmoscopy
- Consider anterior uveitis work-up (see Chap. 6)

Management

- Treat active uveitis and angle-closure glaucoma (see Chap. 6) if present
- Consider laser iridotomy to prevent angle-closure glaucoma

Prognosis

Depends on etiology; poor if glaucoma has developed.

Peripheral Anterior Synechiae (PAS)

Definition

Peripheral adhesions of iris to the cornea or angle structures; extensive PAS (>60% angle involvement) can cause increased intraocular pressure and angle-closure glaucoma.

Etiology

Peripheral iridocorneal apposition due to previous pupillary block, flat/shallow anterior chamber, or inflammation.

Symptoms

Aymptomatic; may have symptoms of angle-closure glaucoma (see Chap. 6).

Signs

Iris adhesions to Schwalbe's line and cornea; may have increased intraocular pressure.

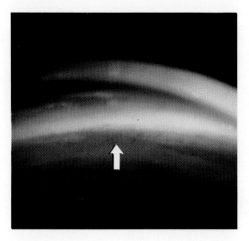

Figure 7–9 Peripheral anterior synechiae demonstrating a broad band of iris (arrow) occluding the angle structures as viewed with gonioscopy; also note that this patient has rubeosis with fine neovascularization.

Differential Diagnosis

See above; any cause of angle-closure glaucoma (see Chap. 6).

Evaluation

■ Complete ophthalmic history and eye exam with attention to cornea, tonometry, anterior chamber, gonioscopy, iris, and ophthalmoscopy

---

Management

- No treatment recommended
- May require treatment of increased intraocular pressure (see Chap. 11) or angle-closure glaucoma (see Chap. 6)
- Consider goniosynechiolysis for recent PAS (<12 months)

Prognosis

Usually good; depends on extent of synechial angle-closure and intraocular pressure control.

Rubeosis Iridis

Definition

Neovascularization of the iris and angle.

Etiology

Secondary to ocular ischemia; most commonly seen with proliferative diabetic retinopathy, central retinal vein occlusion, and carotid occlusive disease; also associated with anterior segment ischemia, chronic retinal detachment, tumors, sickle cell retinopathy, chronic inflammation, and other rarer causes.

Symptoms

Asymptomatic; may have decreased vision or angle-closure symptoms (see Chap. 6).

Signs

Normal or decreased visual acuity, abnormal blood vessels on iris and angle, particularly at pupillary margin and around iridectomies; may have spontaneous hyphema, or retinal lesions; may have signs of angle-closure or neovascular glaucoma (NVG) with increased intraocular pressure, optic nerve cupping, and visual field defects.

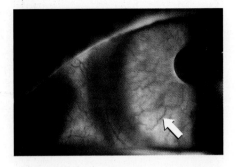

Figure 7–10 Rubeosis iridis (arrow).

Differential Diagnosis

See above.

Evaluation

- Complete ophthalmic history and eye exam with attention to tonometry, gonioscopy, iris, and ophthalmoscopy
- Lab tests: fasting blood glucose (diabetes mellitus), hemoglobin electrophoresis, and sickle cell prep (sickle cell)
- Consider fluorescein angiogram to narrow differential diagnosis and determine cause of ocular ischemia
- Consider medical consultation for systemic diseases including duplex and Doppler scans of carotid arteries to rule out carotid occlusive disease

Management

- Topical steroid (prednisolone acetate 1% qid) and cycloplegic (atropine 1% bid) for inflammation
- May require treatment of increased intraocular pressure (see Chap. 11) and possible glaucoma surgery (see below)
- If retinal ischemia is present and documented with a fluorescein angiogram, consider laser photocoagulation to the areas of nonperfusion

Prognosis

Poor; the rubeotic vessels may regress with appropriate therapy, but most causes of neovascularization are chronic progressive diseases.

Neovascular Glaucoma

Definition

A form of secondary angle-closure glaucoma in which neovascularization of the iris and angle causes occlusion of the trabecular meshwork.

Etiology

Any cause of rubeosis iridis (see above).

Symptoms

Decreased vision and angle-closure symptoms (see Chap. 6).

Signs

Decreased visual acuity; abnormal blood vessels on iris and angle, particularly at pupillary margin and around iridectomies; increased intraocular pressure, optic nerve cupping, and visual field defects; may have corneal edema, spontaneous hyphema, or retinal lesions.

Differential Diagnosis

As for rubeosis iridis (see above).

Evaluation

- Complete ophthalmic history and eye exam with attention to cornea, tonometry, anterior chamber, gonioscopy, iris, and ophthalmoscopy
- Lab tests: fasting blood glucose (diabetes mellitus), hemoglobin electrophoresis and sickle cell prep (sickle cell)
- Consider fluorescein angiogram to narrow differential diagnosis and determine cause of ocular ischemia
- Consider medical consultation for systemic diseases, including duplex and Doppler scans of carotid arteries to rule out carotid occlusive disease

Management

- Topical steroid (prednisolone acetate 1% qid) and cycloplegic (atropine 1% bid) for inflammation
- Choice and order of topical glaucoma medications depend on many factors, including patient's age, intraocular pressure level and control, and amount and progression of optic nerve cupping and visual field defects. Treatment options are presented in the Primary Open-Angle Glaucoma (POAG) section (see Chap. 11); more resistant to treatment than POAG
- If retinal ischemia is present and documented with a fluorescein angiogram, consider laser photocoagulation to the areas of nonperfusion
- Neovascular glaucoma with elevated intraocular pressure despite maximal medical therapy may require glaucoma filtering surgery or a glaucoma drainage implant

Prognosis

Poor; the rubeotic vessels may regress with appropriate therapy, but most causes of neovascularization are chronic progressive diseases.

Heterochromia

Definition

Heterochromia Iridis:

Unilateral; single iris with two colors (iris bicolor).

Heterochromia Iridum:

Bilateral; two eyes with different colors.

Eiology

Congenital:

- **Hypochromic (Involved Eye Lighter):** Congenital Horner's syndrome, Waardenburg's syndrome, Hirschsprung's disease, Parry-Romberg hemifacial atrophy.
- **Hyperchromic (Involved Eye Darker):** Ocular/oculodermal melanocytosis, iris pigment epithelium (IPE) hamartoma.

Acquired:

- **Hypochromic:** Acquired Horner's syndrome, juvenile xanthogranuloma, metastatic carcinoma, Fuchs' heterochromic iridocyclitis, stromal atrophy (glaucoma/inflammation).
- **Hyperchromic:** Siderosis, hemosiderosis, latanoprost (Xalatan; glaucoma medication), iris nevus or melanoma, iridocorneal endothelial (ICE) syndrome, iris neovascularization.

Symptoms

Usually asymptomatic; depends on etiology.

Signs

Iris heterochromia; blepharoptosis, miosis, and anhidrosis in Horner's syndrome; white forelock, premature graying, leucism (cutaneous hypopigmentation), facial anomalies, dystopia canthorum, and deafness in Waardenburg's syndrome; skin, scleral, and choroidal pigmentation in ocular/oculodermal melanocytosis; anterior chamber cell/flare, keratic precipitates, and increased intraocular pressure in uveitis and siderosis; may have intraocular foreign body (siderosis), old hemorrhage (hemosiderosis), or tumor.

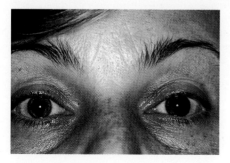

Figure 7–11 Heterochromia.

Differential Diagnosis

See above.

Evaluation

- Complete ophthalmic history and eye exam with attention to cornea, tonometry, anterior chamber, gonioscopy, iris, and ophthalmoscopy
- Consider B-scan ultrasonography if unable to visualize the fundus
- Consider orbital computed tomography (CT) or radiographs to rule out intraocular foreign bodies
- Consider electroretinogram (ERG) to evaluate retinal function in siderosis and hemosiderosis
- Consider medical consultation

Management

- Depends on etiology

Prognosis

Depends on etiology.

Anisocoria

Definition

Inequality in the size of the pupils of >2 mm.

Etiology

Greater Anisocoria in Dark (Abnormal Pupil Is Smaller): Horner's syndrome, Argyll Robertson pupil, iritis, pharmacologic (miotic).

Greater Anisocoria in Light (Abnormal Pupil Is Larger): Adie's tonic pupil, cranial nerve III palsy, pharmacologic (mydriatic/cycloplegic), iris damage (traumatic, ischemic, or surgical), Hutchinson's pupil.

Anisocoria Equal in Light and Dark: Physiologic (difference in pupil size ≤1mm).

Epidemiology

20% of population has physiologic/simple anisocoria

Symptoms

Asymptomatic; may have glare, pain, photophobia, diplopia, and/or blurred vision, depending on etiology.

Signs

Involved pupil may be larger or smaller, round or irregular, reactive or nonreactive; may have other signs depending on etiology

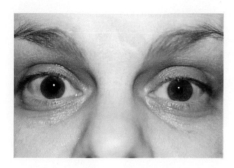

Figure 7–12 Anisocoria demonstrating larger pupil of the right eye.

Evaluation

- Complete ophthalmic history and eye exam with attention to pupils (size in light and dark, pupil response to light and near), lids, motility, and iris
- Gonioscopy and tonometry in traumatic cases to assess associated angle structure damage

- **Greater anisocoria in dark (abnormal pupil is smaller):** Pharmacologic pupil testing (*Note:* testing must be performed before cornea has been manipulated; ie, before any drops, applanation, or other tests have been performed; otherwise the test will be invalid):

(1) Topical cocaine 2–10%:
    dilates = simple anisocoria; no dilation = Horner's syndrome (see below)
(2) Topical hydroxyamphetamine 1% (Paredrine):
    dilates = central or preganglionic Horner's syndrome; no dilation = postganglionic Horner's syndrome

Note: tests cannot be performed on the same day or will be invalid

- **Greater anisocoria in light (abnormal pupil is larger):** Pharmacologic pupil testing:

(1) Topical pilocarpine 0.1% or methacholine 2.5%:
    constricts = Adie's tonic pupil (see below); no constriction = go to #2
(2) Topical pilocarpine 1%:
    constricts = cranial nerve III palsy; no constriction = pharmacologic dilation

- Lab tests: Venereal Disease Research Laboratory (VDRL), fluorescent treponemal antibody absorption test (FTA-ABS) (Argyll Robertson)
- Lumbar puncture for VDRL, FTA-ABS, total protein, and cell counts to rule out neurosyphilis (Argyll Robertson)
- Consider head, neck, and/or chest CT scan or magnetic resonance imaging (MRI) to rule out masses and vascular anomalies

Management

- No treatment recommended
- Consider iris repair in traumatic cases
- May require treatment of underlying cause

Prognosis

Often benign; depends on etiology.

Adie's Tonic Pupil

Definition

Idiopathic, benign form of internal ophthalmoplegia due to lesion in ciliary ganglion or short posterior ciliary nerves with aberrant regeneration of ciliary muscle fibers to iris sphincter

Etiology

Denervation hypersensitivity due to dysfunction of the ciliary ganglion or its neurons.

Epidemiology

Usually occurs in 20- to 40-year-old females (90%); 80% unilateral (may become bilateral over time).

Symptoms

Asymptomatic; may have blurred near vision and photophobia.

Signs

Anisocoria greater in light than dark, dilated pupil with poor light response, segmental palsy with vermiform movements, slow/tonic near response (constriction and redilation), poor accommodation, light-near dissociation; 70% have decreased deep tendon reflexes (Adie's syndrome).

Differential Diagnosis

Sarcoidosis, arteritic ischemic optic neuropathy, botulism, and any cause of light-near dissociation (optic neuropathy, Argyll Robertson pupil, dorsal midbrain syndrome, aberrant regeneration of cranial nerve III, diabetes mellitus, amyloidosis).

Evaluation

- Complete ophthalmic history, neurologic exam, and eye exam with attention to pupils (size in light and dark, pupil response to light and near), iris, and deep tendon reflexes
- Pharmacologic testing with topical pilocarpine 0.1% or methacholine 2.5% (see Anisocoria section); Adie's tonic pupil constricts (normal does not) due to cholinergic supersensitivity

Management

- No treatment recommended

Prognosis

Good; accomodative paresis is usually temporary (months)

Argyll Robertson Pupil

Definition

Small, irregular pupil that reacts briskly to near (accommodation), but not to light; usually bilateral and asymmetric; associated with tertiary syphilis.

Symptoms

Asymptomatic.

Signs

Miotic, irregular pupil, normal near response, absent reaction to light, poor dilation; may have stigmata of congenital syphilis (eg, Hutchinson's triad, fundus changes, skeletal deformities).

Differential Diagnosis

Argyll Robertson-like pupils seen in diabetes mellitus, alcoholism, multiple sclerosis, sarcoidosis.

Evaluation

- Complete ophthalmic history, neurologic exam, and eye exam with attention to pupils, iris, and ophthalmoscopy
- Lab tests: VDRL, FTA-ABS
- Lumbar puncture for VDRL, FTA-ABS, total protein, and cell counts to rule out neurosyphilis
- Medical consultation

Management

- If neurosyphilis present, treat with systemic penicillin G (2.4 million U IV q4h for 10–14 days, then 2.4 million U IM qweek for 3 weeks); or tetracycline for penicillin allergic patients
- Follow serum VDRL to monitor treatment efficacy

Prognosis

Pupil abnormality itself is benign; poor for untreated tertiary syphilis.

Horner's Syndrome

Definition

Group of findings seen in oculosympathetic paresis. Sympathetic damage may occur anywhere along the three-neuron pathway:

Central: Hypothalamus to cilio-spinal center of Budge (C8-T2)

Preganglionic: Spinal cord to superior cervical ganglion

Postganglionic: Along carotid artery to cranial nerve V and VI to orbit and finally to iris dilator muscle

Etiology

Failure of sympathetic nervous system to dilate affected pupil and to stimulate Müller's muscle in the lid.

Central: Cerebrovascular accident, neck trauma, tumor, demyelinating disease (rarely causes isolated Horner's).

Preganglionic: Pancoast's tumor, mediastinal mass, cervical rib, neck trauma, abscess, thyroid tumor, after thyroid or neck surgery.

Postganglionic: Neck lesion, head trauma, migraine, cavernous sinus lesion, carotid dissection, carotid-cavernous fistula, internal cartoid artery aneurysm, nasopharyngeal carcinoma, vascular disease, infections (complicated otitis media).

Congenital Horner's syndrome usually due to birth trauma (brachial plexus injury during delivery).

Symptoms

Asymptomatic; may have droopy eyelid, blurred vision, pain, and other symptoms depending on site and cause of lesion (central usually has other neurologic deficits).

Signs

Triad of ptosis, miosis, and anhidrosis (anhidrosis usually indicates preganglionic lesion); abnormal pupil is smaller and dilates poorly in the dark; may have pain (especially with vascular postganglionic etiologies); in congenital form, get up-side-down ptosis (lower lid elevation) and heterochromia iridum (involved side lighter).

Evaluation

- Complete ophthalmic history, neurologic exam, and eye exam, with attention to lids, motility, pupils, and iris
- **Pharmacologic pupil testing** (*Note:* testing must be performed before cornea has been manipulated; ie, before any drops, applanation, or other tests have been performed; otherwise the test will be invalid):

(1) Topical cocaine 2–10% (place 2 drops in each eye, remeasure pupil after 30 minutes): dilates = normal pupil; no dilation = Horner's syndrome
(2) Topical hydroxyamphetamine 1% (Paredrine): dilates = central or preganglionic Horner's syndrome; no dilation = postganglionic Horner's syndrome

Note: tests cannot be performed on the same day or will be invalid

- Medical or neurology consultation

Management

- Treat underlying cause

Prognosis

Depends on etiology; postganglionic lesions are usually benign; preganglionic and central are usually more serious.

Relative Afferent Pupillary Defect (RAPD; Marcus Gunn Pupil)

Definition

Dilation of one pupil in response to light, due to difference in amount of light perceived by the two eyes when swinging flashlight test is performed.

Etiology

Asymmetric optic nerve disease or widespread retinal damage; mild RAPD may rarely be seen with a dense ocular media opacity, including vitreous hemorrhage and cataract; very rarely seen with amblyopia; optic tract lesions can cause a contralateral RAPD (due to more nasal crossing fibers in the chiasm); most common causes include optic neuropathy, optic neuritis, central retinal vein or artery occlusion, and retinal detachment.

Symptoms

Decreased vision.

Signs

Decreased visual acuity ± color vision, positive RAPD, visual field defect; may have swollen or pale optic nerve, or retinal findings.

Differential Diagnosis

See above.

Evaluation

- Complete ophthalmic history and eye exam with attention to visual acuity, color vision, pupils, iris, and ophthalmoscopy
- Swinging flashlight test: bright light is shined into one eye and then rapidly into the other in an alternating fashion; positive test is when the pupil that the light is shined into dilates instead of constricts; in cases in which the pupil of the involved eye is nonreactive or nonfunctional, observe the fellow, normal eye for a reverse afferent defect (dilation when light is on nonreactive eye, constriction when light is shined on reactive eye)

Management

- Treat underlying cause

Prognosis

Depends on etiology.

Leukocoria

Definition

Variety of disorders that cause the pupil to appear white; usually noted in infancy or early childhood

Symptoms

Decreased vision, white pupil; may notice eye turn or abnormal size of eye.

Signs

Decreased visual acuity, leukocoria; may have positive relative afferent pupillary defect (RAPD), nystagmus, strabismus, buphthalmos, microphthalmos, anterior chamber cell/flare, increased intraocular pressure, cataract, vitritis, retinal detachment, tumor, or other retinal findings; may have systemic findings.

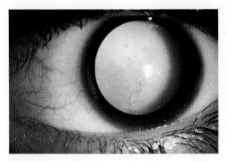

Figure 7–13 Leukocoria in a patient with toxocariasis.

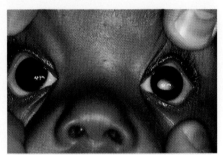

Figure 7–14 Leukocoria due to retinoblastoma in the left eye.

Differential Diagnosis

Cataract, retinoblastoma, retinopathy of prematurity (ROP), persistent hyperplastic primary vitreous (PHPV), Coats' disease, toxocariasis, toxoplasmosis, coloboma, myelinated nerve fibers, Norrie's disease, retinal dysplasia, cyclitic membrane, retinal detachment, incontinentia pigmenti, retinoschisis, and medulloepithelioma.

Evaluation

- Complete ophthalmic history and eye exam, with attention to retinoscopy, pupils, tonometry, anterior chamber, lens, vitreous cells, and ophthalmoscopy
- B-scan ultrasonography to evaluate retrolenticular area, vitreous, and retina
- Consider orbital radiograph, and head and orbital CT scans or MRI to rule out foreign body
- Pediatric consultation

Management

- Treat underlying cause

Prognosis

Usually poor, unless due to mature cataract in an adult.

Congenital Anomalies

Aniridia: Absence of iris, except for small, hypoplastic remnant/stump; patients also have photophobia, nystagmus, glare, decreased visual acuity, amblyopia, and strabismus; associated with glaucoma in 28–50%, lens opacities in 50–85%, corneal pannus, and foveal hypoplasia; seen in 1:100,000 births; mapped to chromosome 11p; three forms:

- **AN1 (autosomal dominant [AD]):** 85% of cases; only ocular findings
- **AN2:** 13% of cases; includes Miller syndrome with both aniridia and Wilms' tumor, and WAGR (Wilms' tumor, aniridia, genitourinary abnormalities, and mental retardation); sporadic, but mapped to chromosome 11p
- **AN3 (autosomal recessive [AR]):** 2% of cases; associated with mental retardation and cerebellar ataxia (Gillespie's syndrome); do not develop Wilms' tumor

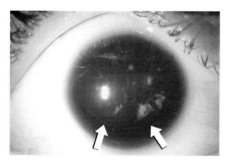

Figure 7–15 Aniridia with entire cataractous lens visible (arrows).

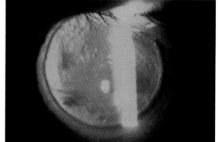

Figure 7–16 Aniridia with the lens equator and zonules visible on retroillumination.

- May require treatment of increased intraocular pressure (see Chap. 11)
- May require cyclocryotherapy or glaucoma filtering surgery if medical treatment fails
- Lensectomy if visually significant cataract develops

Coloboma: Iris sector defect due to failure of embryonic fissure to completely close; usually seen inferiorly; may have other colobomata (lid, lens, retina, choroid, optic nerve); associated with multiple genetic syndromes, including trisomy 22 (cat-eye syndrome), trisomy 18, trisomy 13, and chromosome 18 deletion.

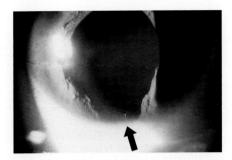

Figure 7–17 Coloboma (arrow).

Persistent Pupillary Membrane: Benign, embryonic, mesodermal remnants (tunica vasculosa lentis) that appear as thin iris strands bridging the pupil; most common ocular congenital anomaly; occurs in 80% of dark eyes and 35% of light eyes; two types:

- **Type 1:** Attached only to the iris
- **Type 2:** Iridolenticular adhesions

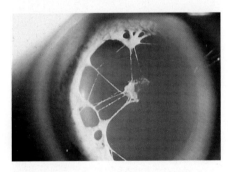

Figure 7–18 Persistent pupillary membrane type 2.

- No treatment required
- If iris strands cross visual axis and are affecting vision, consider Nd:YAG (neodymium:yttrium-aluminum-garnet) laser treatment

Plateau Iris (Configuration/Syndrome): Atypical iris configuration; familial, more common in young, myopic women; 5–8% develop angle-closure glaucoma (plateau iris syndrome)

- May require treatment of increased intraocular pressure (see Chap. 11)
- Consider miotics (pilocarpine 1% qid) or iridoplasty

Mesodermal Dysgenesis Syndromes

Definition

Group of bilateral, congenital, hereditary disorders involving anterior segment structures. Originally thought to be due to faulty cleavage of angle structures and therefore termed angle cleavage syndromes.

Axenfeld's Anomaly (AD): Posterior embryotoxon (anteriorly displaced Schwalbe's line; found in 15% of normal individuals) and prominent iris processes; associated with secondary glaucoma in 50% of patients; mapped to chromosome 4q, 13q.

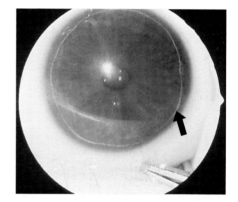

Figure 7–19 Posterior embryotoxon appears as a prominent, white, corneal line inside limbus (arrow).

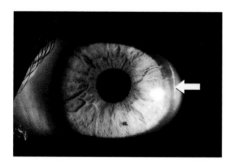

Figure 7–20 Axenfeld's anomaly with abnormal iris and posterior embryotoxon (arrow).

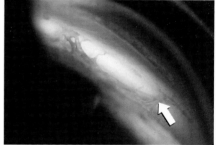

Figure 7–21 Gonioscopy view of Axenfeld's anomaly demonstrating iris adhesions to the cornea (arrow).

Alagille's Syndrome: Axenfeld's anomaly and pigmentary retinopathy, corectopia, esotropia, and systemic abnormalities, including absent deep tendon reflexes, abnormal facies, pulmonic valvular stenosis, peripheral arterial stenosis, and skeletal abnormalities. Abnormal electroretinogram (ERG) and electrooculogram (EOG)

Rieger's Anomaly: Axenfeld's anomaly and iris hypoplasia with holes; associated with secondary glaucoma in 50% of patients; mapped to chromosome 4q, 13q.

Rieger's Syndrome (AD): Combination of Rieger's anomaly with mental retardation and systemic abnormalities, including dental, craniofacial, genitourinary, and skeletal problems; mapped to chromosome 4q, 13q.

Peter's Anomaly: Corneal leukoma (due to central defect in Descemet's membrane and absence of endothelium) and iris adhesions with or without cataract; usually sporadic; 80% bilateral; associated with secondary glaucoma in 50% of patients, congenital cardiac defects, cleft lip/palate, craniofacial dysplasia, and skeletal abnormalities; mapped to chromosome 11p.

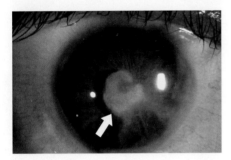

Figure 7–22   Peter's anomaly demonstrating corneal leukoma (arrow).

Symptoms

Asymptomatic; may have decreased vision or notice iris abnormalities or a white spot on eye.

Signs

Normal or decreased visual acuity; may have systemic abnormalities and signs of glaucoma, including increased intraocular pressure, optic nerve cupping, and visual field defects.

Differential Diagnosis

Iridocorneal endothelial (ICE) syndromes, posterior polymorphous dystrophy, aniridia, coloboma, ectopia lentis et pupillae.

Evaluation

■ Complete ophthalmic history and eye exam with attention to cornea, tonometry, anterior chamber, gonioscopy, iris, lens, and ophthalmoscopy

- Check visual fields in patients with elevated intraocular pressure or optic nerve cupping to rule out glaucoma
- B-scan ultrasonography in Peter's anomaly if unable to visualize the fundus

---

Management

- May require treatment of increased intraocular pressure (see Chap. 11)
- May require penetrating keratoplasty, cataract extraction, and treatment of amblyopia for Peter's anomaly

---

Prognosis

Poor for Peter's anomaly or when associated with glaucoma; otherwise good.

Iridocorneal Endothelial (ICE) Syndromes

Definition

Unilateral, nonhereditary, slowly progressive abnormality of the corneal endothelium causing a spectrum of diseases with features including corneal edema, iris distortion, and secondary angle-closure glaucoma.

Essential Iris Atrophy: Iris atrophy with holes and corectopia, ectropion uveae, polycoria, and focal stromal effacement.

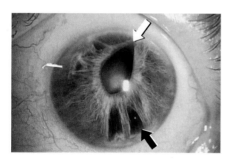
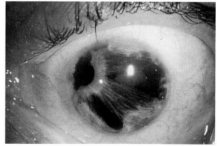

Figure 7–23 Essential iris atrophy demonstrating iris atrophy (black arrow) and corectopia (white arrow).

Figure 7–24 Advanced essential iris atrophy.

Chandler's Syndrome: Variant of above with mild or no iris changes, irregular corneal endothelium with beaten metal appearance, corneal edema common, intraocular pressure may not be elevated.

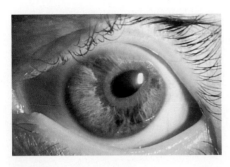

Figure 7–25 Chandler's syndrome.

Iris Nevus (Cogan-Reese) Syndrome: Pigmented pedunculated iris nodules, flattening of iris stroma, pupil abnormalities, and ectropion uveae.

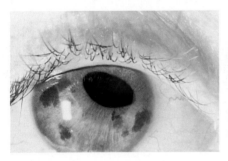

Figure 7–26 Iris nevus (Cogan-Reese) syndrome.

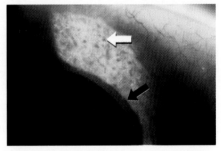

Figure 7–27 Iris nevus (Cogan-Reese) syndrome with small, pigmented iris nodules (white arrow) and ectropion uveae (black arrow).

Mechanism

Altered, abnormal corneal endothelium proliferates across the angle and onto the iris, forming a membrane that obstructs the trabecular meshwork, distorts the iris, and may form nodules by contracting around the iris stroma.

Epidemiology

Mostly young or middle-aged females; increased risk of secondary angle-closure glaucoma.

Symptoms

Asymptomatic; may have decreased vision, glare, monocular diplopia or polyopia; may notice iris changes.

Signs

Normal or decreased visual acuity, beaten-metal appearance of corneal endothelium, corneal edema, increased intraocular pressure, peripheral anterior synechiae, iris changes (see above).

Differential Diagnosis

Posterior polymorphous dystrophy, mesodermal dysgenesis syndromes, Fuchs' endothelial dystrophy, iris nevi or melanoma, aniridia, iridodialysis.

Evaluation

- Complete ophthalmic history and eye exam with attention to cornea, tonometry, anterior chamber, gonioscopy, iris, lens, and ophthalmoscopy
- Check visual fields in patients with elevated intraocular pressure or optic nerve cupping to rule out glaucoma

Management

- No treatment recommended
- May require treatment of increased intraocular pressure (see Chap. 11)
- May require penetrating keratoplasty or glaucoma surgery

Prognosis

Chronic, progressive process; poor when associated with glaucoma.

Tumors

Cyst: Can be primary (more common; usually peripheral from stroma or iris pigment epithelium) or secondary (usually post-traumatic or surgical due to ingrowth of surface epithelium); may cause segmental elevation of iris and angle-closure; rarely detaches and becomes free-floating in anterior chamber; may also form at pupillary margin from chronic use of strong miotic medications; complications include distortion of pupil, occlusion of visual axis, and secondary glaucoma.

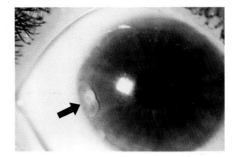

Figure 7–28 Peripheral iris cysts (arrow).

■ May require treatment of increased intraocular pressure (see Chap. 11)
■ Consider surgical excision if vision is affected and/or secondary glaucoma exists

Iris Nevus: Single or multiple, flat, pigmented, benign lesions; pigment spots/freckles occur in 50% of population; rare before 12 years of age; nevus differentiated from melanoma by size (<3 mm in diameter), thickness (<1 mm thick), and the absence of vascularity, ectropion uveae, secondary cataract, secondary glaucoma, and signs of growth.

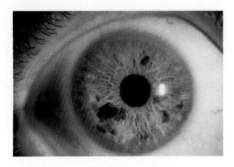

Figure 7–29 Iris nevi.

■ Serial anterior segment photographs to document any evidence of growth
■ Follow closely for evidence of elevation of intraocular pressure
■ Consider iris fluorescein angiogram to differentiate between nevus and melanoma: nevus has filigree filling pattern that hyperfluoresces early and leaks late or is angiographically silent; melanoma has irregular vessels that fill late

Iris Nodules: Collections of cells on iris surface; several different types:

■ **Brushfield spots:** Ring of small, white-gray peripheral iris spots associated with Down's syndrome; occurs in 24% of normal individuals
■ **Lisch nodules:** Bilateral, lightly pigmented, gelatinous, melanocytic hamartomas seen in 92% of patients with neurofibromatosis (NF) type 1 (very rare in NF-2); usually involve inferior half of iris; do not involve iris stroma.

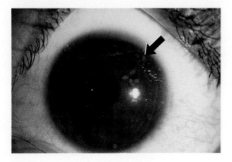

Figure 7–30 Lisch nodules (arrow) in a patient with neurofibromatosis.

- **Inflammatory nodules:** Due to collections of monocytes and inflammatory debris seen in granulomators uveitis; Two types:

(1) *Busacca nodules:* Nodules on anterior iris surface
(2) *Koeppe nodules:* Nodules at pupillary border

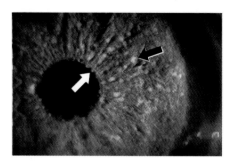

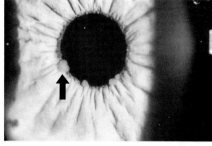

Figure 7–31 Busacca (black arrow) and Koeppe (white arrow) nodules.

Figure 7–32 Koeppe nodules (arrow).

Iris Pigment Epithelium (IPE) Tumors: Very rare tumors of the iris pigment epithelium (adenoma or adenocarcinoma); appear as darkly pigmented, friable nodules.

- Treatment with chemotherapy, radiation, and surgical excision should be performed by a tumor specialist

Juvenile Xanthogranuloma (JXG): Yellow iris lesions composed of histiocytes; may bleed, causing spontaneous hyphema.

Malignant Melanoma: Dark or amelanotic (pigmentation variable), elevated lesion that usually involves inferior iris and replaces the iris stroma; may be diffuse (associated with heterochromia and secondary glaucoma), tapioca (dark tapioca appearance), ring-shaped, or localized; some have feeder vessels; may involve angle structures, cause sectoral cataract, produce hyphemas, or cause secondary glaucoma; 1–3% of all malignant melanomas of the uveal tract involve the iris; predilection for Caucasians and patients with light irides, rare in African Americans; many patients have history of nevus that undergoes growth; prognosis good; 4% mortality.

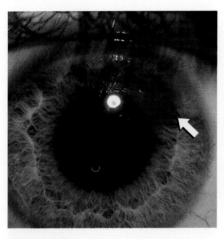

Figure 7–33 Malignant melanoma of the iris (arrow).

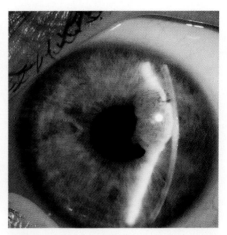

Figure 7–34 Amelanotic melanoma of the iris.

- Consider B-scan ultrasonography or ultrasound biomicroscopy to rule out ciliary body involvement
- Treatment with chemotherapy, radiation, surgical excision, and enucleation; should be performed by a tumor specialist
- May require treatment of increased intraocular pressure (see Chap. 11); glaucoma filtering surgery is not recommended

Metastatic Tumors: Rare; usually amelanotic, and from primary carcinoma of the breast, lung, or prostate; often found after primary lesion is discovered.

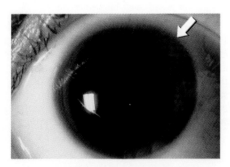

Figure 7–35 Metastatic carcinoid of the iris appears as an orange-brown peripheral lesion (arrow).

- Treatment with chemotherapy, radiation, and surgical excision; should be performed by a tumor specialist
- May require treatment of increased intraocular pressure (see Chap. 11); glaucoma filtering surgery is not recommended

Lens

Congenital Cataract

Definition

Lenticular opacity usually categorized by etiology or location:

Capsular: Opacity of the lens capsule, usually anteriorly

Lamellar/Zonular: Opacity surrounds nucleus in concentric ring

Lenticular/Nuclear: Opacity of the lens nucleus

Polar: Central opacity located near the lens capsule, anteriorly or posteriorly

Sutural: Y-shaped opacity in the center of the lens

Etiology

HEREDITARY/SYNDROMES:

Chromosomal abnormalities (Down's syndrome, Turner's syndrome, and others).

Lowe's Oculocerebrorenal Syndrome (X-Linked): Small discoid lens, posterior lenticonus, and glaucoma; systemic findings include acidosis, aminoaciduria, renal rickets, hypotonia, mental retardation; female carriers have posterior, white, punctate cortical opacities and subcapsular, plaque-like opacities.

INFECTIOUS:

Congenital Rubella Syndrome:

Cataracts, glaucoma, microcornea, microphthalmos, iris hypoplasia, and retinopathy with characteristic fine, granular, salt-and-pepper appearance (most common finding); other complications include prematurity, mental retardation, neurosensory deafness, congenital heart disease, growth retardation, hepatosplenomegaly, interstitial pneumonitis, and encephalitis.

Congenital Varicella Syndrome: Cataract, chorioretinitis, optic nerve atrophy or hypoplasia, nystagmus, and Horner's syndrome; systemic findings include hemiparesis, bulbar palsies, dermatomal cicatricial skin lesions, developmental delay, and learning difficulties.

METABOLIC:

Galactosemia: Bilateral, oil-droplet cataracts from accumulation of galactose metabolites (galactitol) due to hereditary enzymatic deficiency; usually galactose-1-phosphate uridyltransferase, also galactokinase; associated with mental retardation, hepatosplenomegaly, cirrhosis, malnutrition, and failure to thrive

Hypocalcemia: Diffuse lamellar cataracts.

Also, **Birth Trauma, Idiopathic, and Persistent Hyperplastic Primary Vitreous (PHPV).**

Epidemiology

Congenital cataracts occur in approximately 1 of 2000 live births; Roughly one third are isolated, one third are familial (usually dominant), and one third are associated with a syndrome; most unilateral cases are not metabolic or genetic.

Symptoms

Decreased vision; may notice white pupil and eye turn.

Signs

Decreased visual acuity, leukocoria, amblyopia; may have strabismus (usually with unilateral cataracts), nystagmus (usually does not appear until 2–3 months of age; rarely when cataracts develop after age 6 months).

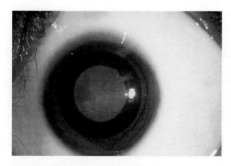

Figure 8–1 Congenital cataract with central white discoid appearance.

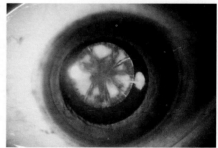

Figure 8–2 Congenital zonular cataract.

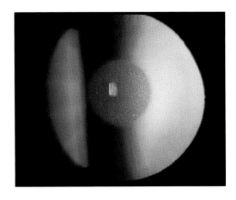

Figure 8–3 Appearance of congenital nuclear cataract as viewed with retroillumination.

Differential Diagnosis

See leukocoria (see Chap. 7).

Evaluation

- Complete ophthalmic history with attention to family history of eye disease, trauma, maternal illnesses during pregnancy, systemic diseases in the child, and birth problems
- Complete eye exam with attention to cycloplegic refraction, retinoscopy, gonioscopy, lens (size and density of the opacity as viewed with retroillumination), and ophthalmoscopy
- May require examination under anesthesia (EUA)
- Keratometry and A-scan biometry when intraocular lens implantation is anticipated
- Lab tests: TORCH titers (toxoplasmosis, other infections [syphilis], rubella, cytomegalovirus infection, and herpes simplex), fasting blood sugar (hypoglycemia), urine-reducing substances after milk feeding (galactosemia), calcium (hypocalcemia), and urine amino acids (Lowe's syndrome)
- B-scan ultrasonography if unable to visualize the fundus (can perform through the lids of a crying child)
- Pediatric consultation

Management

- Dilation (tropicamide 1% [Mydriacyl] ± phenylephrine 2.5% [Mydfrin] tid) may be used as a temporary measure before surgery to allow light to pass around the cataract; however, surgery should not be delayed
- If the cataract obscures the visual axis (media opacity >3 mm) or is causing secondary ocular disease (glaucoma or uveitis), cataract extraction should be performed within days to a week after diagnosis in

Management *Continued*

infants because delay may lead to amblyopia; postoperatively, the child requires proper aphakic correction with contact lens or spectacles if bilateral; depending on age and etiology, intraocular lens implantation should be considered
- If the cataract is not causing amblyopia, glaucoma, or uveitis, the child is observed closely for progression
- Patching/occlusion therapy for amblyopia (see Chap. 12)
- Almost all patients with visually significant, unilateral, congenital cataracts have strabismus and may require muscle surgery after cataract extraction
- Restrict dietary galactose in galactosemia

Prognosis

Depends on age and duration of visually significant cataract prior to surgery; poor if amblyopia exists.

Acquired Cataract

Definition

Lenticular opacity usually categorized by etiology or location:

Cortical Degeneration: Asymmetrically located, radial, spoke-like opacities or punctate vacuoles extending from the lens periphery toward the lens poles; caused by swelling and liquefaction of the younger cortical fiber cells.

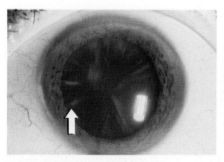

Figure 8–4 Cortical cataract demonstrating white cortical spoking (arrow).

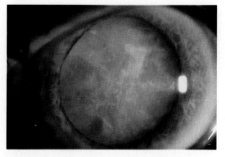

Figure 8–5 Mature cataract with white, liquified cortex.

Nuclear Sclerosis: Centrally located lens discoloration; caused by deterioration of the older fiber cells near the center of the lens.

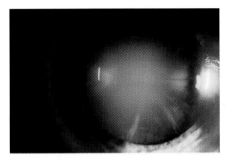

Figure 8–6 Cataract with 2$^+$ yellow-green nuclear sclerosis.

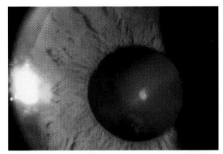

Figure 8–7 Brunescent nuclear sclerotic cataract.

Figure 8–8 Hypermature (morgagnian) cataract demonstrating a dense brown nucleus (arrow) sinking inferiorly in a white, liquified cortex.

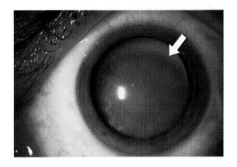

Subcapsular Cataract

■ **Anterior Subcapsular (ASC):** Caused by metaplasia of the central zone lens epithelial cells beneath the anterior lens capsule.

Figure 8–9 Anterior subcapsular star-pattern cataract due to phenothiazine.

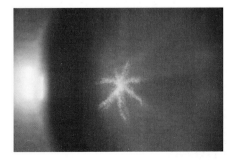

■ **Posterior Subcapsular (PSC):** Asymmetric granular opacities at the posterior surface of the lens; caused epithelial (Wedl) cells migrating to the posterior pole.

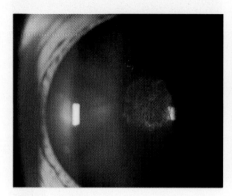

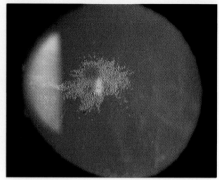

Figure 8–10 Posterior subcapsular cataract.

Figure 8–11 Posterior subcapsular cataract due to topical steroid use, as viewed with retroillumination.

Etiology

Most commonly senile; also secondary to a variety of causes:

Systemic Disease: Many different systemic diseases can cause cataracts, including:

■ **Diabetes Mellitus:** "Sugar" cataracts are cortical or posterior subcapsular opacities that occur earlier in diabetic patients than in age-matched controls, progress rapidly, and are related to poor glucose control more than duration of disease
■ **Hypocalcemia:** Lens opacities are usually small white dots, but can aggregate into larger flakes
■ **Myotonic Dystrophy:** Central, iridescent, crystal deposits; may develop a posterior subcapsular cataract later (see Chap. 2); mapped to chromosome 19q
■ Also **Fabry's disease, atopic dermatitis, and ectodermal dysplasia**
■ **Wilson's Disease:** Sunflower cataract due to copper deposition (chalcosis lentis); green/brown surface opacity in the central lens with short stellate processes rather than a full flower-petal pattern

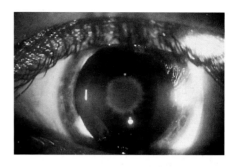

Figure 8–12 Sunflower cataract in a patient with Wilson's disease.

Other Eye Diseases: Uveitis, glaucoma, retinal detachment, myopia, intraocular tumors, retinitis pigmentosa (posterior subcapsular cataracts), Refsum's disease (posterior subcapsular cataracts), Stickler's syndrome (cortical cataracts).

Toxic: Steroids (posterior subcapsular cataracts), miotics; ionizing (x-rays, gamma rays, and neutrons), infrared, ultraviolet, and short-wave radiation; electricity, and chemicals.

Trauma: Blunt or penetrating; intraocular foreign bodies (iron, copper); and postoperative.

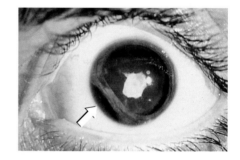

Figure 8–13 Dense, white, central cataract due to trauma; also note iridodialysis (arrow).

Epidemiology

Senile cataracts represent senescent lens changes, related in part to ultraviolet-B radiation. In the Framingham Eye Study, the prevalence of senile cataracts was 4.5% in adults 52 to 64 years old, 18.0% in 65- to 74-year-olds, and 45.9% in 75- to 85-year-olds. African American men and women were more likely to have cataracts in every age category. Cataract is the leading cause of blindness worldwide.

Symptoms

Painless, progressive loss of vision, decreased contrast and color sensitivity, glare; rarely monocular diplopia.

Signs

Decreased visual acuity (distance vision usually affected more than near vision in nuclear sclerosis, and near vision affected more than distance vision in posterior subcapsular), focal or diffuse lens opacification (yellow, green, brown, or white; often best appreciated with retroillumination), induced myopia; intumescent cataracts may cause the iris to bow forward and lead to secondary angle-closure (see Chap. 6); hypermature cataracts may leak lens proteins and cause phacolytic glaucoma (see Lens-Induced Secondary Glaucoma section).

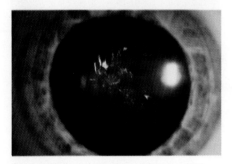

Figure 8–14 Polychromatic, refractile, cholesterol deposits within the crystalline lens.

Differential Diagnosis

See above; senile cataract is a diagnosis of exclusion; rule out secondary causes.

Evaluation

- Complete ophthalmic history with attention to systemic diseases, medications, prior use of steroids, trauma, radiation treatment, other ocular diseases, congenital problems, and functional visual status.
- Complete eye exam with attention to refraction, cornea, gonioscopy, lens, and ophthalmoscopy
- Consider brightness acuity tester (BAT) and potential acuity meter (PAM) testing (PAM is used to estimate visual potential, especially when posterior segment pathology exists)
- B-scan ultrasonography if unable to visualize the fundus
- Keratometry and A-scan biometry to calculate the intraocular lens (IOL) implant power
- Consider specular microscopy and pachymetry if cornea guttata or corneal edema exists

Management

- Cataract extraction and insertion of an intraocular lens is indicated when visual symptoms interfere with daily activities and the patient desires improved visual function, when the cataract causes other ocu-

Management Continued

lar diseases (eg, phacolytic glaucoma, uveitis), or when the cataract prevents examination or treatment of a pre-existing ocular condition (eg, diabetic retinopathy, glaucoma).

- Dilation (tropicamide 1% [Mydriacyl] ± phenylephrine 2.5% [Mydfrin] tid) may help the patient see around a central opacity in those rare instances when the patient cannot undergo or declines cataract surgery

Prognosis

Very good; success rate for routine cataract surgery is >95%.

Posterior Capsular Opacification (Secondary Cataract)

After cataract extraction, up to 50% of adult patients develop posterior capsule opacification, causing decreased vision and glare. This is caused by epithelial cell proliferation (Elschnig's pearls) and fibrosis of the capsule; may be treated with neodymium:yttrium-aluminum-garnet (Nd:YAG) laser posterior capsulotomy. Complications of Nd:YAG capsulotomy include increased intraocular pressure, intraocular lens (IOL) damage or dislocation, retinal detachment, cystoid macular edema, and hyphema. Newer IOL materials may reduce the incidence of posterior capsular opacification.

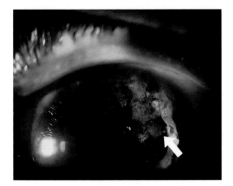

Figure 8–15 Secondary cataract composed of Elschnig's pearls (arrow).

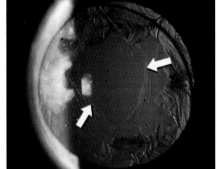

Figure 8–16 Posterior capsule opening (arrows) following Nd:YAG laser capsulotomy when viewed with retroillumination.

Aphakia

Definition
Absence of crystalline lens; usually secondary to surgery, rarely traumatic (total dislocation of crystalline lens [see Fig. 8–26]), or very rarely congenital.

Symptoms
Asymptomatic; may have loss of accommodation and decreased vision.

Signs
Decreased visual acuity, no lens, iridodonesis; may have a visible surgical wound, peripheral iridectomy, vitreous in anterior chamber, complications from surgery (bullous keratopathy, increased intraocular pressure, iritis, posterior capsule opacification, cystoid macular edema), or evidence of ocular trauma (see appropriate sections).

Evaluation
- Complete ophthalmic history and eye exam with attention to refraction, tonometry, gonioscopy, iris, lens, and ophthalmoscopy
- Consider specular microscopy and pachymetry if cornea guttata or corneal edema exists

Management
- Proper aphakic correction with contact lens; consider aphakic spectacles if bilateral
- Consider secondary IOL implantation
- Treat complications if present

Prognosis
Usually good; increased risk of retinal detachment, especially for high myopes.

Pseudophakia

Definition
Presence of intraocular lens (IOL) implant after crystalline lens has been removed; may be inserted primarily or secondarily.

Symptoms

Asymptomatic; may have decreased vision, loss of accommodation, edge glare, monocular diplopia or polyopia, or induced myopia with decentered IOL.

Signs

IOL implant (may be in anterior chamber, iris plane, capsular bag, or ciliary sulcus with or without suture fixation to iris or sclera); may have a visible surgical wound, peripheral iridectomy, complications from surgery (bullous keratopathy, iris capture, decentered IOL, increased intraocular pressure, iritis, hyphema, opacified posterior capsule, cystoid macular edema [CME]).

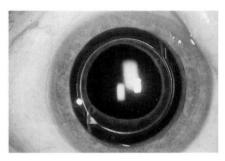 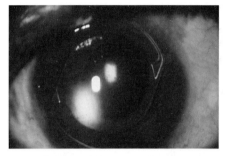

Figure 8–17 Pseudophakia demonstrating posterior chamber intraocular lens well-centered in the capsular bag.

Figure 8–18 Pseudophakia demonstrating anterior chamber intraocular lens.

Evaluation

■ Complete ophthalmic history and eye exam with attention to refraction, cornea, gonioscopy, IOL position, posterior capsule integrity and clarity, and ophthalmoscopy

Management

■ No treatment recommended
■ May require correction of refractive error (usually reading glasses)
■ Treat complications if present

Prognosis

Usually good; increased risk of retinal detachment, especially for high myopes.

Exfoliation

Definition

True exfoliation is delamination, or schisis, of the anterior lens capsule into sheet-like lamellae.

Epidemiology

Rare; caused by infrared and thermal radiation, classically seen in glass blowers; also senile form.

Symptoms

Asymptomatic.

Signs

Splitting of anterior lens capsule, appears as scrolls; may have posterior subcapsular cataract.

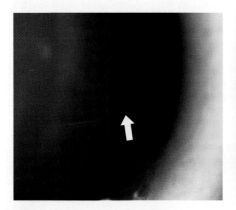

Figure 8–19 True lens exfoliation demonstrating scrolling of split anterior lens capsule (arrow).

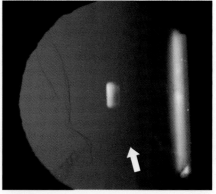

Figure 8–20 Same patient as shown in Figure 8–19, demonstrating appearance of lens capsule exfoliation (arrow) as viewed with retroillumination.

Differential Diagnosis

Pseudoexfoliation syndrome.

Work-Up

- Complete ophthalmic history and eye exam with attention to lens

Management

- No treatment recommended
- Prevention by use of protective goggles
- May require cataract extraction

Prognosis

Good.

Pseudoexfoliation Syndrome (PXS)

Definition

Pseudoexfoliation is a generalized basement membrane disorder that causes abnormal accumulation of small, gray-white fibrillar aggregates (resembling amyloid) on the lens capsule, iris, anterior segment structures, and systemically; may involve the skin, heart, and lungs.

Epidemiology

Pseudoexfoliation is often unilateral; usually asymmetric; found in all racial groups, common in Scandinavians, South African Blacks, Navaho Indians, and Australian aborigines; almost absent in Eskimos; age-related, rare in individuals <50 years old, incidence increases after 60 years of age (4–6% in patients >60 years old); up to 60% develop ocular hypertension or glaucoma (see below); in the United States, 20% have elevated intraocular pressure at initial examination, and 15% develop it within 10 years.

Symptoms

Asymptomatic.

Signs

Loss of pupillary ruff, iris transillumination defects, pigment deposits on the iris, trabecular meshwork, and anterior to Schwalbe's line (Sampaolesi's line); target pattern of exfoliative material on lens capsule (central disc and peripheral ring with intervening clear area); white exfoliation material is also seen on zonules, anterior hyaloid, iris, and pupillary margin; shallow anterior chamber due to forward migration of lens-iris diaphragm; may have iridodenesis, phacodonesis, cataract (40%), or increased intraocular pressure.

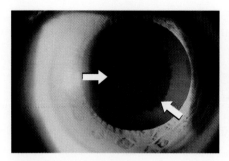

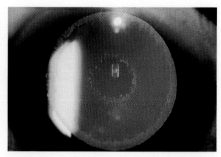

Figure 8–21 Exfoliative material on the anterior lens surface in typical pattern of central disc and peripheral ring (arrows) in a patient with pseudoexfoliation syndrome.

Figure 8–22 Central disc and peripheral ring of exfoliative material as seen with retroillumination.

Evaluation

- Complete ophthalmic history and eye exam with attention to tonometry, gonioscopy, iris, lens, and ophthalmoscopy
- Consider visual fields in patients with elevated intraocular pressure or optic nerve cupping to rule out glaucoma

Management

- No treatment recommended
- May require treatment of increased intraocular pressure (see Chap. 11)

Prognosis

Good; poorer if glaucoma exists; increased incidence of complications at cataract surgery due to weak zonules and increased lens mobility.

Pseudoexfoliation Glaucoma (PXG)

Definition

A form of secondary open-angle glaucoma associated with the pseudoexfoliation syndrome.

Epidemiology

Most common cause of secondary open-angle glaucoma; 2% of US population >50 years old; up to 60% with pseudoexfoliation syndrome (PXS) develop ocular hypertension or glaucoma; 50% bilateral, often asymmetric; age-related (rare in individuals <50 years old, increases after age 60 years old).

Mechanism

Trabecular meshwork dysfunction due to dispersion of pigment or exfoliative material.

Symptoms

Asymptomatic; may have decreased vision or visual field defects in late stages.

Signs

Intraocular pressure elevation can be very high and asymmetric; similar ocular signs as pseudoexfoliation syndrome (see above).

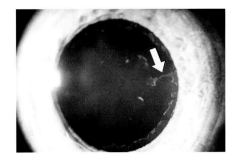

Figure 8–23 Patient with pseudoexfoliation glaucoma demonstrating peripheral ring of exfoliative material on the lens surface with bridging band (arrow) connecting to the central disc.

Differential Diagnosis

Primary open-angle glaucoma, other secondary open-angle glaucomas.

Evaluation

- Complete ophthalmic history and eye exam with attention to cornea, tonometry, anterior chamber, gonioscopy, iris, lens, and ophthalmoscopy
- Check visual fields
- Stereo optic nerve photos are useful for comparison at subsequent evaluations

Management

- Choice and order of topical glaucoma medications depend on many factors, including patient's age, intraocular pressure level and control, and amount and progression of optic nerve cupping and visual field defects. Treatment options are presented in the Primary Open-Angle Glaucoma (POAG) section (see Chap. 11); more resistant to treatment than primary open-angle glaucoma
- Laser trabeculoplasty is effective, but action may be short-lived
- May require glaucoma filtering procedure if medical treatment fails

Prognosis

Poorer than primary open-angle glaucoma; increased incidence of angle-closure; lens removal has no effect on progression of disease; increased incidence of complications at cataract surgery due to weak zonules and increased lens mobility.

Lens-Induced Secondary Glaucomas

Definition

Secondary glaucomas due to lens-induced abnormalities.

Mechanism

Lens Particle: Retained cortex or nucleus after cataract surgery or penetrating trauma causes inflammatory reaction and obstructs trabecular meshwork; more anterior segment inflammation than phacolytic.

Phacoanaphylactic: Immunologic sensitization to lens proteins after cataract surgery or penetrating injury is followed by a latent period and then a zonal granulomatous reaction.

Phacolytic: Lens proteins from hypermature cataract leak through intact capsule and are ingested by macrophages; can occur with intact, dislocated lens; lens proteins and macrophages obstruct trabecular meshwork.

Phacomorphic: Enlarged, cataractous lens pushes the iris forward, causing secondary angle-closure (see Chap. 6).

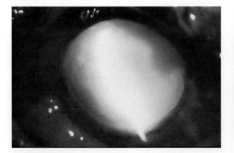

Figure 8–24 Phacolytic glaucoma.

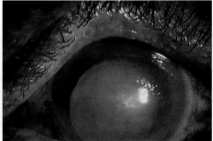

Figure 8–25 Phacomorphic angle-closure glaucoma due to intumescent cataract pushing the iris forward and thereby obstructing the trabecular meshwork.

Symptoms

Decreased vision, pain, photophobia, red eye; may have halos around lights and signs of angle-closure (see Chap. 6).

Signs

Decreased visual acuity, increased intraocular pressure, ciliary injection, anterior chamber cell/flare, peripheral anterior synechiae, cataract or residual lens material, signs of recent surgery or trauma including surgical wounds, sutures, and signs of an open globe (see Chap. 4).

Differential Diagnosis

See above; other secondary glaucomas, uveitis, endophthalmitis.

Evaluation

- Complete ophthalmic history and eye exam with attention to cornea, tonometry, anterior chamber, gonioscopy, iris, lens, and ophthalmoscopy
- B-scan ultrasonography if unable to visualize the fundus

Management

- Medical treatment of increased intraocular pressure. Treatment options are presented in the Primary Open-Angle Glaucoma (POAG) and Angle-Closure Glaucoma sections (see Chaps. 11 and 6, respectively)
- Topical steroid (prednisolone acetate 1% up to q1h) and cycloplegic (cyclopentolate 1% or scopolamine 0.25% bid–tid)
- Definitive treatment consists of surgical lens extraction for lens particle and phacoanaphylactic or removal of retained lens fragments
- May require glaucoma filtering procedure

Prognosis

Good if definitive treatment is performed early and pressure control is achieved.

Dislocated Lens (Ectopia Lentis)

Definition

Congenital, developmental, or acquired displacement of the crystalline lens; may be incomplete (subluxation) or complete dislocation (luxation) of the lens into the anterior chamber or vitreous.

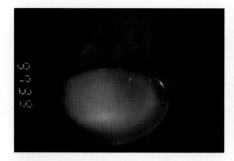

Figure 8–26 Dislocated crystalline lens resting on the retina.

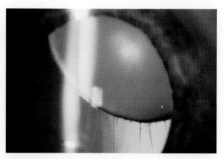

Figure 8–27 Subluxed lens (up and out) due to trauma; note broken inferior zonular fibers.

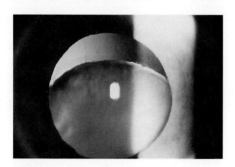

Figure 8–28 Subluxed lens (downward) due to trauma.

Etiology

Ectopia Lentis et Pupillae (autosomal recessive [AR]): Associated with oval or slit-like pupils; pupil displacement is in opposite direction of the lens displacement.

Homocystinuria (AR): Lens dislocation is not present at birth; progressive thereafter, typically in a down and inward direction; >90% have dislocated lenses by the 3rd decade; enzymatic disorder of methionine metabolism with elevated levels of homocystine and methionine; patients develop seizures, osteoporosis, mental retardation, and thromboembolism.

Hyperlysinemia: Inability to metabolize lysine; lens subluxation, muscular hypotony, and mental retardation.

Marfan's Syndrome (autosomal dominant [AD]): Usually bilateral; occurs in about two thirds of Marfan's patients due to a defective zonular apparatus; direction of lens displacement is typically up and out; other signs include marfanoid habitus with disproportionate growth of extremities, arachnodactyly, joint laxity, pectus deformities, scoliosis, and increasing dilatation of the ascending aorta with aortic insufficiency (may cause death); mapped to chromosome 15q.

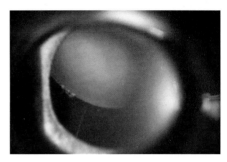

Figure 8–29 Subluxed lens (upward) in a patient with Marfan's syndrome.

Microspherophakia: Small spherical lens seen as isolated anomaly or as part of various syndromes (dominant spherophakia, Weill-Marchesani syndrome, Lowe's syndrome).

Simple Ectopia Lentis (AD): Often present at birth; lens is small and spherical (microphakic and spherophakic); direction of lens displacement is typically up and out.

Sulfite Oxidase Deficiency (AR): Error of sulfur metabolism with ectopia lentis, seizures, and mental retardation.

Also, Aniridia, Ehlers-Danlos syndrome, Trauma, Syphilis, Megalocornea.

Epidemiology

Most common cause of lens subluxation/luxation is trauma (22–50%); associated with cataract and rhegmatogenous retinal detachment; most frequent cause of heritable lens dislocation is Marfan's syndrome.

Symptoms

Asymptomatic; may have decreased vision, diplopia, symptoms of angle-closure.

Signs

Normal or decreased visual acuity, subluxated or luxated lens, phacodonesis, iridodonesis; may have increased intraocular pressure, anterior chamber cell/flare, vitreous in AC, iris transillumination defects, angle abnormalities, and other signs of ocular trauma.

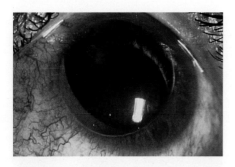

Figure 8–30 Dislocated lens in the anterior chamber.

Differential Diagnosis

See above.

Evaluation

- Complete ophthalmic history and eye exam with attention to refraction, corneal diameter, tonometry, gonioscopy, iris, and lens
- Consider B-scan ultrasonography if unable to visualize the fundus
- Lab tests: Venereal Disease Research Laboratory (VDRL), fluorescent treponema antibody absorption test (FTA-ABS), lumbar puncture if syphilis suspected
- Medical consultation for systemic diseases

Management

- No treatment recommended
- Correct any refractive error
- Consider lens extraction
- May require treatment of angle-closure (see Chap. 6); miotics may exacerbate a pupillary block and should be avoided
- Microspherophakia causing pupillary block is treated with a cycloplegic (scopolamine 0.25% tid or atropine 1% bid); may also require laser iridotomy
- Treat underlying disorder (eg, dietary restriction in homocystinuria, IV penicillin for syphilis)

Prognosis

Depends on etiology.

Congenital Anomalies

Definition

Coloboma: Inferior lens notch due to incomplete embryonic fissure closure during development and focal absence of zonular support; other ocular colobomata (iris, ciliary body) usually exist; ciliary body tumors may cause a secondary coloboma.

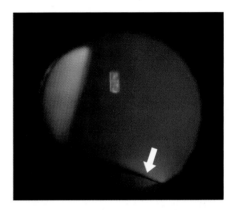

Figure 8–31 Lens coloboma appears as inferior flattening or truncation of lens due to lack of zonular attachments when viewed with retroillumination (arrow).

Lenticonus: Cone-shaped lens due to bulging from a thin lens capsule; either anteriorly or posteriorly, rarely in both directions:

- **Anterior:** Usually males; bilateral; may be associated with Alport's syndrome (AD)(basement membrane disease associated with acute hemorrhagic nephropathy, deafness, anterior lenticonus, anterior polar and/or cortical cataracts, and albipunctatus-like spots in the fundus).

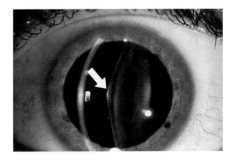

Figure 8–32 Anterior lenticonus in a patient with Alport's syndrome; note peaked slit beam as it crosses anterior lens surface (arrow).

- **Posterior:** More common; slight female predilection; may have associated cortical lens opacities.

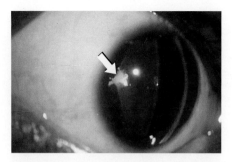

Figure 8–33 Posterior lenticonus with polar cataract (arrow).

Lentiglobus: Globe-shaped lens caused by bulging from thin lens capsule; rare.

Microspherophakia: Small spherical lens; isolated anomaly or part of various syndromes (Weill-Marchesani syndrome, Lowe's syndrome).

Mittendorf Dot: A small white spot on the posterior lens capsule that represents a remnant of the posterior tunica vasculosa lentis where the former hyaloid artery attached.

Symptoms

Asymptomatic (Mittendorf dot, coloboma); may have decreased vision (lenticonus, lentiglobus, and microspherophakia), diplopia, or angle-closure symptoms (microspherophakia).

Signs

Normal or decreased visual acuity; may have amblyopia, strabismus, nystagmus; myopia and an "oil-droplet" fundus reflex on retroillumination in lenticonus and lentiglobus; may have dislocated lens and increased intraocular pressure in microspherophakia.

Differential Diagnosis

See above.

Evaluation

■ Complete ophthalmic history and eye exam with attention to cycloplegic refraction, retinoscopy, gonioscopy, lens, and ophthalmoscopy

Management

- ■ Correct any refractive error
- ■ Patching/occlusion therapy for amblyopia (see Chap. 12)

Management Continued

- Microspherophakia causing pupillary block is treated with a cyclo-plegic (scopolamine 0.25% tid or atropine 1% bid); may also require laser iridotomy or lens extraction

Prognosis

Usually good; poorer if amblyopia exists.

Vitreous

Amyloidosis

Granular, glass-wool opacities often with strands attached to the retina that form in the vitreal cortex near retinal blood vessels; bilateral involvement indicates familial amyloidosis (autosomal dominant [AD]); may significantly reduce vision.

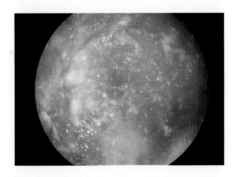

Figure 9–1 Amyloidosis.

■ No treatment recommended unless opacities become so severe that they affect vision, then consider pars plana vitrectomy by a vitreoretinal specialist; recurs even after vitrectomy

Asteroid Hyalosis

Multiple, yellow-white, round, birefringent particles composed of calcium-phosphate soaps attached to the vitreous framework. Common degenerative process seen in elderly patients over 60 years of age (0.5% of population). Usually asymptomatic, does not interfere with vision, but does affect view of fundus; usually unilateral (75%); associated with diabetes mellitus (30%).

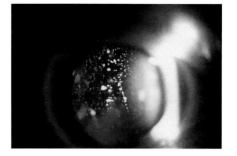

Figure 9–2 Asteroid hyalosis.

- No treatment usually recommended
- Consider pars plana vitrectomy if asteroids become so severe that they affect vision or interfere with the diagnosis or treatment of retinal disorders; should be performed by a vitreoretinal specialist

Persistent Hyperplastic Primary Vitreous (PHPV)

Definition

Sporadic, unilateral (90%), developmental anomaly with abnormal regression of the tunica vasculosa lentis (hyaloid artery) and primary vitreous.

Symptoms

Decreased vision; may have eye turn.

Signs

Leukocoria, strabismus, microphthalmos, nystagmus, pink-white retrolenticular/intravitreal membrane often with radiating vessels; lens is clear early but becomes cataractous; associated with shallow anterior chamber (AC) (more shallow with age), elongated ciliary processes extending toward membrane, large radial blood vessels that often cover iris; may have angle-closure (see Chap. 6), vitreous hemorrhage, or retinal detachment.

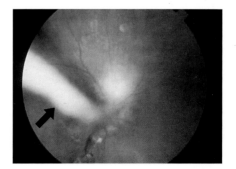

Figure 9–3 Persistent hyperplastic primary vitreous with fibrovascular stalk (arrow) emanating from the optic disc.

Differential Diagnosis

Leukocoria (see Chap. 7).

Evaluation

- Complete ophthalmic history and eye exam with attention to tonometry, lens, and ophthalmoscopy
- B-scan ultrasonography if unable to visualize the fundus
- Check orbital computed tomography (CT) scan for intraocular calcifications

Management

- Correct any refractive error
- Retinal surgery with pars plana vitrectomy, lensectomy, and membrane peel advocated early (within first few months of life); should be performed by a vitreoretinal specialist
- Patching/occlusion therapy for amblyopia (see Chap. 12)

Prognosis

Poor prognosis without treatment; earlier treatment improves prognosis.

Posterior Vitreous Detachment (PVD)

Definition

Syneresis (liquefaction) of the vitreous gel that causes dehiscence of the posterior hyaloid from the retina (internal limiting membrane) and collapse of the vitreous toward the vitreous base away from the macula and optic disc. Can be localized, partial, or total.

Epidemiology

Most commonly caused by aging (53% by 50 years old, 65% by 65 years old); By age 70, majority of the posterior vitreous is liquefied (synchysis senilis); female predilection; occurs earlier after trauma, vitritis, cataract surgery, neodymium: yttrium-aluminum-garnet (Nd:YAG) laser posterior capsulotomy, and in patients with myopia, diabetes mellitus, hereditary vitreoretinal degenerations, and retinitis pigmentosa.

Symptoms

Acute onset of floaters and photopsias, especially with eye movement.

Signs

Circular vitreous condensation often over disc (Weiss ring), anterior displacement of the posterior hyaloid, vitreous opacities, vitreous pigment cells (tobacco dust), focal intraretinal, preretinal, or vitreous hemorrhage.

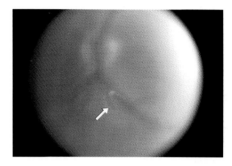

Figure 9–4 Horseshoe-shaped posterior vitreous detachment (arrow).

Differential Diagnosis

Vitreous hemorrhage (see below), vitritis, fungal cyst.

Evaluation

- Complete ophthalmic history and eye exam with attention to anterior vitreous, Hruby lens examination, 78/90 diopter or contact lens fundus exam, and careful depressed peripheral retinal examination to identify any retinal breaks

Management

- No treatment recommended
- Instruct patient on retinal detachment warning signs: photopsias, increased floaters, and shadow in the visual field; instruct patient to return immediately if warning signs occur to rule out retinal tear or detachment
- Repeat dilated retinal exam 1–3 months after acute posterior vitreous detachment to rule out retinal tear or detachment
- Treat retinal breaks if present (see Chap. 10)

Prognosis

Good; 10–15% risk of retinal break in acute, symptomatic posterior vitreous detachments; 70% risk of retinal break if vitreous hemorrhage is present.

Synchesis Scintillans

Golden brown, refractile crystals that are freely mobile within vitreous cavity; associated with liquid vitreous, so the crystals settle in the most dependent area of the vitreous body; rare syndrome that occurs after chronic vitreous hemorrhage, uveitis, or trauma; composed of cholesterol crystals.

- No treatment recommended
- Consider pars plana vitrectomy if synchesis scintillans becomes so severe that it affects vision or interferes with the diagnosis or treatment of retinal disorders; should be performed by a vitreoretinal specialist

Vitreous Hemorrhage (VH)

Definition

Blood in the vitreous space.

Etiology

Retinal break, posterior vitreous detachment, ruptured retinal arterial macroaneurysm, juvenile retinoschisis, familial exudative vitreoretinopathy, Terson's syndrome (blood dissects through the lamina cribrosa into the eye due to subarachnoid hemorrhage and elevated intracranial pressure, often bilateral with severe headache), trauma, retinal angioma, retinopathy of blood disorders, Valsalva retinopathy, and neovascularization from various disorders including diabetic retinopathy, Eales' disease, hypertensive retinopathy, radiation retinopathy, sickle cell retinopathy, and retinopathy of prematurity.

Symptoms

Sudden onset of floaters and decreased vision.

Signs

Decreased visual acuity, vitreous cells (red blood cells), poor or no view of fundus, poor or absent red reflex; old vitreous hemorrhage appears gray-white.

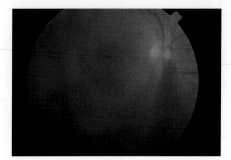

Figure 9–5 Vitreous hemorrhage.

Differential Diagnosis

Vitritis, asteroid hyalosis, pigment cells, pars planitis.

Evaluation

- Complete ophthalmic history and eye exam with attention to visual acuity, tonometry, ophthalmoscopy
- B-scan ultrasonography to rule out retinal detachment if unable to visualize the fundus

Management

- Conservative treatment and follow for resolution of vitreous hemorrhage
- Bedrest and elevation of head of bed may settle hemorrhage inferiorly to allow visualization of fundus
- Avoid aspirin and aspirin-containing products (and other anticoagulants)
- Consider pars plana vitrectomy if there is persistent vitreous hemorrhage for >6 months, intractable increased intraocular pressure, decreased vision in fellow eye, or retinal detachment; should be performed by a vitreoretinal specialist
- Treat underlying medical condition

Prognosis

Usually good.

Retina / Choroid

Trauma

Choroidal Rupture: Tear in choroid, Bruch's membrane, and retinal pigment epithelium (RPE) usually seen after blunt trauma. Acutely, the rupture site may be obscured by hemorrhage. Anterior ruptures are usually parallel to the ora serrata, posterior ruptures are usually crescent-shaped and concentric to the optic nerve. Patient may have decreased vision if commotio or hemorrhage is present, or if rupture is located in the macula; increased risk of developing a subretinal neovascular membrane (SRNVM).

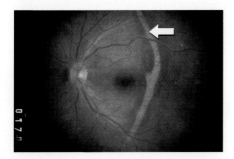

Figure 10–1 Choroidal rupture (arrow) with surrounding subretinal hemorrhage.

- No treatment recommended, unless neovascular membrane occurs (laser photocoagulation)
- Monitor for SRNVM with Amsler grid

Commotio Retinae (Berlin's Edema): Gray-white discoloration of the outer retina due to photoreceptor outer segment disruption following blunt eye trauma; can affect any area of the retina and may be accompanied by hemorrhages or choroidal rupture; can cause acute decrease in vision if located within the macula that resolves as the retinal discoloration disappears; may cause permanent loss of vision if fovea is damaged.

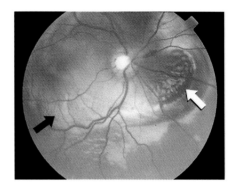

Figure 10-2 Commotio retinae demonstrating retinal whitening (black arrow); note subretinal hemorrhage (white arrow) from underlying choroidal rupture.

- Fluorescein angiogram: early blocked fluorescence in the areas of commotio
- No treatment recommended

Purtscher's Retinopathy: Multiple patches of retinal whitening, large cotton-wool spots, and hemorrhages that surround the optic disc following multiple long bone fractures with fat emboli or severe compressive injuries to the chest or head; may have optic disc edema and a positive relative afferent pupillary defect (RAPD); resolves over weeks to months.

- No treatment recommended

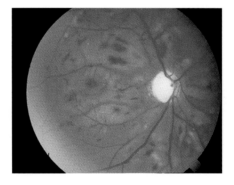

Figure 10-3 Purtscher's retinopathy.

Retinal Break: Full-thickness tear in the retina, often horseshoe-shaped, that usually occurs along the vitreous base, posterior border of lattice degeneration, or at cystic retinal tufts (areas with strong vitreoretinal adhesions). Giant retinal tears (tears >90 degrees in circumferential extent), avulsion of vitreous base, and retinal dialysis (circumferential separation of the retina at the ora serrata, usually in superonasal quadrant) are more common after trauma. Associated with pigmented vitreous cells ("tobacco-dust"), vitreous hemorrhages, operculum (often located over the break), and posterior vitreous detachment. Patients usually report photopsias and floaters that shift with eye movement. Liquefied vitreous can pass through the tear into the subretinal space, causing a retinal detachment even months to years after the tear forms; chronic tears have a ring of pigment around the break.

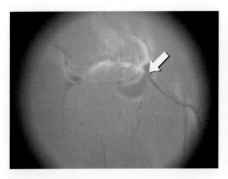

Figure 10–4 Horseshoe-shaped retinal tear with overlying retinal vessel (arrow).

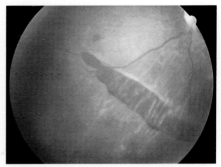

Figure 10–5 Giant retinal tear.

- If asymptomatic, close follow-up
- If symptomatic, treatment with cryopexy along edge of tear (do not treat bare retinal pigment epithelium) or two to three rows of laser photocoagulation demarcation around the tear
- Retinal surgery required if retinal detachment, retinal dialysis, avulsion of the vitreous base, or giant retinal tear exists; should be performed by a retina specialist

Hemorrhages

Preretinal Hemorrhage: Hemorrhage located between retina and posterior vitreous face (subhyaloid) or under internal limiting membrane of the retina (sub-ILM). Often amorphous or boat-shaped, with flat upper border and curved lower border, that obscures the underlying retina; caused by trauma, neovascularization (diabetic retinopathy, radiation retinopathy, breakthrough bleeding from a choroidal neovascular membrane [CNVM]), hypertensive retinopathy, Valsalva retinopathy, posterior vitreous detachment, shaken-baby syndrome, or retinal breaks, and less frequently by vascular occlusion, retinopathy of blood disorders, and leukemia.

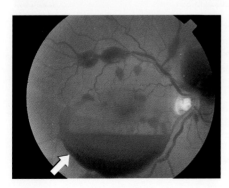

Figure 10–6 Preretinal hemorrhage in boat-shaped configuration (arrow).

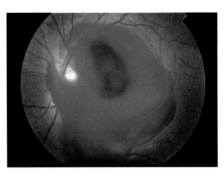

Figure 10–7 Valsalva retinopathy demonstrating vitreous, preretinal, and retinal hemorrhages.

Intraretinal Hemorrhage: Bilateral intraretinal hemorrhages are associated with systemic disorders (eg, diabetes mellitus and hypertension); unilateral intraretinal hemorrhages generally occur in venous occlusive diseases.

- **Flame-shaped hemorrhage:** Located in the superficial retina oriented with the nerve fiber layer; feathery borders; usually seen in hypertensive retinopathy and vein occlusion; may be peripapillary in glaucoma, especially in normal-tension glaucoma (called splinter hemorrhage) and disc edema.
- **Dot/blot hemorrhage:** Located in the outer plexiform layer, confined by the anteroposterior orientation of the photoreceptor, bipolar, and Müller's cells; round dots or larger blots; usually seen in diabetic retinopathy.

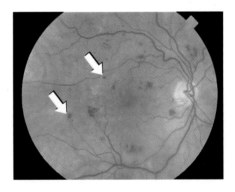

Figure 10–8 Intraretinal dot and blot hemorrhages (arrows) in a patient with nonproliferative diabetic retinopathy.

- **Roth spot:** Hemorrhage with white center that represents an embolus with lymphocytic infiltration; classically associated with subacute bacterial endocarditis (seen in 1–5% of such patients); also occurs in leukemia, severe anemia, collagen vascular diseases, diabetes mellitus, and multiple myeloma (see Fig. 10–26).

Subretinal Hemorrhage: Amorphous hemorrhage located under the neurosensory retina or RPE; appears dark and is deep to the retinal vessels; associated with trauma, subretinal and choroidal neovascular membranes, and macroaneurysms (see Fig. 10–42).

All three types of hemorrhages may occur together in several disorders including age-related macular degeneration (ARMD), acquired retinal macroaneurysms, Eales' disease, and capillary hemangioma.

Cotton-Wool Spot (CWS)

Asymptomatic, yellow-white, fluffy lesions in the superficial retina (see Fig. 10–76); believed to result from focal retinal ischemia; nonspecific finding seen in several systemic diseases including acquired immunodeficiency syndrome (AIDS), anemia, hypertension, leukemia, collagen vascular diseases, cardiac valvular diseases, acute pancreatitis, and diabetes mellitus (most common cause); also associated with vascular occlusions, radiation retinopathy, and high-altitude retinopathy.

- Treat underlying medical condition (identified in 95% of cases)

Branch/Central Retinal Artery Occlusion (BRAO/CRAO)

Definition

Disruption of the vascular perfusion in the central retinal artery (CRAO) or in its branches (BRAO), leading to focal or global retinal ischemia.

Etiology

BRAO: Mainly due to embolism from cholesterol (carotid arteries), calcifications (heart valves), platelet-fibrin (arteriosclerosis), or septic (heart valve vegetations seen in bacterial endocarditis or IV drug abuse).

CRAO: Due to emboli (only visible in 20% of cases) or thrombus at the lamina cribrosa; other causes include temporal arteritis, leukoemboli in collagen vascular diseases, fat emboli following trauma, vasospasm, hypercoagulation disorders, syphilis, sickle cell disease, amniotic fluid emboli, mitral valve prolapse, particles (talc) from IV drug abuse, and compressive lesions; associated with optic disc drusen, papilledema, and primary open-angle glaucoma.

Epidemiology

Usually occurs in elderly patients; associated with hypertension (67%), carotid occlusive disease (25%), diabetes mellitus (33%), and cardiac valvular disease (25%). CRAO more common (57%) than BRAO (38%) or cilioretinal artery occlusion (5%) (in 32% of eyes, a cilioretinal artery is present).

Symptoms

BRAO: Sudden, unilateral, painless, partial loss of vision, with a visual field defect depending on the location of the occlusion.

CRAO: Sudden, unilateral, painless loss of vision.

May have history of amaurosis fugax (fleeting episodes of loss of vision), prior cerebrovascular accident (CVA), or transient ischemic attacks (TIAs).

Signs

BRAO: Visual field defect with normal or decreased visual acuity; focal, wedge-shaped area of retinal whitening within the distribution of a branch arteriole; usually in superotemporal quadrant; emboli (60%) or Hollenhorst plaques composed of cholesterol may be seen at retinal vessel bifurcations.

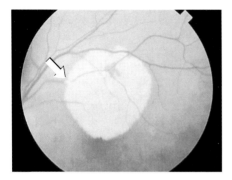

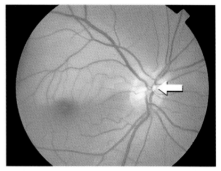

Figure 10–9 Branch retinal artery occlusion with Hollenhorst plaque (arrow).

Figure 10–10 Superior hemiretinal artery occlusion with Hollenhorst plaque (arrow).

CRAO: Decreased visual acuity in the count fingers (CF) to light perception (LP) range; positive relative afferent pupillary defect (RAPD); diffuse retinal whitening and arteriole constriction with segmentation (box-carring) of blood flow; visible emboli (20%); cherry-red spot in the macula (thin fovea allows visualization of the underlying choroidal circulation). In ciliary retinal artery sparing CRAO (10%), small wedge-shaped area of perfused retina may be present temporal to the optic disc. *Note:* Ophthalmic artery obstruction usually does *not* produce a cherry-red spot due to underlying choroidal ischemia.

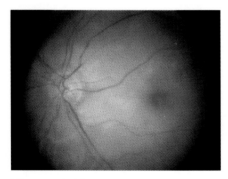

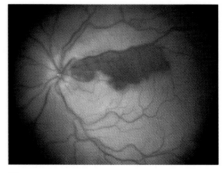

Figure 10–11 Central retinal artery occlusion with cherry-red spot and surrounding retinal edema.

Figure 10–12 Central retinal artery occlusion with patent cilioretinal artery sparing the macula.

Differential Diagnosis

Ophthalmic artery occlusion, commotio retinae, cherry-red spot due to inherited metabolic or lysosomal storage diseases.

Evaluation

- Complete ophthalmic history and eye exam with attention to pupils, 78/90 diopter or contact lens fundus exam, and ophthalmoscopy (retinal vasculature and arteriole bifurcations)
- Check visual fields
- Check blood pressure
- Lab tests: fasting blood glucose (FBS) and complete blood count (CBC) with differential; consider platelets, prothrombin time/partial thromboplastin time (PT/PTT), antinuclear antibody (ANA), rheumatoid factor (RF), serum protein electrophoresis, hemoglobin electrophoresis, Venereal Disease Research Laboratory (VDRL), and fluorescent treponemal antibody absorption test (FTA-ABS). In patients >50 years old, check erythrocyte sedimentation rate (ESR) to rule out temporal arteritis. If positive, start temporal arteritis treatment immediately (see Chap. 11)
- Fluorescein angiogram: delayed retinal vascular filling and capillary nonperfusion
- B-scan ultrasonography or orbital computed tomography (CT) to rule out compressive lesion
- Medical consultation for complete cardiovascular evaluation including electrocardiogram, echocardiogram, and carotid Doppler studies

Management

- **BRAO:** Same treatment as CRAO (see below), but treatment controversial due to good prognosis and questionable benefit of treatment.

OCULAR EMERGENCY:

- **CRAO:** Treat immediately *before* starting work-up (if patient presents within 24 hours of visual loss)

  - Digital ocular massage
  - Systemic acetazolamide (Diamox 500 mg IV or PO)
  - Topical β-blocker (timolol 0.5% 1 gtt q15min × 2, repeat as necessary)
  - Anterior chamber paracentesis
  - Consider admission to hospital for carbogen treatment (95% O_2–5% CO_2 for 10 minutes q2h for 24–48 hours)
  - Unproven treatments include hyperbaric oxygen, antifibrinolytic drugs, retrobulbar vasodilators

Prognosis

Retinal pallor fades and circulation is restored over several weeks.

BRAO: Good prognosis; 90% have ≥20/40 vision.

CRAO: Poor prognosis; most have persistent severe visual loss with constricted retinal arterioles and optic atrophy. Rubeosis (20%) and disc/retinal neovascularization rare.

Branch/Central/Hemiretinal Vein Occlusion (BRVO/CRVO/HRVO)

Definition

Occlusion of the central retinal vein (CRVO) or a branch retinal vein (BRVO) usually caused by a thrombus; hemiretinal occlusion (HRVO) occurs when the superior and inferior retinal drainage does not merge into a central retinal vein (20%) and is occluded (more like CRVO than BRVO).

Etiology

Associated with hypertension (60%), coronary artery disease, diabetes mellitus, peripheral vascular disease, hypercoagulable states (eg, macroglobulinemia, cryoglobulinemia), systemic lupus erythematosus, syphilis, sarcoid, homocystinuria, malignancies (eg, multiple myeloma, polycythemia vera, leukemia), optic nerve drusen, external compression, and open-angle glaucoma (40%). In younger patients, associated with oral contraceptive pills, collagen vascular disease, acquired immunodeficiency syndrome, protein S/protein C/antithrombin III deficiency, or activated protein C resistance (factor V Leiden polymerase chain reaction [PCR] assay).

Epidemiology

Usually in elderly patients (90% are >50 years old); slight male predilection. Two types: nonischemic (64%) and ischemic (defined as ≥5 [BRVO] or ≥10 [CRVO] disc areas of capillary nonperfusion on fluorescein angiography).

Symptoms

BRVO: Sudden, unilateral, painless, visual field defect.

CRVO: Sudden, unilateral, painless loss of vision.

Patients may have normal vision, especially when macula is not involved.

Signs

BRVO: Visual field defect (entire superior or inferior hemifield in HRVO); dilated, tortuous retinal veins with superficial, retinal hemorrhages, and cotton-wool spots in a wedge-shaped area radiating from an arteriovenous crossing (usually arterial over-crossing where an arteriole and venule share a common vascular sheath). The closer the obstruction is to the optic disc, the greater the

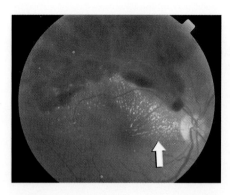

Figure 10–13 Branch retinal vein occlusion with exudates forming partial macular star (arrow).

retinal area involved. Microaneurysms or macroaneurysms, macular edema (50%), and/or epiretinal membranes (20%) may develop.

CRVO: Decreased visual acuity ranging from 20/100 to hand motion (HM); positive relative afferent pupillary defect (RAPD); dilated, tortuous retinal veins with superficial, retinal hemorrhages, and cotton-wool spots in all four quadrants extending to periphery; optic disc hyperemia, disc edema, and macular edema common. Ischemic disease can produce rubeosis (20% in CRVO, rare in BRVO), disc/retinal neovascularization (border of perfused/nonperfused retina), neovascular glaucoma, and vitreous hemorrhages. Collateral optociliary shunt vessels between retinal and ciliary circulations (50%) occur late. Impending CRVO may have absence of spontaneous venous pulsations (but this also occurs in normal individuals).

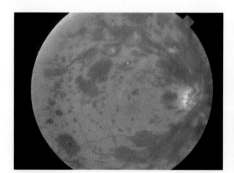

Figure 10–14 Central retinal vein occlusion.

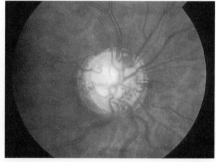

Figure 10–15 Optociliary shunt vessels in a patient with an old central retinal vein occlusion.

Differential Diagnosis

Venous stasis retinopathy, ocular ischemic syndrome, hypertensive retinopathy, leukemic retinopathy, retinopathy of anemia, diabetic retinopathy, papilledema, papillophlebitis (in young patients).

Evaluation

- Complete ophthalmic history and eye exam with attention to pupils, tonometry, gonioscopy, 78/90 diopter or contact lens fundus exam, and ophthalmoscopy
- Check visual fields
- Check blood pressure
- Consider lab tests: fasting blood glucose, CBC with differential, platelets, PT/PTT, ANA, RF, angiotensin converting enzyme (ACE), ESR, serum protein electrophoresis, FTA-ABS, and VDRL. In a patient <40 years old, check human immunodeficiency virus (HIV) status, protein S/protein C/antithrombin III deficiency, lupus anticoagulant, anticardiolipin antibody titer, and activated protein C resistance (Factor V Leiden PCR assay)
- Fluorescein angiogram: delayed retinal vascular filling, increased transit time (>20 seconds increases risk of rubeosis), and capillary nonperfusion (ischemic defined as ≥5 [BRVO] or ≥10 [CRVO] disc areas of capillary nonperfusion)
- B-scan ultrasonography or orbital CT scan to rule out compressive lesion
- Medical consultation for complete cardiovascular evaluation including electrocardiogram, echocardiogram, and carotid Doppler studies

Management

- Panretinal (CRVO) or quadrantic (BRVO) laser photocoagulation (500 μm spots) when rubeosis (≥2 clock-face increments ["clock hours"] of iris or any angle neovascularization), disc/retinal neovascularization, or neovascular glaucoma develops in ischemic CRVO or BRVO (Branch Vein Occlusion Study-BVOS conclusion and Central Retinal Vein Occlusion Study-CVOS conclusion)
- Macular grid/focal photocoagulation (100 μm spots) when macular edema lasts >3–6 months and vision is <20/40 in BRVO (BVOS conclusion). No benefit in CRVO (CVOS conclusion).
- Consider aspirin (325 mg PO qd)
- Treat underlying medical conditions

Prognosis

BRVO: Good; 50% have ≥20/40 vision unless foveal ischemia or chronic macular edema is present.

CRVO: Nonischemic has better prognosis. Risk of neovascularization depends on amount of ischemia.

Venous Stasis Retinopathy

Milder form of central retinal vein occlusion (CRVO) representing patients with better perfusion; dot/blot/flame hemorrhages, dilated/tortuous vasculature, microaneurysms, usually bilateral; more benign course; associated with hypervis-

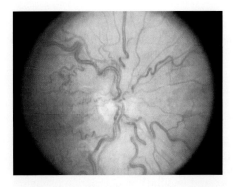

Figure 10–16 Dilated, tortuous, retinal vessels in a patient with hyperviscosity syndrome.

cosity syndromes including polycythemia vera, multiple myeloma, and Waldenström's macroglobulinemia.

Ocular Ischemic Syndrome

Widespread ischemia of the eye due to carotid occlusive disease that causes gradual loss of vision (90%) over weeks, with accompanying dull eye pain/headache (40%); patients may also report amaurosis fugax; usually in patients age 50–70 years old; 80% unilateral; male predilection (2:1); associated with atherosclerosis, heart disease, hypertension, and diabetes mellitus. Signs include retinal arterial narrowing and venous dilatation, retinal hemorrhages, microaneurysms, cotton-wool spots, disc/retinal neovascularization, and spontaneous pulsations of the retinal arteries; conjunctival injection, corneal edema, anterior chamber (AC) cell/flare, iris atrophy, and rubeosis are also common. Poor prognosis; 5-year mortality rate is 40%.

- Fluorescein angiogram: delayed or patchy choroidal filling, arterial vascular staining, and increased transit time
- Medical consultation for complete cardiovascular evaluation including duplex and Doppler scans of carotid arteries: (≥90% obstruction of the ipsilateral internal or common carotid arteries)
- Consider carotid endarterectomy if carotid obstruction exists
- Panretinal laser photocoagulation when disc/retinal neovascularization develops

Retinopathy of Prematurity (ROP)

Definition

Abnormal retinal vasculature development in premature infants, especially after supplemental oxygen therapy.

Epidemiology

Premature birth (<36 weeks' gestation), low birth weight (<1250 g; incidence 40–77% if <1000 g), supplemental oxygen therapy (>50 days), and a complicated hospital course.

Symptoms

Asymptomatic; later may have decreased vision; may notice white pupil and/or eye turn.

Signs

Shallow anterior chamber, corneal edema, iris atrophy, poor pupillary dilation, posterior synechiae, ectropion uveae, leukocoria, and retrolental fibroplasia. International classification of ROP describes the retinal changes in 5 stages:

Stage 1: Thin, circumferential, white, flat, demarcation line between posterior vascularized and peripheral avascular retina (beyond line)

Stage 2: Elevation and organization of line forms pink-white ridge, no fibrovascular growth seen

Stage 3: Extraretinal fibrovascular proliferation along ridge

Stage 4: Dragging of vessels, subtotal traction retinal detachment (4A is extrafoveal, 4B involves fovea)

Stage 5: Total retinal detachment (almost always funnel detachment)

"Plus" disease: Shunted blood causes vascular engorgement in the posterior pole with tortuous arteries, dilated veins, pupillary rigidity due to iris vascular engorgement, and vitreous haze.

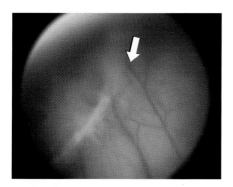

Figure 10–17 Retinopathy of prematurity demonstrating extraretinal fibrovascular proliferation along the ridge (arrow; Stage 3 ROP).

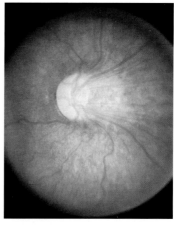

Figure 10–18 Retinopathy of prematurity demonstrating dragged vessels (Stage 4 ROP).

Describe extent of retina involved by number of clock hours and location by zone:

Zone 1: Inner zone (posterior pole) corresponding to the area enclosed by a circle around the optic disc with radius equal to twice the distance from the disc to the macula (diameter of 60 degrees)

Zone 2: The area between Zone 1 and a circle centered on the optic disc and tangent to the nasal ora serrata

Zone 3: Remaining temporal crescent of retina (last area to become vascularized)

Differential Diagnosis

Coats' disease, Eales' disease, familial exudative vitreoretinopathy, sickle cell retinopathy, juvenile retinoschisis, persistent hyperplastic primary vitreous, incontinentia pigmenti (Bloch-Sulzberger syndrome), and leukocoria (see Chap. 7).

Evaluation

- Screen all infants at 4–6 weeks chronological age who weighed <1250–1750 g at birth, and larger premature infants on supplemental oxygen for >50 days
- Complete ophthalmic history with attention to birth history and birth weight
- Complete eye exam with attention to iris, lens, and ophthalmoscopy (retinal vasculature and retinal periphery)
- Pediatric consultation

Management

- Treat when reach threshold disease = Stage 3 Plus disease with at least 5 contiguous or 8 cumulative clock hours involvement in Zone 1 or 2
- Indirect argon green or diode laser photocoagulation (500 μm spots) to entire avascular retina in Zone 1 and peripheral Zone 2; laser is at least as effective as cryotherapy (Laser-ROP study conclusion) *or*
- Cryotherapy to entire avascular retina in Zone 2, but not ridge (Cryotherapy for ROP [CRYO-ROP] study conclusion)
- Tractional retinal detachment or rhegmatogenous retinal detachment (cicatricial ROP, Stages 4–5) require vitreoretinal surgery with pars plana vitrectomy, lensectomy, membrane peel, and possible scleral buckle; should be performed by a retina specialist
- Follow very closely (every 1–2 weeks depending on location and severity of the disease) until extreme periphery vascularized, then monthly; beware "rush" disease = Plus disease in Zone 1 or posterior Zone 2, which has a significant risk of rapid progression to Stage 5 within a few days.

Prognosis

Depends on the amount and stage of ROP; 80–90% will spontaneously regress; Stage 5 disease carries a poor prognosis (functional success in only 3%); may develop high myopia, glaucoma, cataracts, keratoconus, band keratopathy, and retinal detachment.

Coats' Disease/Leber's Miliary Aneurysms

Unilateral (90%), progressive, developmental retinal vascular abnormality; usually occurs in young males (10:1) <20 years old. Retinal microaneurysms (MA), lipid exudation, "light-bulb" vascular dilatations, and capillary nonperfusion are seen primarily in the temporal quadrants, especially on fluorescein angiogram where microaneurysm leakage is common. Spectrum of disease from milder form seen in older patients with equal sex predilection and often bilateral (Leber's miliary aneurysms) to severe form with localized exudative retinal detachments and yellowish subretinal masses, and is included in the differential diagnosis of leukocoria (Coats' disease).

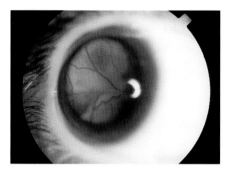

Figure 10–19 Coats' disease demonstrating leukocoria due to exudative retinal detachment.

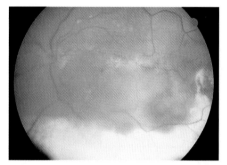

Figure 10–20 Coats' disease with massive exudative retinal detachment.

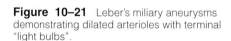

Figure 10–21 Leber's miliary aneurysms demonstrating dilated arterioles with terminal "light bulbs".

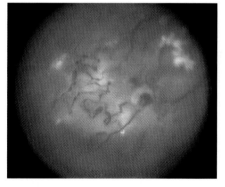

- Fluorescein angiogram: capillary nonperfusion, microaneurysms, light-bulb vascular dilatations, and macular edema
- Scatter laser photocoagulation to posterior or cryotherapy to anterior areas of abnormal vasculature and areas of nonperfusion. May require multiple treatment sessions.

Eales' Disease

Idiopathic, bilateral, peripheral obliterative vasculopathy seen in young adults age 20–30 years old. Patients usually notice floaters and decreased vision and have vitreous hemorrhages, areas of vascular sheathing, vitreous cells, peripheral retinal nonperfusion, microaneurysms, intraretinal hemorrhages, white sclerotic ghost vessels, and disc (NVD)/iris (NVI)/retinal (NVE) neovascularization; may have signs of iritis with keratic precipitates and anterior chamber cell/flare; variable prognosis.

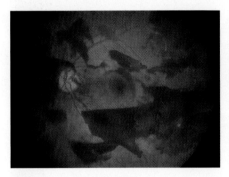
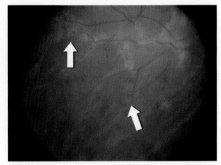

Figure 10–22 Eales' disease with preretinal and retinal hemorrhages.

Figure 10–23 Eales' disease with peripheral vascular abnormalities (arrows).

- Fluorescein angiogram: peripheral retinal nonperfusion, microaneurysms, neovascularization
- Scatter laser photocoagulation to nonperfused retina when neovascularization develops

Juxtafoveal Telangiectasia (JXT)

Group of disorders with abnormal telangiectatic capillaries confined to the juxtafoveal region (1–199 μm from center of fovea). Several forms:

Type 1A (Unilateral Congenital Parafoveal Telangiectasia): Seen in men in the 4th decade; yellow exudate seen at outer edge of telangiectasis usually temporal to the fovea; decreased vision ranging from 20/25 to 20/40 from macular edema and exudate. May represent mild presentation of Coats' disease in an adult.

Type 1B (Unilateral Idiopathic Parafoveal Telangiectasia): Seen in middle-aged men; minimal exudate usually confined to edge of the foveal avascular zone; usually asymptomatic with vision better than 20/25.

Type 2 (Bilateral Acquired Parafoveal Telangiectasia): Onset of symptoms in the 5–6th decades with equal sex distribution; mild blurring of central vision early, slowly progressive loss of central vision over years; blunting or grayish discoloration of the foveal reflex, right-angle retinal venules, and stellate retinal pigment epithelial hyperplasia/atrophy; leakage from telangiectatic vessels, but no exudates; associated with choroidal neovascular membranes (CNVM), hemorrhagic macular detachments, and retinochoroidal anastomosis.

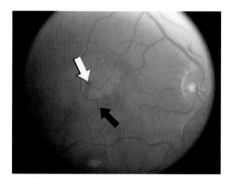 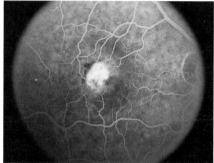

Figure 10–24 Juxtafoveal telangiectasia type 2 with abnormal foveal reflex, intraretinal hemorrhages (white arrow), and retinal pigment epithelium (RPE) changes (black arrow).

Figure 10–25 Fluorescein angiogram of patient shown in Figure 10–24, demonstrating hyperfluorescent leakage from telangiectatic vessels and blockage from the hemorrhages.

Type 3 (Bilateral Perifoveal Telangiectasis with Capillary Occlusion): Rare form; seen in adults in the 5th decade; slowly progressive loss of vision due to the marked aneurysmal dilatation and obliteration of the perifoveal telangiectatic capillary network; no leakage from telangiectasis; associated with optic nerve pallor and hyperactive deep tendon reflexes.

- Fluorescein angiogram: right-angle venules and variable leakage from the telangiectatic vessels (depending on type)
- **Type 1A:** Consider focal laser photocoagulation to peripheral lesions
- **Type 1B, 2, and 3:** No treatment recommended

Retinopathies Associated with Blood Abnormalities

Retinopathy of Anemia: Superficial, flame-shaped, intraretinal hemorrhages, cotton-wool spots, and rarely exudates, retinal edema, and vitreous hemorrhage in patients with anemia (hemoglobin <8 g/100 mL). Retinopathy is worse when associated with thrombocytopenia. Roth spots are seen in pernicious anemia and aplastic anemia.

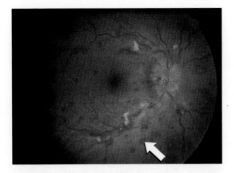

Figure 10–26 Retinopathy of anemia demonstrating Roth spots (arrow).

- Resolves with treatment of anemia
- Medical or hematology consultation

Leukemia/Leukemic Retinopathy: Superficial, flame-shaped, intraretinal (24%), preretinal, and vitreous hemorrhages (2%), microaneurysms, Roth spots (11%), cotton-wool spots (16%), dilated/tortuous vessels, perivascular sheathing, and disc edema; rarely direct leukemic infiltrates (3%); direct choroidal involvement appears with choroidal infiltrates, choroidal thickening, and an overlying serous retinal detachment. Sea-fan–shaped retinal neovascularization can occur late. Retinopathy is due to the associated anemia, thrombocytopenia, and hyperviscosity.

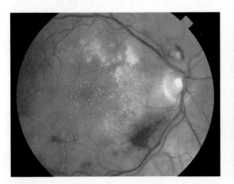 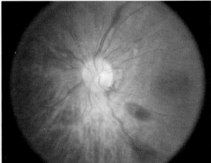

Figure 10–27 Leukemic retinopathy with macular edema, cotton-wool spots, hemorrhages, and Roth spots.

Figure 10–28 Leukemic retinopathy.

- Resolves with treatment of underlying hematologic abnormality
- Treat direct leukemic infiltrates with chemotherapy and/or radiation therapy; should be performed by an experienced tumor specialist
- Medical or oncology consultation

Sickle Cell Retinopathy: Nonproliferative and proliferative vascular changes due to the sickling hemoglobinopathies; proliferative changes (response to retinal ischemia) are more common with SC (most severe) and S-Thal variants; patients are usually asymptomatic, but may have decreased vision, visual field defects, floaters, photopsias, scotomas, and dyschromatopsia; more common in people of African and Mediterranean descent. Follows orderly progression:

Stage I: Background (nonproliferative) stage with venous tortuosity, "salmon patch" hemorrhages (pink intraretinal hemorrhages), iridescent spots (schisis cavity with refractile elements), cotton-wool spots, hairpin vascular loops, macular infarction, angioid streaks, black "sunburst" chorioretinal scars, comma-shaped conjunctival and optic nerve head vessels, and peripheral arteriole occlusions

Stage II: Arteriovenous (AV) anastomoses stage with peripheral "silver-wire" vessels and shunt vessels between arterioles and medium-sized veins at border of perfused and nonperfused retina

Stage III: Neovascular (proliferative) stage with sea-fan peripheral neovascularization (spontaneously regresses in 60% of cases); sea-fans grow along retinal surface in a circumferential pattern

Stage IV: Vitreous hemorrhage stage with vitreous traction bands contracting around the sea-fans, causing vitreous hemorrhages (most common in SC variant, 23%)

Stage V: Retinal detachment stage with tractional/rhegmatogenous retinal detachments from contraction of the vitreous traction bands

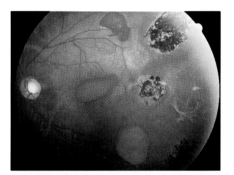

Figure 10–29 Nonproliferative sickle cell retinopathy demonstrating salmon-patch hemorrhages, iridescent spots, and black sunbursts.

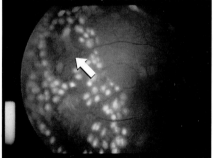

Figure 10–30 Proliferative sickle cell retinopathy demonstrating sea-fans (arrow) following laser treatment.

- Lab tests: sickle cell prep, hemoglobin electrophoresis
- Fluorescein angiogram: capillary nonperfusion near hairpin loops, enlarged foveal avascular zone, peripheral nonperfusion, arteriovenous anastomoses, and sea-fan neovascularization
- When active peripheral neovascularization develops, scatter laser photocoagulation (500 μm spots) to nonperfused retina
- If neovascularization persists, then complete panretinal photocoagulation and consider adding direct laser photocoagulation to neovascularization or feeder vessel (increases risk of complications including vitreous hemorrhage)

- Triple freeze-thaw cryotherapy for peripheral neovascularization is controversial
- Retinal surgery for retinal detachment and chronic vitreous hemorrhage (>6 months); should be performed by a retinal specialist; consider exchange transfusion preoperatively (controversial)
- Medical or hematology consultation

Diabetic Retinopathy (DR)

Definition

Retinal vascular complication of diabetes mellitus classified into nonproliferative (NPDR) and proliferative (PDR) forms.

Epidemiology

Leading cause of blindness in US population aged 20–64 years old. Insulin-dependent diabetes (IDDM, Type I) usually occurs before age 40 years; 98% of patients with IDDM get DR after 15 years; severity worsens with increasing duration of diabetes mellitus.

Non-insulin-dependent diabetes (NIDDM, Type II) usually diagnosed after age 40 years; more common form (90%); DR commonly exists at the time of diagnosis (60%) in NIDDM. Risk of DR increases with hypertension, chronic hyperglycemia, renal disease, hyperlipidemia, and pregnancy.

Symptoms

Asymptomatic, may have decreased or fluctuating vision.

Signs

NPDR: Grading of NPDR and risk of progression to PDR depends on the amount and location of hard and soft exudates, intraretinal hemorrhages, microaneurysms (MA), venous beading, and intraretinal microvascular abnormalities (IRMA). Cotton-wool spots, dot and blot hemorrhages, posterior subcapsular cataracts, and induced myopia/hyperopia (from lens swelling due to high blood sugar) are common.

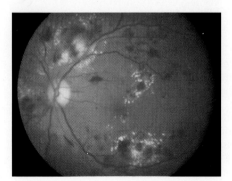

Figure 10–31 Nonproliferative diabetic retinopathy with hemorrhages, microaneurysms, and exudates.

PDR: Neovascularization of the disc (NVD) or elsewhere in the retina (NVE), preretinal and vitreous hemorrhages, and tractional retinal detachments define proliferative disease; may develop neovascularization of the iris (NVI) and subsequent neovascular glaucoma (NVG).

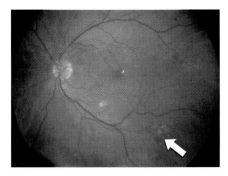

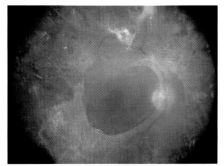

Figure 10–32 Proliferative diabetic retinopathy demonstrating florid neovascularization of the disc and elsewhere (arrow).

Figure 10–33 Proliferative diabetic retinopathy demonstrating neovascularization, fibrosis, and traction retinal detachment.

Figure 10–34 Proliferative diabetic retinopathy following laser treatment.

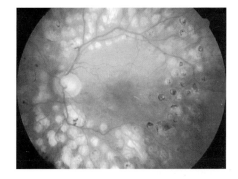

Differential Diagnosis

Hypertensive retinopathy, radiation retinopathy, retinopathy associated with blood disorders, Eales' disease.

Evaluation

- Complete ophthalmic history and eye exam with attention to tonometry, gonioscopy (NVG), iris (NVI), lens, 78/90 diopter or contact lens fundus exam, and ophthalmoscopy (retinal vascular abnormalities, optic disc [NVD], and midperiphery [NVE])
  - IDDM Type I: Examine 5 years after onset of diabetes mellitus, then annually if no retinopathy is seen

- NIDDM Type II: Examine at diagnosis of diabetes mellitus, then annually if no retinopathy is seen
- During pregnancy: Examine before pregnancy, each trimester, and 3–6 months post partum
- Fluorescein angiogram: capillary nonperfusion, neovascularization, and macular edema
- Lab tests: fasting blood glucose, hemoglobin A_{1C}, blood urea nitrogen (BUN), and creatinine
- Medical consultation with attention to blood pressure, cardiovascular system, renal system, and glucose control

Management

- Tight control of blood glucose levels (Diabetes Control and Complications Trial–DCCT conclusion)
- Laser photocoagulation using transpupillary delivery and argon green (focal/panretinal photocoagulation) or krypton red laser (panretinal photocoagulation, especially when vitreous hemorrhage or cataract is present), depending on stage of diabetic retinopathy:
  - **Clinically significant macular edema (CSME—Table 10–1):** Macular grid photocoagulation (50–100 μm spots) to areas of diffuse leakage and focal treatment to focal leaks regardless of visual acuity (Early Treatment Diabetic Retinopathy Study–ETDRS conclusion)
  - **High-risk characteristics (HR) of PDR (see Table 10–1):** Scatter panretinal photocoagulation, 1200–1600 burns, 1 burn width apart (500 μm gray-white spots) in two to three sessions (Diabetic Retinopathy Study–DRS conclusion). Treat inferior/nasal quadrants first to allow further treatment in case of subsequent vitreous hemorrhage during treatment
  - Additional indications for considering panretinal photocoagulation: Rubeosis, neovascular glaucoma, widespread retinal ischemia on fluorescein angiogram, NVE alone in Type I IDDM, poor patient compliance
  - Patients approaching high-risk PDR should have focal treatment before panretinal photocoagulation; if high-risk characteristics exist, do not delay panretinal photocoagulation for focal treatment
- Pars plana vitrectomy, endolaser, and removal of any fibrovascular complexes in patients with non-clearing vitreous hemorrhage for >6 months or vitreous hemorrhage for >1 month in Type I IDDM (Diabetic Retinopathy Vitrectomy Study–DRVS conclusions); other indications for vitreoretinal surgery include monocular patient with vitreous hemorrhage, bilateral vitreous hemorrhage, diabetic macular edema due to posterior hyaloidal traction, tractional retinal detachment (TRD) with rhegmatogenous component, or TRD involving macula; should be performed by a retina specialist

Prognosis

Early treatment allows better control. Prognosis is good for NPDR without CSME. After adequate treatment, diabetic retinopathy often becomes quiescent

Table 10–1 Diabetic Retinopathy Definitions

> ### Clinically Significant Macular Edema (CSME)
> Retinal thickening ≤ 500 μm from center of fovea *or*
> Hard exudates with adjacent thickening ≤ 500 μm from center of fovea *or*
> Retinal thickening ≥1 disc size in area ≤ 1 disc diameter from center of fovea
>
> ### High-Risk (HR) Characteristics of Proliferative Diabetic Retinopathy (PDR)
> Neovascularization of the disc (NVD) ≥ standard photo 10A used in DRS (one
> quarter to one third disc area) *or*
> Any NVD *and* vitreous hemorrhage (VH) or preretinal hemorrhage *or*
> Neovascularization elsewhere (NVE) ≥ standard photo 7 (one half disc area) *and*
> VH or preretinal hemorrhage

for extended periods of time. Complications include cataracts (often posterior sub-capsular) and neovascular glaucoma.

Hypertensive Retinopathy

Definition

Retinal vascular changes secondary to chronic or acutely (malignant) elevated systemic blood pressure.

Epidemiology

Hypertension defined as blood pressure >140/90 mm Hg; 60 million Americans over 18 years of age have hypertension; more prevalent in African Americans.

Symptoms

Asymptomatic; rarely, decreased vision.

Signs

Retinal arteriole narrowing/straightening, copper or silver-wire arteriole changes (arteriolosclerosis), arteriovenous crossing changes (nicking), cotton-wool spots, microaneurysms, flame hemorrhages, hard exudates (may be in a circinate or macular star pattern), Elschnig spots (yellow [early] or hyperpigmented [late] patches of retinal pigment epithelium overlying infarcted choriocapillaris lobules), Siegrist streaks (linear hyperpigmented areas over choroidal vessels), arterial macroaneurysms, and disc hyperemia or edema with dilated tortuous vessels (in malignant hypertension).

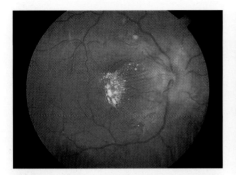 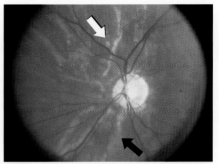

Figure 10–35 Hypertensive retinopathy with disc edema, macular star, and retinal folds in a patient with acute, malignant hypertension.

Figure 10–36 Hypertensive retinopathy demonstrating attenuated arterioles, choroidal ischemia, Elschnig spots (white arrow), and Siegrist streaks (black arrow).

Differential Diagnosis

Diabetic retinopathy, radiation retinopathy, vein occlusion, leukemic retinopathy, retinopathy of anemia, collagen vascular disease.

Evaluation

- Complete ophthalmic history and eye exam with attention to 78/90 diopter or contact lens fundus exam and ophthalmoscopy (retinal vasculature and arteriovenous crossings)
- Check blood pressure
- Fluorescein angiogram: retinal arteriole narrowing/straightening, microaneurysms, capillary nonperfusion, and macular edema
- Medical consultation with attention to cardiovascular and cerebrovascular systems

Management

- Treat underlying hypertension

Prognosis

Usually good.

Toxemia of Pregnancy

Severe hypertension, proteinuria, edema (pre-eclampsia), and seizures (eclampsia) seen in 2–5% of obstetric patients in the third trimester; patients have decreased vision, photopsias, and floaters usually just before or after delivery; signs include bullous exudative retinal detachments, focal arteriolar narrowing, cotton-wool spots, retinal hemorrhages, hard exudates, Elschnig spots, and disc edema.

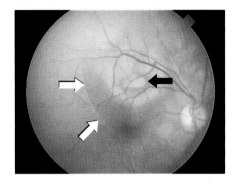

Figure 10–37 Toxemia of pregnancy with serous retinal detachment (white arrows) and yellow-white patches (black arrow).

- Usually resolves without sequelae after treating hypertension and delivery
- Obstetrics consultation

Acquired Retinal Arterial Macroaneurysm

Focal dilatation of retinal artery (>100 μm); more common in women >60 years old with hypertension or atherosclerosis. Usually asymptomatic; may cause sudden loss of vision from vitreous hemorrhage; macroaneurysms nasal to the optic disc are less likely to cause symptoms. Subretinal, intraretinal, preretinal, or vitreous hemorrhages from rupture of aneurysm, and surrounding circinate exudates are common. May spontaneously sclerose, forming a Z-shaped kink at old site.

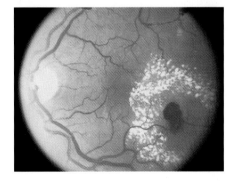

Figure 10–38 Acquired retinal arterial macroaneurysm with circinate exudate.

- Fluorescein angiogram: immediate uniform filling of the macroaneurysm with late leakage

■ Most require no treatment; laser photocoagulation to microvascular changes around leaking aneurysm if decreased acuity is present (direct treatment controversial because it may cause a vitreous hemorrhage, distal ischemia, or a branch retinal artery occlusion [BRAO]).

Radiation Retinopathy

Definition

Alteration in optic disc and retinal vascular permeability after receiving ionizing radiation.

Epidemiology

Usually requires >30–35 Gy (3000–3500 rads) total radiation dose; appears 1–2 years after ionizing radiation; diabetics and patients receiving chemotherapy have a lower threshold.

Symptoms

Decreased vision.

Signs

Microaneurysms, telangiectasia, cotton-wool spots, hard exudates, retinal hemorrhages, macular edema, vascular sheathing, disc edema, retinal/disc/iris neovascularization.

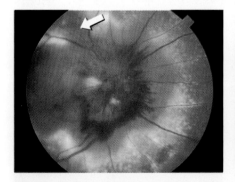 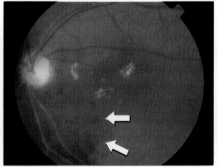

Figure 10–39 Radiation papillopathy; note regressed malignant melanoma temporally (arrow).

Figure 10–40 Radiation retinopathy with sclerotic vessels overlying regressed malignant melanoma (arrows).

Differential Diagnosis

Diabetic retinopathy, hypertensive retinopathy, retinal vascular occlusion.

Evaluation

- Complete ophthalmic history with attention to radiated field, total dose delivered, and fractionation schedule
- Complete eye exam with attention to tonometry, gonioscopy, iris, lens, 78/90 diopter or contact lens fundus exam, and ophthalmoscopy
- Fluorescein angiogram: capillary nonperfusion, macular edema, and neovascularization

Management

- Focal grid laser photocoagulation (50–100 μm spots) to areas of leakage
- Panretinal photocoagulation with 1200–1600 applications (500 μm spots) if neovascularization develops

Prognosis

Fair; complications include cataract, macular edema, choroidal neovascular membrane, optic atrophy, vitreous hemorrhage, and neovascular glaucoma.

Age-Related Macular Degeneration (ARMD)

Definition

Progressive degenerative disease of the retinal pigment epithelium, Bruch's membrane, and choriocapillaris; classified into two types: nonexudative/dry (90%) and exudative/wet (10%).

Etiology

Risk factors include increasing age (>75 years old), positive family history, cigarette smoking, hyperopia, light iris color, hypertension, and cardiovascular disease; nutritional factors and light toxicity may also play a role in pathogenesis.

Epidemiology

Leading cause of blindness in US population >65 years old, as well as most common cause of blindness in the Western world; 6.4% of patients 65–74 years old and 19.7% of patients >75 years old had signs of ARMD in the Framingham Eye Study; more prevalent in Caucasians; slight female predilection.

Symptoms

Initially asymptomatic or may have decreased vision, metamorphopsia in the nonexudative form; may have sudden, profound loss of vision or scotoma in the exudative form.

Signs

Nonexudative: Normal or decreased visual acuity; abnormal Amsler grid (central/paracentral scotomas or metamorphopsia); small, hard and larger, soft drusen, geographic atrophy of the retinal pigment epithelium, pigment clumping, and blunted foveal reflex.

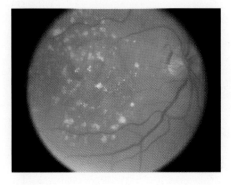

Figure 10–41 Dry, age-related macular degeneration demonstrating drusen and pigmentary changes.

Exudative: Gray-green choroidal neovascular membrane (CNVM), lipid exudates, subretinal hemorrhage/fluid, pigment epithelial detachment (PED), retinal pigment epithelial tears, and fibrovascular disciform scars.

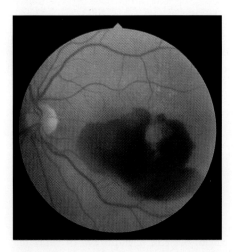

Figure 10–42 Wet, age-related macular degeneration demonstrating subretinal hemorrhage from choroidal neovascular membrane.

Differential Diagnosis

Dominant drusen, pattern dystrophy, Best's disease, central serous retinopathy, Stargardt's disease, cone dystrophy, drug toxicity, and choroidal neovascularization from other causes, including presumed ocular histoplasmosis syndrome, angioid streaks, myopic degeneration, choroidal rupture, retinal dystrophies, and optic nerve drusen.

Evaluation

- Complete ophthalmic history and eye exam with attention to Amsler grid and 78/90 diopter or contact lens fundus exam
- Fluorescein angiogram: window defects (geographic atrophy) and punctate hyperfluorescence (drusen) in nonexudative form; early hyperfluorescence and progressive leakage from CNVM in exudative form; fluorescein angiogram required to determine CNVM location, map foveal avascular zone, and within 96 hours of treatment to guide laser application
- Consider indocyanine green (ICG) angiogram if CNVM is poorly demarcated or obscured by hemorrhage on fluorescein angiogram

---

Management

- **Nonexudative:** Follow with Amsler grid qd and examine every 6 months; examine sooner if patient experiences a change in vision
- **Exudative:** Focal laser photocoagulation of CNVM depends on size, location, and visual acuity based on the results of the Macular Photocoagulation Study (MPS, Table 10–2). *Note:* only patients with a classic CNVM met eligibility criteria for the MPS study (classic CNVM: discrete, well-demarcated area of hyperfluorescence that appears in the early phase of the fluorescein angiogram and continues to increase in fluorescence in transit views, and leaks in late views); argon green or krypton red laser with a transpupillary delivery system used to form confluent (200–500 μm spots) white burns over entire CNVM
  - **Extrafoveal:** Treat entire CNV and 100 μm beyond all boundaries in all patients
  - **Juxtafoveal:** Treat entire CNV and 100 μm beyond on nonfoveal side, and up to CNV border on foveal side in all patients
  - **Subfoveal:** Treat entire CNV and 100 μm beyond all boundaries *only* in patients with poor vision (<20/400) or small lesions (<2 disc areas)
- Low vision aids and registration with blind services for patients who are legally blind (<20/200 best corrected visual acuity or <20 degree visual field in better seeing eye)
- Treatments being evaluated in clinical trials include surgical removal of CNVM, radiation therapy, photodynamic therapy, and thalidomide

---

Table 10–2   Macular Photocoagulation Study (MPS) Definitions

Extrafoveal = 200 to 2500 μm from center of foveal avascular zone (FAZ)
Juxtafoveal = 1 to 199 μm from center of FAZ *or* choroidal neovascular membrane (CNVM) 200 to 2500 μm from center of FAZ with blood or blocked fluorescence within 200 μm of FAZ center
Subfoveal = under center of FAZ

Prognosis

Variable prognosis; worse for exudative form; severe visual loss (defined as loss of >6 lines) occurs in 88% of exudative and 12% of nonexudative cases. Chance of severe visual loss is decreased with laser treatment except in subfoveal group; up to 50% recurrence rate after treatment; risk of fellow eye developing CNVM is 4–12% annually; presence of large, soft drusen and focal retinal pigment epithelium hyperpigmentation increases risk of developing exudative form (MPS conclusion).

Myopic Degeneration/Pathologic Myopia

Progressive retinal degeneration seen in high myopia (>−6.00 diopters, axial length >26.5 mm) and pathologic myopia (axial length >32.5 mm) with scleral thinning, posterior staphyloma, lacquer cracks (yellow streaks), peripapillary temporal crescent, tilted optic disc, Fuchs' spots (dark spots [RPE hyperplasia] in macula), and chorioretinal atrophy; increased incidence of posterior vitreous detachment, premature cataract formation, glaucoma, lattice degeneration, giant retinal tears, retinal detachments, and CNVM.

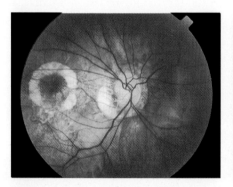
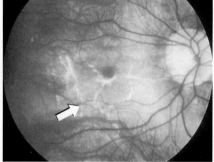

Figure 10–43 Myopic degeneration with peripapillary and macular atrophy.

Figure 10–44 Myopic degeneration with lacquer cracks (arrow).

- Correct any refractive error; contact lenses help reduce image minification and prismatic effect
- Follow for signs of complications (CNVM, retinal detachment, glaucoma, cataracts)

Angioid Streaks

Definition

Breaks in calcified, thickened Bruch's membrane.

Etiology

Idiopathic or associated with systemic diseases (50%) including pseudoxanthoma elasticum (PXE, 60%; redundant skin folds in the neck, gastrointestinal bleeding, hypertension), Paget's disease (8%; extraskeletal calcification, osteoarthritis, deafness, vertigo, increased serum alkaline phosphatase and urine calcium levels), senile elastosis, calcinosis, sickle cell disease (5%), thalassemia, hereditary spherocytosis, and Ehlers-Danlos syndrome (blue sclera, hyperextendable joints, elastic skin); also associated with optic disc drusen, Bassen-Kornzweig syndrome, and retinitis pigmentosa.

Symptoms

Asymptomatic; may have decreased vision, metamorphopsia if subretinal neovascular membrane develops.

Signs

Normal or decreased visual acuity; irregular, deep, dark red-brown streaks radiating from the optic disc in a spoke-like pattern; often have "peau d'orange" retinal pigmentation, peripheral salmon spots, and pigmentation around the streaks; may have subretinal hemorrhage/fluid, retinal pigment epithelial detachments, macular degeneration, and central/paracentral scotomas if SRNVM develops.

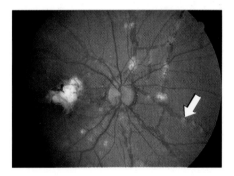

Figure 10–45 Angioid streaks appear as dark red, branching lines (arrow) radiating from the optic nerve.

Differential Diagnosis

Age-related macular degeneration, lacquer cracks, myopic degeneration, choroidal rupture, choroidal folds.

Evaluation

- Complete ophthalmic history and eye exam with attention to 78/90 diopter or contact lens fundus exam, and ophthalmoscopy
- Check Amsler grid if SRNVM is present
- Lab tests: sickle cell prep, hemoglobin electrophoresis, serum alkaline phosphatase, urine calcium, stool guaiac, skin biopsy
- Fluorescein angiogram to evaluate for SRNVM if suspected clinically
- Medical consultation to rule out systemic diseases

Management

- Treat SRNVM similar to MPS guidelines (see Age-Related Macular Degeneration section)
- Polycarbonate safety glasses because trauma can cause hemorrhages
- Treat underlying medical condition

Prognosis

Good unless SRNVM develops (high recurrence rates).

Central Serous Retinopathy (CSR)/ Idiopathic Central Serous Choroidopathy (ICSC)

Definition

Idiopathic leakage of fluid from the choroid into the subretinal space due to retinal pigment epithelium dysfunction.

Epidemiology

Usually occurs in males (10:1) age 20–50 years old; more common in Caucasians, Hispanics, and Asians; rare in African Americans; associated with type-A personality, stress, hypochondriasis, pregnancy, steroid use, and organ transplantation.

Symptoms

Decreased vision, micropsia, metamorphopsia, and mild dyschromatopsia; may be asymptomatic.

Signs

Normal or decreased visual acuity ranging from 20/20 to 20/200 (visual acuity improves with pinhole or plus lenses); induced hyperopia, abnormal Amsler grid (central/paracentral scotomas or metamorphopsia); single or multiple, round or oval-shaped, shallow, serous retinal detachment or pigment epithelial detachment (PED) with deep yellow spots at the level of the retinal pigment epithelium; areas of retinal pigment epithelium atrophy may be seen in chronic form.

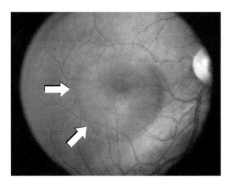

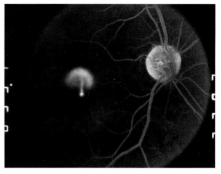

Figure 10–46 Idiopathic central serous retinopathy with large serous retinal detachment (arrows).

Figure 10–47 Same patient as shown in Figure 10–46, demonstrating classic smokestack appearance on fluorescein angiogram.

Differential Diagnosis

Age-related macular degeneration (especially in patients >50 years old), Vogt-Koyanagi-Harada syndrome, uveal effusion syndrome, toxemia of pregnancy, optic nerve pit, pigment epithelial detachment from other causes including neovascular membrane.

Evaluation

- Complete ophthalmic history and eye exam with attention to Amsler grid, 78/90 diopter or contact lens fundus exam, and ophthalmoscopy
- Fluorescein angiogram: focal dot of hyperfluorescence early that leaks in a classic smoke-stack pattern (10%) or gradually pools in the pigment epithelial detachment (90%); more than one site may be present simultaneously (30%); often see punctate window defects in other areas in both eyes (OU)

Management

- No treatment required
- Treatment considered for patients who require quicker visual rehabilitation for occupational reasons (monocular, pilots, etc), poor vision in fellow eye due to central serous retinopathy, no resolution after 4–6 months, recurrent episodes with poor vision
- Low intensity, direct laser photocoagulation to leakage site (must be >500 μm from center of macula) shortens duration by 2 months, but has no effect on final acuity or recurrence rate

Prognosis

Good; 94% regain ≥20/30 acuity; 95% of pigment epithelial detachments resolve spontaneously in 3–4 months, acuity improves over 21 months; recurrences common (45%); 5% develop subretinal neovascular membranes.

Cystoid Macular Edema (CME)

Definition

Accumulation of extracellular fluid in the macular region with characteristic cystic spaces in the outer plexiform layer and a petalloid pattern on fluorescein angiogram.

Etiology

Post-surgery (especially in older patients and if the posterior capsule is violated with vitreous loss; CME following cataract surgery is called Irvine-Gass syndrome), post-laser treatment (neodymium:yttrium-aluminum-garnet [Nd:YAG] laser capsulotomy, especially if performed within 3 months of cataract surgery), uveitis, diabetic retinopathy, juxtafoveal/retinal telangiectasia, vein occlusions, retinal vasculitis, epiretinal membrane, hereditary retinal dystrophies (dominant CME, retinitis pigmentosa), drug toxicity (epinephrine in aphakic patients), hypertensive retinopathy, collagen vascular diseases, hypotony, and chronic inflammation.

Symptoms

Decreased or washed-out vision.

Signs

Decreased visual acuity, loss of foveal reflex, thickened fovea, foveal folds, intraretinal cystoid spaces, epiretinal membrane, lipid exudates; may have signs of uveitis or surgical complications including open posterior capsule, vitreous to the wound, peaked pupil, and iris incarceration in wound.

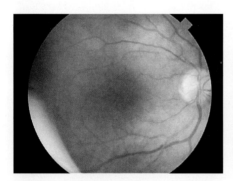
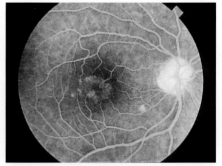

Figure 10–48 Cystoid macular edema with decreased foveal reflex.

Figure 10–49 Same patient as shown in Figure 10–48, demonstrating petalloid appearance on fluorescein angiogram.

Differential Diagnosis

Macular hole (Stage 1), foveal retinoschisis, central serous retinopathy, choroidal neovascular membrane.

Evaluation

■ Complete ophthalmic history and eye exam with attention to cornea, anterior chamber, iris, lens, 78/90 diopter or contact lens fundus exam, and ophthalmoscopy

■ Fluorescein angiogram: early, perifoveal, punctate hyperfluorescence and characteristic late leakage in a petalloid pattern. *Note:* No leakage seen in cystoid macular edema from juvenile retinoschisis, nicotinic acid (niacin) maculopathy, Goldmann-Favre disease, and some forms of retinitis pigmentosa

Management

■ Topical nonsteroidal anti-inflammatory drops ([NSAIDs], Voltaren, or Acular qid) and/or topical steroid (prednisolone acetate 1% qid for 1 month, then taper slowly)

■ If no response, consider oral NSAIDs (indomethacin 25 mg PO tid for 6–8 weeks), oral steroid (prednisone 40–60 mg PO qd for 1–2 weeks, then taper slowly), and/or oral acetazolamide (Diamox 250 mg PO bid)

■ Consider sub-Tenon's steroid injection (triamcinolone acetonide 40 mg/mL) in patients who do not respond to oral medications

■ If vitreous is present to the wound and vision is <20/80, consider Nd:YAG laser vitreolysis or perform pars plana vitrectomy and sectioning of vitreous strands (Vitrectomy-Aphakic Cystoid Macular Edema Study conclusion)

Prognosis

Usually good; spontaneous resolution in weeks to months (post-surgical); prognosis poorer for chronic CME (>6 months), may develop macular hole.

Macular Hole

Definition

Retinal hole in the fovea.

Etiology

Idiopathic; other risk factors are cystoid macular edema, trauma, post-surgical, and post-inflammatory.

Epidemiology

Senile (idiopathic) macular holes (83%) usually occur in women (3:1) aged 60–80 years old; traumatic holes rare (5%); 25–30% bilateral.

Symptoms

Decreased vision.

Signs

Decreased visual acuity ranging from 20/40 in Stage 1 to 20/200 in Stage 3/4; fundus findings can be classified into 4 stages:

Stage 1: Premacular hole (impending hole) with foveal detachment, absent foveal reflex, macular cyst (1A = yellow spot, 1B = yellow ring)

Stage 2: Early, eccentric full-thickness hole

Stage 3: Full-thickness hole (≥400 μm) with yellow deposits at level of retinal pigment epithelium (Klein's tags), operculum, cuff of subretinal fluid, cystoid macular edema, and positive Watzke's sign (subjective interruption of slit beam on biomicroscopy)

Stage 4: Stage 3 and posterior vitreous detachment (PVD)

Retinal detachments rare except in high myopes.

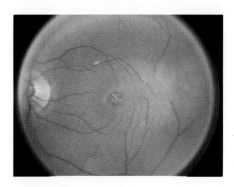

Figure 10–50 Macular hole.

Differential Diagnosis

Epiretinal membrane with pseudo-hole, solar retinopathy, central serous retinopathy, vitreomacular traction syndrome, cystoid macular edema.

Evaluation

- Complete ophthalmic history and eye exam with attention to visual acuity, Amsler grid, Watzke's test, 78/90 diopter or contact lens fundus exam, and ophthalmoscopy

Management

- No treatment recommended for Stage 1 holes because spontaneous hole closure can occur

> ### Management Continued
>
> - Pars plana vitrectomy, membrane peel, gas fluid exchange, and gas injection for full-thickness holes of recent onset (<1½ years); use of adjuvant agents including autologous serum, platelets, and tissue glue—still controversial; should be performed by a retina specialist

Prognosis

Good for recent onset holes; surgery has successful anatomic results in 60–90% depending on duration, of which 73% have improved acuity; poor prognosis for holes >1 year's duration.

Epiretinal Membrane/Macular Pucker

Definition

Cellular proliferation along the internal limiting membrane and retinal surface. Contraction of this membrane causes the retinal surface to become wrinkled (pucker/cellophane maculopathy).

Etiology

Risk factors include prior retinal surgery, intraocular inflammation, vitreous hemorrhage, trauma, laser photocoagulation, and cryotherapy; often idiopathic.

Epidemiology

Incidence increases with increasing age; occurs in 2–10% of population >50 years old and in 20% >75 years old; 10–20% bilateral; slight female predilection (3:2).

Symptoms

Asymptomatic; decreased vision, metamorphopsia, macropsia, or monocular diplopia if macular pucker exists.

Signs

Normal or decreased visual acuity; abnormal Amsler grid; thin, translucent membrane appears as mild sheen (cellophane) along macula; may have dragged vessels, retinal striae, pseudo-holes, and cystoid macular edema.

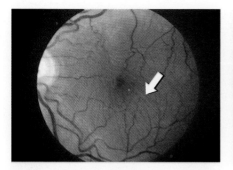

Figure 10–51 Epiretinal membrane and macular pucker with retinal striae (arrow).

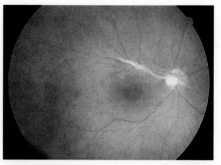

Figure 10–52 Epiretinal membrane with macular pucker and dragged vessels.

Differential Diagnosis

Traction retinal detachment from diabetic retinopathy, sickle cell retinopathy, or radiation retinopathy; choroidal folds.

Evaluation

- Complete ophthalmic history and eye exam with attention to 78/90 diopter or contact lens fundus exam, and ophthalmoscopy

Management

- Treatment rarely required
- Pars plana vitrectomy and membrane peel in patients with reduced acuity (eg, <20/60) or intractable symptoms; should be performed by a retina specialist

Prognosis

Good; 75% of patients have improvement in symptoms and acuity after surgery.

Myelinated Nerve Fibers

Abnormal myelination of ganglion cell axons anterior to the lamina cribrosa; appears as yellow-white patches with feathery borders in the superficial retina (nerve fiber layer); typically unilateral (80%) and occurs adjacent to the optic nerve, but can be located anywhere in the posterior pole; obscures underlying retinal vasculature and can be confused with cotton-wool spots, astrocytic hamartomas, commotio retinae, or rarely retinal artery occlusion if extensive. Patients are usually asymptomatic, but scotomas corresponding to the areas of myelination can be demonstrated on visual fields; slight male predilection.

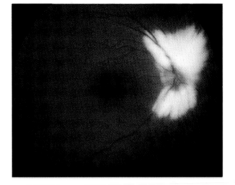

Figure 10–53 Myelinated nerve fibers.

- No treatment required
- Consider visual fields

Solar/Photic Retinopathy

Bilateral decreased vision (20/40 to 20/100), metamorphopsia, photophobia, dyschromatopsia, after-images, scotomas, headaches, and orbital pain 1–4 hours after unprotected, long-term sun gazing. Retinal damage ranges from no changes to yellow spot with surrounding pigmentary changes in the foveolar region in the early stages. Late changes include lamellar holes or depressions in the fovea. Vision can improve over 3–6 months, with residual scotomas and metamorphopsia. Similar problems may occur from lasers, welding arcs, and extended exposure to operating-room microscope lights (unilateral).

- No effective treatment

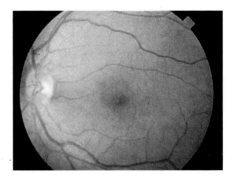

Figure 10–54 Solar retinopathy. Note pigmentary changes in the macula.

Toxic/Drug Maculopathies

Aminoglycosides (Gentamicin/Tobramicin/Amikacin): Acute, severe, permanent visual loss after intraocular injection of toxic doses. Retinal toxic reaction with marked retinal whitening (especially in macula) and retinal hemorrhages seen after injecting 0.1 mg of gentamicin (also described after diffusion through cataract wound from subconjunctival injection). Optic atrophy and pigmentary changes occur later. Visual prognosis is poor.

- Fluorescein angiogram: sharp zones of capillary nonperfusion corresponding to the areas of ischemic retina
- No effective treatment

Canthaxanthine: Usually asymptomatic or produces mild metamorphopsia and decreased vision while this oral tanning agent is being taken. Refractile yellow spots in a wreath-like pattern around the fovea (gold-dust retinopathy). Seen with cumulative doses >35 g.

- Check visual fields (central 10 degrees)
- Decrease or discontinue the medication if toxicity develops

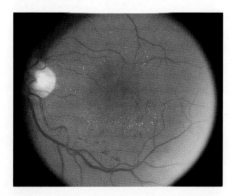

Figure 10–55 Crystalline maculopathy due to canthaxanthine.

Chloroquine (Aralen)/Hydroxychloroquine (Plaquenil): Produces central/paracentral scotomas, nyctalopia, photopsias, dyschromatopsia, and photophobia. Early changes include loss of foveal reflex and abnormal macular pigmentation; "bull's eye" maculopathy, peripheral bone spicules, vasculature attenuation, and disc pallor appear later; may also develop whorl-like subepithelial corneal deposits (corneal verticillata, vortex keratopathy). Doses >3.5 mg/kg/day or 300 g total (chloroquine), and >6.5 mg/kg/day or 700 g total (hydroxychloroquine) may produce the maculopathy; often progresses after medications are discontinued.

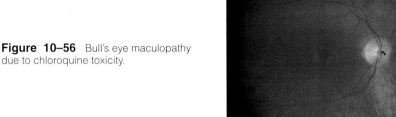

Figure 10–56 Bull's eye maculopathy due to chloroquine toxicity.

- Fluorescein angiogram: hypofluorescence with ring of hyperfluorescence corresponding to the bull's eye lesion, often visible before fundus lesion
- Check color vision, red Amsler grid, and visual fields (central 10 degrees with red test object)
- Electro-oculogram (EOG) (reduced [<1.6] light-to-dark [Arden] ratio)
- Re-examine every 6 months while patient is taking medications
- Decrease or discontinue the medication if toxicity develops

Talc: Refractive yellow deposits near or in arterioles seen in IV drug abusers; Similar picture occurs in IV drug abusers injecting suspensions of crushed methylphenidate (Ritalin) tablets.

- No effective treatment

Tamoxifen: Produces decreased vision. Refractile yellow-white spots scattered throughout the posterior pole, cystoid macular edema, and retinal pigmentary changes; may develop whorl-like, white, subepithelial corneal deposits. Seen with doses >30 mg/day.

- Decrease or discontinue the medication if toxicity develops

Thioridazine (Mellaril): Produces nyctalopia, decreased vision, ring/paracentral scotomas, and brown discoloration of vision. Pigment granularity in the midperiphery appears first, then progresses and coalesces into large areas of pigmentation or chorioretinal atrophy with short-term, high-dose use. A variant nummular retinopathy with chorioretinal atrophy posterior to the equator occurs with chronic use. Doses >800 mg/day (300 mg recommended) can produce retinopathy; may progress after medication is withdrawn.

- Check color vision and visual fields
- Electroretinogram (ERG) (reduced amplitude, abnormal dark adaptation)
- Decrease or discontinue the medication if toxicity develops

Lipid Storage Diseases

Sphingolipid storage diseases cause accumulation of ceramide in liposomes, especially in retinal ganglion cells, giving a characteristic cherry-red spot in the macula.

Farber's Disease (Glycolipid) (Autosomal Recessive [AR]): Mild cherry-red spot, failure to thrive, subcutaneous nodules, hoarse cry, progressive arthropathy, and early mortality by 6–18 years of age.

Mucolipidosis (Mucopolysaccharidoses) (AR): Cherry-red spot, nystagmus, myoclonus, corneal clouding, optic atrophy, cataracts, Hurler-like facies, hepatosplenomegaly, and failure to thrive.

Niemann-Pick Disease (Ceramide Phosphatidyl Choline) (AR): Prominent cherry-red spot, corneal stromal opacities, splenomegaly, bone marrow foam cells, and hyperlipidemia.

Sandhoff's Disease (Gangliosidosis Type II) (AR): Prominent cherry-red spot and optic atrophy with associated lipid storage problems in the kidney, liver, pancreas, and other gastrointestinal organs.

Tay-Sachs Disease (Gangliosidosis Type I) (AR): Prominent cherry-red spot, blindness, deafness, convulsions. Mainly in Ashkenazic Jewish children.

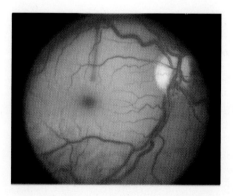

Figure 10–57 Cherry-red spot in an infant with Tay-Sachs disease.

Peripheral Retinal Degenerations

Lattice Degeneration: Occurs in 8–10% of general population; more common in myopes; oval, circumferential area of retinal thinning and overlying vitreous liquefaction found anterior to the equator. Appears as criss-crossing, white lines (sclerotic vessels) with variable overlying retinal pigmentation. Atrophic holes (25%) common; retinal tears can occur with posterior vitreous separation pulling on the atrophic, thinned retina; increased risk of retinal detachment.

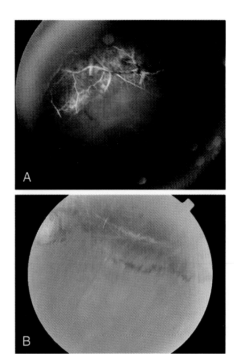

Figure 10–58 Lattice degeneration.

- Asymptomatic lattice degeneration, atrophic holes, and retinal tears do not require treatment; *consider* prophylactic treatment in patients with high myopia, aphakia, history of retinal detachment in the fellow eye, or strong family history of retinal detachment. Prophylactic treatment before cataract extraction is controversial.
- Symptomatic lesions (photopsias/floaters) should receive prophylactic treatment with either cryopexy (anterior lesions) or two to three rows of laser photocoagulation around tears or holes (posterior lesions)

Pavingstone/Cobblestone Degeneration: Occurs in 22–27% of general population; round, discrete, yellow-white lesions with darkly pigmented borders found anterior to the equator; correspond to areas of thinned outer retina with loss of choriocapillaris and retinal pigment epithelium; usually found inferiorly; normal vitreous over lesions. May protect against retinal detachment due to adherence of thinned retina and choroid.

- No treatment recommended

Peripheral Cystoid Degeneration: Clusters of tiny intraretinal cysts (in the outer plexiform layer) just posterior to ora serrata; retinoschisis precursor; no increased risk of retinal detachment.

- No treatment recommended

Snail Track Degeneration: Chains of fine, white dots seen circumferentially in the peripheral retina; associated with myopia; atrophic holes may develop in the areas of degeneration, increasing the risk of retinal detachment.

- Asymptomatic snail track degeneration, atrophic holes, and tears do not require treatment; *consider* prophylactic treatment in patients with high myopia, aphakia, history of retinal detachment in the fellow eye, or strong family history of retinal detachment. Prophylactic treatment before cataract extraction is controversial.
- Symptomatic lesions (photopsias/floaters) should receive prophylactic treatment with either cryopexy (anterior lesions) or two to three rows of laser photocoagulation around tears or holes (posterior lesions)

Retinoschisis

Definition
Splitting of the retina. Two types:

Acquired: Senile, degenerative process with splitting between the inner nuclear and outer plexiform layers.

Juvenile: Congenital process with splitting of the nerve fiber layer.

Epidemiology
Acquired: More common; seen in 4–7% of general population especially in patients >50 years old; 75% bilateral; also associated with hyperopia.

Juvenile (X-Linked Recessive): Mapped to chromosome Xp22; rarely autosomal; 98% bilateral.

Symptoms
Acquired: Usually asymptomatic, may have visual field defect with sharp borders.

Juvenile: Decreased vision; may have eye turn.

Signs
Acquired: Bilateral, smooth, convex, elevated schisis cavity usually in inferotemporal quadrant; height of elevation constant even with change in head position; white dots and retinal vessels (sclerotic in periphery) are seen in the elevated retinal layer; outer layer breaks are common; inner layer breaks, vitreous hemorrhage, and rhegmatogenous retinal detachments are rare.

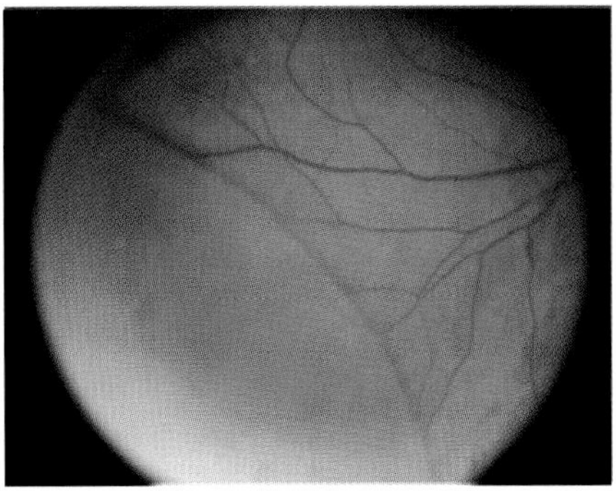

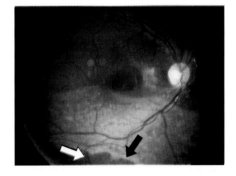

Figure 10–59 Acquired retinoschisis.

Juvenile: Decreased visual acuity ranging from 20/40 to 20/80, nystagmus, and strabismus are often seen; foveal schisis with fine, radiating folds from fovea, spoke-like foveal cysts, pigment mottling, and microcystic foveal elevation (looks like cystoid macular edema) common; may have vitreous hemorrhage, vitreous veils, retinal vessels bridging inner and outer layers; peripheral schisis (50%) with peripheral pigmentation and loss of retinal vessels, especially in inferotemporal quadrant, often seen.

Figure 10–60 Juvenile retinoschisis with foveal and peripheral schisis (black arrow); note bridging retinal vessel (white arrow).

Differential Diagnosis

Retinal detachment, Goldmann-Favre disease, hereditary macular disease.

Evaluation

- Complete ophthalmic history and eye exam with attention to color vision, 78/90 diopter or contact lens fundus exam, ophthalmoscopy, and depressed peripheral retinal exam
- Check visual fields
- Electroretinogram (ERG) (decreased b-wave, normal a-wave), electro-oculogram (EOG) (normal to subnormal in advanced cases), and dark adaptation (normal to subnormal) in juvenile form
- Fluorescein angiogram: macular cysts seen in foveal schisis do not leak fluorescein

Management

- No treatment recommended; follow closely if breaks are identified
- If symptomatic retinal detachment occurs, may require retinal surgery to repair
- If vitreous hemorrhage occurs, treat conservatively (occlusive patching in child); rarely, pars plana vitrectomy required

Prognosis

Good; usually stationary for years.

Retinal Detachment (RD)

Definition

Separation of the neurosensory retina from the retinal pigment epithelium; two different types:

Rhegmatogenous Retinal Detachment (RRD): From Greek rhegma = rent; retinal detachment due to full-thickness retinal break (tear/hole/dialysis) that allows vitreous fluid access to subretinal space.

Non-Rhegmatogenous Retinal Detachment: Retinal detachment not due to retinal break. Two types:

- **Serous/exudative:** Retinal detachment due to subretinal transudation of fluid from tumor, inflammatory process, or degenerative lesion
- **Traction (TRD):** Retinal detachment due to fibrovascular proliferation and subsequent contraction pulling on retina

Etiology

Rhegmatogenous Retinal Detachment: Lattice degeneration (30%), posterior vitreous detachment (especially with vitreous hemorrhage), myopia, trauma (5–10%), and previous ocular surgery (especially with vitreous loss) increase risk of rhegmatogenous retinal detachments; retinal dialysis and giant retinal tears (>3 clock hours in extent) common after trauma.

Serous/Exudative Retinal Detachment: Vogt-Koyanagi-Harada syndrome, Harada's disease, uveal effusion syndrome, choroidal tumors, central serous retinopathy, posterior scleritis, hypertensive retinopathy, Coats' disease, optic nerve pit, retinal coloboma, and toxemia of pregnancy most common.

Traction Retinal Detachment: Diabetic retinopathy, sickle cell retinopathy, retinopathy of prematurity, proliferative vitreoretinopathy, toxocariasis, and familial exudative vitreoretinopathy most common.

Symptoms

Acute onset of photopsias, floaters ("shade" or "cob-webs"), shadow across visual field, decreased vision; may be asymptomatic.

Signs

Rhegmatogenous Retinal Detachment: Undulating, mobile, convex, with corrugated folds; retinal break usually seen; may have "tobacco-dust" (Shafer's sign: pigment cells in the vitreous), vitreous hemorrhage, or operculum; chronic rhegmatogenous retinal detachments may have pigmented demarcation lines and intraretinal cysts. Configuration of detachment helps localize retinal break:

(1) Superotemporal/nasal detachment: break within 1–1.5 clock hours of highest border
(2) Superior detachment that straddles 12 o'clock: break between 11 and 1 o'clock
(3) Inferior detachment with one higher side: break within 1–1.5 clock hours of highest border
(4) Inferior detachment equally high on either side: break between 5 and 7 o'clock

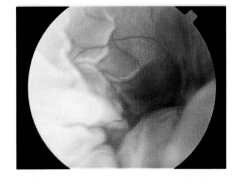

Figure 10–61 Rhegmatogenous retinal detachment.

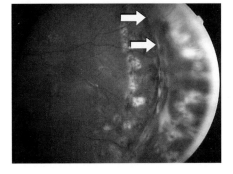

Figure 10–62 Appearance of retina overlying scleral buckle (arrows) following retinal detachment surgery; note laser scars on buckle and retinal periphery.

Serous/Exudative Retinal Detachment: Smooth, serous elevation; subretinal fluid shifts with changing head position.

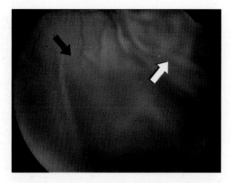

Figure 10–63 Exudative retinal detachment (black arrow) secondary to malignant melanoma (white arrow).

Traction Retinal Detachment: Smooth, concave, usually localized, does not extend to the ora serrata; often with fibrovascular proliferation and pseudo-holes.

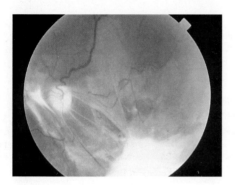

Figure 10–64 Traction retinal detachment due to proliferative vitreoretinopathy following penetrating ocular trauma.

Differential Diagnosis

Retinoschisis, choroidal detachment.

Evaluation

- Complete ophthalmic history and eye exam with attention to visual acuity, pupils, ophthalmoscopy, and depressed peripheral retinal exam to identify any retinal breaks
- B-scan ultrasonography if unable to visualize the fundus: smooth, convex, freely mobile (rhegmatogenous retinal detachment), or tented with vitreous adhesions (traction retinal detachment), retina appears as highly reflective echo in the vitreous cavity that is attached at the optic nerve head and ora serrata

Management

- **Asymptomatic Rhegmatogenous Retinal Detachment,** *not* **Threatening Macula:** May follow closely by retina specialist, usually consider treatment (see below); should be performed by a retina specialist
- **Symptomatic Rhegmatogenous Retinal Detachment:** Pneumatic retinopexy or retinal surgery with scleral buckle, cryotherapy, pars plana vitrectomy, drainage, endolaser, and/or other surgical maneuvers. Macular threatening ("Mac on") rhegmatogenous retinal detachment is treated emergently (within 24 hours); if macula is already detached ("Mac off"), treat urgently (within 48 to 96 hours)
- **Serous/Exudative Retinal Detachment:** Treat underlying condition; rarely requires surgical intervention
- **Traction Retinal Detachment:** Retinal surgery to release the vitreoretinal traction depending on clinical situation

Prognosis

Variable (depends on underlying condition); 5–10% of rhegmatogenous retinal detachment repairs develop proliferative vitreoretinopathy (PVR).

Choroidal Detachment

Smooth, bullous, orange-brown elevation of retina and choroid. Two forms:

Choroidal Effusion: Often asymptomatic with decreased intraocular pressure, may have shallow anterior chamber; associated with acute ocular hypotony, post-surgical (excessive filtration through filtering bleb, wound leak, cyclodialysis cleft, post-scleral buckling surgery), posterior scleritis, Vogt-Koyanagi-Harada syndrome, trauma (open globe), intraocular tumors, or uveal effusion syndrome.

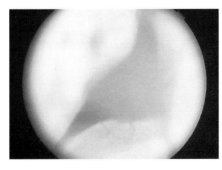

Figure 10–65 Choroidal detachment.

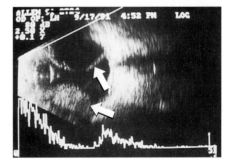

Figure 10–66 B-scan ultrasonogram of patient shown in Figure 10–65, demonstrating the choroidal detachment (arrows).

Choroidal Hemorrhage: Causes pain (often severe), decreased vision, red eye, intraocular inflammation, and increased intraocular pressure; classically occurring acutely during anterior segment surgery, but may be delayed up to 1–7 days after surgery or after rupture of choroidal neovascular membrane (CNVM).

- B-scan ultrasonography: smooth, convex, elevated membrane limited in the equatorial region by the vortex veins and anteriorly by the scleral spur; appears thicker and less mobile than retina
- Treat intraoperative choroidal hemorrhage with immediate closure of surgical wound and if massive hemorrhage, perform sclerotomies to allow drainage of blood
- Topical cycloplegic (atropine 1% bid) and steroid (prednisolone acetate 1% qid)
- May require treatment of increased intraocular pressure (see Chap. 11)
- Consider surgical drainage when "kissing" (temporal and nasal choroid touch), severe intraocular pressure elevation despite maximal medical treatment, or corneal decompensation
- Treat underlying condition

Proliferative Vitreoretinopathy (PVR)

Fibrotic membranes composed of retinal pigment epithelial, glial, and inflammatory cells that form after retinal surgery (8–10%); the membranes contract and pull on the retinal surface (6–8 weeks after surgery); may be preretinal or subretinal; primary cause of redetachment after successful retinal detachment surgery. Risk factors include previous retinal surgery, vitreous hemorrhage, choroidal detachment, giant retinal tears, penetrating trauma, excessive cryotherapy, and failure to reattach the retina at primary surgery. Final anatomic reattachment rates 72–96%, visual prognosis variable (14–37% achieve > 20/100 vision).

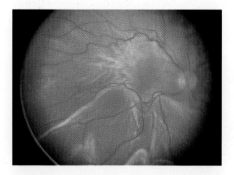

Figure 10–67 Retinal detachment with proliferative vitreoretinopathy.

- Retinal surgery to remove fibrotic membranes and reattach retina using silicon oil or intraocular C_3F_8 gas injection (The Silicon Oil Study conclusions); should be performed by a retina specialist

Neuroretinitis/Leber's Idiopathic Stellate Neuroretinitis

Definition

Optic disc edema and macular star formation with no other systemic abnormalities.

Etiology

Due to pleomorphic gram-negative bacillus *Bartonella henselae* (formerly known as *Rochalimaea*); associated with cat-scratch disease.

Symptoms

Mild, unilateral decreased vision, rarely pain with eye movement; may have viral prodrome (52%) with fever, malaise, lymphadenopathy, upper respiratory, gastrointestinal, or urinary tract infection.

Signs

Decreased visual acuity, visual field defects (cecocentral/central scotomas), positive relative afferent pupillary defect (RAPD), optic disc edema with macular star, peripapillary exudative retinal detachment, vitreous cells, rare anterior chamber cell/flare, yellow-white lesions at level of retinal pigment epithelium.

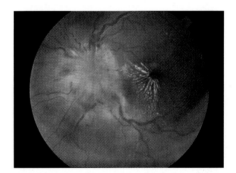

Figure 10–68 Leber's idiopathic stellate neuroretinitis demonstrating optic disc edema and partial macular star.

Differential Diagnosis

Hypertensive retinopathy, diabetic retinopathy, anterior ischemic optic neuropathy (AION), retinal vein occlusion, syphilis, diffuse unilateral subacute neuroretinitis (DUSN), acute macular neuroretinopathy, viral retinitis, sarcoidosis, toxocariasis, toxoplasmosis, tuberculosis, papilledema.

Evaluation

- Complete ophthalmic history and eye exam with attention to pupils, 78/90 diopter and contact lens fundus exam, and ophthalmoscopy

- Fluorescein angiogram: leakage from optic disc capillaries, no perifoveal leakage
- Lab tests: Venereal Disease Research Laboratory (VDRL), fluorescent treponemal antibody absorption test (FTA-ABS), purified protein derivative (PPD), indirect fluorescent antibody test for *Bartonella henselae (Rochalimaea)*
- Check blood pressure

Management

- No treatment recommended
- Use of systemic antibiotics (doxycycline, tetracycline, ciprofloxacin, trimethoprim [Bactrim]) and steroids is controversial

Prognosis

Good; 67% regain ≥20/20 vision, and 97% >20/40 vision; usually spontaneous recovery; disc edema resolves over 8–12 weeks, macular star over 6–12 months; optic atrophy may develop.

Infections

Acute Retinal Necrosis (ARN): Fulminant retinitis/vitritis due to the herpes zoster virus (HZV), herpes simplex virus (HSV), or, rarely, cytomegalovirus (CMV) seen in healthy, as well as immunocompromised, patients. Slight male predilection (2:1); patients have pain, decreased vision, and floaters after a recent herpes simplex or zoster infection. Starts with small, yellow lesions that spread rapidly into large, confluent areas of white, retinal necrosis with retinal vascular occlusions and small satellite lesions; 36% bilateral (BARN); associated with granulomatous anterior uveitis and retinal vasculitis. In the cicatricial phase (1–3 months later), retinal detachments (50–75%) with multiple holes and giant tears are common; poor visual prognosis (only 30% achieve >20/200 vision).

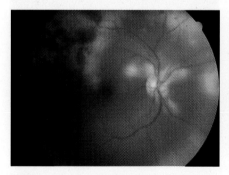

Figure 10–69 Acute retinal necrosis.

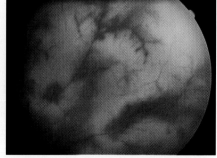

Figure 10–70 Acute retinal necrosis in same patient as shown in Figure 10–69, 2 days later.

- Lab tests: HZV and HSV (type 1 and 2) immunoglobulin G and M titers
- Systemic antivirals (acyclovir 5–10 mg/kg IV in three divided doses qd for 1 week, then 800 mg PO 5x/day for 1–2 months); follow blood urea nitrogen (BUN) and creatinine levels for nephrotoxicity
- 24 hours *after* acyclovir started, oral steroids (prednisone 60–100 mg PO qd for 1–2 months with slow taper); check PPD, blood glucose, and chest radiographs before starting systemic steroids
- Add H_2-blocker (ranitidine [Zantac] 150 mg PO bid) when giving systemic steroids
- 24 hours *after* acyclovir started, topical steroid (prednisolone acetate 1% q2–6h) and cycloplegic (atropine 1% bid) for 1–2 weeks
- If treatment fails, fulminant course, or patient is HIV-positive, then consider IV ganciclovir and/or foscarnet, as well as intravitreal foscarnet injections (see doses in Cytomegalovirus section)
- Role of anticoagulation is controversial
- Consider three to four rows of laser photocoagulation to demarcate active areas of retinitis and necrosis to prevent retinal breaks and retinal detachments (controversial)
- Laser demarcation or retinal surgery for retinal detachments; usually requires use of silicon oil
- Medical consultation

Candidiasis: Endogenous endophthalmitis caused by fungal *Candida* species (*C. albicans* or *C. tropicalis*) with white, fluffy, chorioretinal infiltrates and overlying vitreous haze; vitreous puff-balls, anterior chamber cell/flare, hypopyon, Roth spots, and hemorrhages occur less often. Occurs in IV drug abusers and debilitated or immunocompromised patients who have decreased vision and floaters.

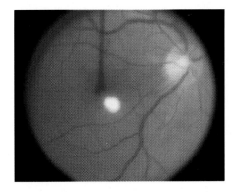

Figure 10–71 Candidiasis.

- Lab tests: sputum, urine, blood, and stool cultures for fungi
- Systemic antifungal (fluconazole 100 mg PO bid or amphotericin B 0.25–1.0 mg/kg IV over 6h) if disseminated disease is present
- If moderate to severe inflammation, pars plana vitrectomy and intraocular injection of antifungal (amphotericin B 0.005 mg/0.1 mL) and steroid (dexamethasone 0.4 mg/0.1 mL)
- Topical steroid (prednisolone acetate 1% qid) and cycloplegic (scopolamine 0.25% bid to qid)
- Medical consultation to treat systemic source of infection

Cysticercosis: Subretinal or intravitreal, round, mobile, translucent, yellow-white cyst due to *Cysticercus cellulosae,* the larval form of the tapeworm *Taenia solium*; asymptomatic until the parasite grows and causes painless, progressive, decreased vision and visual field defects. Worm death may incite an inflammatory response. Can also have central nervous system (CNS) involvement with seizures, hydrocephalus, and headaches.

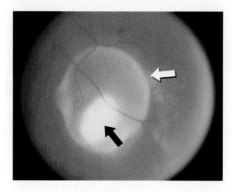

Figure 10–72 Cysticercosis with cyst (white arrow) surrounding the tapeworm (black arrow).

- B-scan ultrasonography: highly reflective echoes from the cyst walls and often the worm within the cystic space
- Lab tests: enzyme-linked immunosorbent assay (ELISA) for anticysticercus immunoglobulin G
- No antihelminthic medication is effective for intraocular infection
- Consider direct laser photocoagulation of worm
- Pars plana vitrectomy for removal of intravitreal cysticercus
- Neurology consultation to rule out CNS involvement

Cytomegalovirus (CMV): Well-circumscribed, hemorrhagic retinitis with thick, yellow-white retinal necrosis, vascular sheathing (severe sheathing with frosted-branch appearance may occur outside of area of retinitis), mild anterior chamber cell/flare, vitreous cells, and retinal hemorrhages. Brush-fire appearance with indolent, granular, yellow advancing border and peripheral, atrophic region is also common. Retinal detachments (15–50%) with multiple, small, peripheral breaks commonly occur in atrophic areas. Patients are usually asymptomatic, but may have floaters, paracentral scotomas, metamorphopsia, and decreased acuity. Bilateral on presentation in 40%; 15–20% become bilateral after treatment. Most common retinal infection in acquired immunodeficiency syndrome (AIDS; 15–46%) especially when CD4 <50 cells/mm^3.

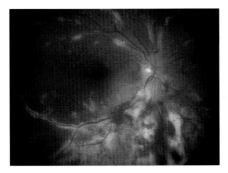

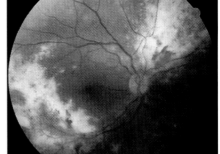

Figure 10–73 Cytomegalovirus retinitis.   **Figure 10–74** Cytomegalovirus retinitis.

- Lab tests: human immunodeficiency virus (HIV) test, CD4 count, urine for CMV; consider CMV polymerase chain reaction (PCR) assay
- If first episode, induction therapy with either:
  - Ganciclovir (Cytovene 5–7.5 mg/kg IV bid for 2–4 weeks then maintenance with 5–10 mg/kg IV qd); follow CBC for neutropenia (worsened by zidovudine [formerly AZT]) and thrombocytopenia; if bone marrow suppression is severe, add recombinant granulocyte colony stimulating factor (G-CSF) (filgrastim [Neupogen]) or recombinant granulocyte-macrophage colony stimulating factor (GM-CSF) (sargramostim [Leukine])
  - Foscarnet (Foscavir, 90 mg/kg IV bid or 60 mg/kg IV tid for 2 weeks, then maintenance with 90–120 mg/kg IV qd); infuse slowly with 500–1000 mL normal saline or 5% dextrose; push liquids to avoid dehydration; follow electrolytes (potassium, phosphorus, calcium, and magnesium), BUN, and creatinine for nephrotoxicity; avoid other nephrotoxic medications
    Note: Foscarnet-Ganciclovir CMV Retinitis Trial showed equal efficacy between foscarnet and ganciclovir; possible survival advantage with IV foscarnet
  - Cidofovir (Vistide, 3–5 mg/kg IV every week for 2 weeks, then maintenance with 3–5 mg/kg IV q2wk) and probenecid (1 g PO before infusion, 2 mg PO after infusion); does not work in patients with ganciclovir resistance; follow BUN and creatinine for nephrotoxicity
- Alternatively, combination of intravitreal surgical implantation of a ganciclovir pellet (releases 1 μg per hour, lasts ~6–8 months) and oral ganciclovir (1000–2000 mg PO tid) for systemic CMV prophylaxis; good choice in new onset, unilateral cases; do not use in recurrent cases; should be performed by retina specialist
- Recurrence/progression can be re-induced with same regimen or new drug regimen (mean time to relapse ~60 days in Foscarnet-Ganciclovir CMV Retinitis Trial)
- Treatment failures should be induced with new drug or a combination of drugs (use lower dosages due to the higher risk of toxic side effects); combination treatment is effective against disease progression (Cytomegalovirus Retreatment Trial conclusion)
- Intravitreal injections can be used if there is an intolerance to antiviral therapy or progressive retinitis despite systemic treatment (should be performed by retina specialist):
  - Ganciclovir (Cytovene, 200–2000 μg/0.1 mL 2 to 3 times a week for 2–3 weeks then maintenance with 200–2000 μg/0.1 mL once a week)

- Foscarnet (Foscavir, 2.4 mg/0.1 mL or 1.2 mg/0.05 mL 2 to 3 times a week for 2–3 weeks, then maintenance with 2.4 mg/0.1 mL 1 to 2 times a week)
- Follow monthly with serial photography (60-degree, nine peripheral fields) to document inactivity/progression
- Retinal detachments that threaten the macula with no macular retinitis may be treated with pars plana vitrectomy, endolaser, and silicon oil tamponade; peripheral shallow detachments may be followed closely (especially inferiorly) or demarcated with two to three rows of laser photocoagulation
- Medical consultation

Diffuse Unilateral Subacute Neuroretinitis (DUSN): Unilateral, indolent, multifocal, diffuse pigmentary changes with gray-yellow outer retinal lesions that reflect the movement of a subretinal nematode: *Ancylostoma caninum* (dog hook- worm, 400–1000 µm, endemic in southeastern United States, South America, and the Caribbean) or *Baylisascaris procyonis* (raccoon intestinal worm, 1500–2000 µm, endemic in northern and midwestern United States). Usually minimal intraocular inflammation; occurs in healthy patients with decreased vision (often out of proportion to retinal findings); may have a positive relative afferent pupillary defect (RAPD). Chronic infection causes poor vision (20/200), visual field defects, optic nerve pallor, and narrowed retinal vessels in a retinitis pigmentosa-like pattern.

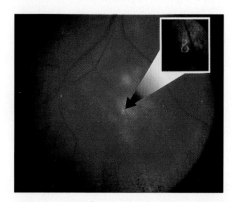

Figure 10–75   Diffuse unilateral subacute neuroretinitis demonstrating subretinal nematode (inset).

- Complete history with attention to travel and animal exposure
- Fluorescein angiogram: lesions hypofluorescent early and stain late, more advanced disease shows widespread window defects
- Lab tests: stool for ova and parasites
- Electroretinogram (ERG) (subnormal, loss of b-wave) helps differentiate from optic nerve abnormalities
- Only effective treatment is direct laser photocoagulation of the worm
- Systemic antihelminthic medications (thiabendazole, diethylcarbamazine, pyrantel pamoate) are controversial, since worm death may increase inflammation

Human Immunodeficiency Virus (HIV): Asymptomatic, nonprogressive, microangiopathy characterized by multiple cotton-wool spots (50–70%), Roth spots (40%), retinal hemorrhages, and microaneurysms in the posterior pole that resolves without treatment within 1–2 months. Seen in up to 50% of patients.

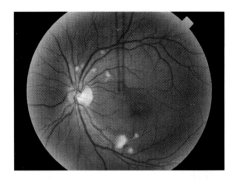

Figure 10–76 Human immunodeficiency virus retinopathy demonstrating cotton-wool spots and one intraretinal hemorrhage.

- Lab tests: HIV test, CD4 count
- No treatment necessary
- Medical consultation

Pneumocystis carinii Choroidopathy: Asymptomatic, multifocal, round, creamy, yellow choroidal infiltrates located in the posterior pole caused by disseminated infection from the opportunistic organism *Pneumocystis carinii*; enlarge slowly with minimal vitreous inflammation; may be bilateral; resolution takes weeks to months after therapy is initiated; has become very rare with the elimination of aerosolized pentamidine prophylaxis.

- Lab tests: induced sputum or bronchoalveolar lavage (BAL) for histopathologic staining
- Fluorescein angiogram: early hypofluorescence with late staining of lesions
- Systemic antibiotics (trimethoprim 20 mg/kg and sulfamethoxazole 100 mg/kg divided equally IV qid) or pentamidine isethionate (slow infusion 4 mg/kg IV qd) for 14–21 days
- Medical consultation

Presumed Ocular Histoplasmosis Syndrome (POHS): Small, round, yellow-brown, punched-out chorioretinal lesions ("histo spots") in midperiphery and posterior pole, and juxtapapillary atrophic changes caused by the dimorphic fungus, *Histoplasma capsulatum*; endemic in the Ohio and Mississippi river valleys; no vitritis; histo spots occur in 2–3% of population in endemic areas; rare in African Americans; usually asymptomatic; macular disciform lesions can occur due to choroidal neovascular membranes (CNVM); better visual prognosis than CNVM due to age-related macular degeneration, 30% recurrence rate; associated with HLA-B7.

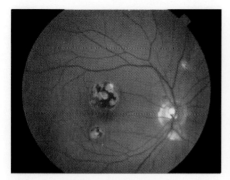

Figure 10–77 Presumed ocular histoplasmosis syndrome demonstrating macular and peripapillary lesions.

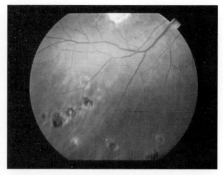

Figure 10–78 Presumed ocular histoplasmosis syndrome demonstrating peripheral histo spots.

- Check Amsler grid
- Fluorescein angiogram: early hypofluorescence and late staining of histo spots, also identifies CNVM if present
- Lab tests: histoplasmin antigen skin testing (not necessary)
- Extra and juxtafoveal CNVM (see Table 10–2) can be treated with focal laser photocoagulation (MPS-OHS conclusion)
- Subfoveal CNVM should *not* be treated with laser (14% regress spontaneously), removal with subretinal surgery is being evaluated in the Subretinal Surgery Trial
- Oral steroid treatment (prednisone 60–100 mg PO qd with slow taper) is controversial

Progressive Outer Retinal Necrosis Syndrome (PORN): Multifocal, patchy, retinal opacification that starts in the posterior pole and spreads rapidly to involve the entire retina due to the herpes zoster virus (HZV); minimal anterior chamber cell/flare, vitreous cells, or retinal vasculitis (differentiates from acute retinal necrosis); occurs in immunocompromised patients; poor response to therapy; may develop retinal detachments.

- Lab tests: HZV immunoglobulin G and M titers
- Systemic antivirals (acyclovir 5–10 mg/kg IV in divided doses tid for 1 week, then 800 mg PO 5x/d for 1–2 months); follow BUN and creatinine for nephrotoxicity
- 24 hours *after* acyclovir started, oral steroids (prednisone 60–100 mg PO qd for 1–2 months with slow taper); check PPD, blood glucose, and chest radiographs before starting systemic steroids
- Add H_2-blocker (ranitidine [Zantac] 150 mg PO bid) when giving systemic steroids
- 24 hours *after* antivirals started, topical steroids (prednisolone acetate 1% q2–6h) and cycloplegic (scopolamine 0.25% bid to qid) for 1–2 weeks
- If treatment fails or fulminant course, consider IV ganciclovir and/or foscarnet, as well as intravitreal foscarnet injections (see CMV section for doses)
- Laser demarcation or retinal surgery for retinal detachments; usually requires use of silicon oil
- Medical consultation

Rubella: Congenital syndrome classically characterized by congenital cataracts, glaucoma, and rubella retinopathy with salt-and-pepper pigmentary changes; also associated with microphthalmia, iris transillumination defects, bilateral deafness, congenital heart disease, growth retardation, and bone and dental abnormalities; 80% bilateral; vision is generally good (20/25); may rarely develop choroidal neovascular membrane (CNVM).

■ Fluorescein angiogram: mottled hyperfluorescence

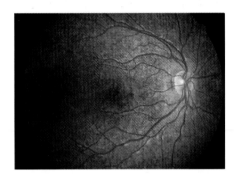

Figure 10–79 Rubella retinopathy demonstrating salt-and-pepper fundus appearance.

Syphilis (Luetic Chorioretinitis): Extensive iritis/retinitis/vitritis (panuveitis) seen in secondary syphilis (6 weeks to 6 months after primary infection) due to the spirochete *Treponema pallidum*. Signs include anterior chamber cell/flare, keratic precipitates, vitritis, multifocal, yellow-white chorioretinal infiltrates, salt-and-pepper pigmentary changes, flame-shaped retinal hemorrhages, and vascular sheathing; called "great mimic," since it can resemble many other retinal diseases; associated with sectoral interstitial keratitis, papillitis, and rarely CNVM. Variant called acute syphilitic posterior placoid chorioretinitis (ASPPC) with large, placoid, yellow lesions with faded centers. Mucocutaneous manifestations of secondary syphilis are often evident.

■ Lab tests: Venereal Disease Research Laboratory (VDRL, reflects current activity) and fluorescent treponemal antibody absorption (FTA-ABS)
■ Lumbar puncture for VDRL, FTA-ABS, total protein, and cell counts to rule out neurosyphilis
■ Penicillin G (2.4 million U IV q4h for 10–14 days then 2.4 million U IM every week for 3 weeks); tetracycline if patient is allergic to penicillin
■ Long-term tetracycline (250–500 mg PO qd) or doxycycline (100 mg PO qd) in HIV-positive or immunocompromised patients
■ Follow serum VDRL to monitor treatment efficacy
■ Medical consultation

Toxocariasis: Unilateral, multifocal, subretinal, yellow-white granulomas; associated with papillitis, serous/traction retinal detachments, dragged macula and retinal vessels, vitritis, dense vitreous infiltrates, and chronic endophthalmitis; caused by the second-stage larval form of the roundworm *Toxocara canis*. Gray-white chorioretinal scars remain after active infection. Usually occurs in children (included in differential diagnosis of leukocoria) and young adults; associated

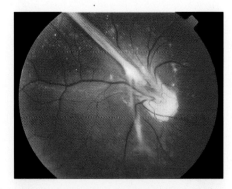

Figure 10–80 Toxocariasis.

with pica (eating dirt) and close contact with puppies; children with visceral larva migrans do not develop ocular involvement.

- Lab tests: ELISA for *Toxocara* antibody titers
- Topical steroid (prednisolone acetate 1% q2–6h) and cycloplegic (scopolamine 0.25% bid to qid) for active anterior segment inflammation
- Sub-Tenon's steroid injection (triamcinolone acetonide 40 mg/mL) and oral steroids (prednisone 60–100 mg PO qd) for severe inflammation. Check PPD, blood glucose, and chest radiographs before starting systemic steroids
- Add H_2-blocker (ranitidine [Zantac] 150 mg PO bid) when taking systemic steroids
- Systemic antihelminthic medications (thiabendazole, diethylcarbamazine, pyrantel pamoate) controversial, since worm death may increase inflammation
- Retinal surgery for retinal detachment (successful in 70–80%)

Toxoplasmosis: Acquired (eating poorly cooked meat) or congenital (transplacental transmission) necrotizing retinitis caused by the parasite *Toxoplasma gondii.* Congenital toxoplasmosis appears as an atrophic, chorioretinal scar (often located in the macula) with gray-white punctate peripheral lesions; associated with microphthalmia, nystagmus, strabismus, intracranial calcifications, microcephaly, and hydrocephalus. Acquired toxoplasmosis (especially in immunocompromised patients) and re-activated congenital lesions present with decreased vision, photophobia, floaters, vascular sheathing, full-thickness retinal necrosis, fluffy yellow-white retinal lesion adjacent to old scars, overlying vitreous reaction, and anterior chamber cell/flare. May have peripapillary form with disc edema and no chorioretinal lesions (simulating optic neuritis).

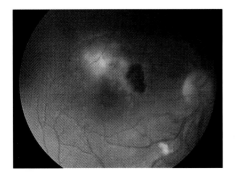

Figure 10–81 Toxoplasmosis demonstrating active, fluffy white lesion adjacent to old, darkly pigmented scar.

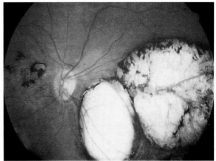

Figure 10–82 Congenital toxoplasmosis demonstrating inactive chorioretinal macular and peripheral scars.

- Lab tests: ELISA or indirect immunofluorescence assay (IFA) for *Toxoplasma* immunoglobulin G or M (definitive test) except in immunocompromised patients
- **Posterior pole lesions:** sulfadiazine (2 g PO loading dose, then 1 g PO qid for maintenance), pyrimethamine (Daraprim, 75–100 mg PO loading dose then 25 mg PO qd for maintenance), and folinic acid (leucovorin 5 mg PO 2–3 times a week); give plenty of fluids to prevent sulfadiazine renal crystals
- **Peripheral lesions:** clindamycin (300 mg PO qid) and sulfadiazine (2 g PO loading dose, then 1 g PO qid for maintenance) or trimethoprim-sulfamethoxazole (Bactrim, 1 double-strength tablet PO bid). *Note:* Immunocompetent patients may not require treatment.
- Treat with antibiotic combinations for 4–6 weeks; immunocompromised patients may require indefinite treatment and should be treated regardless of location of lesion
- If lesion is near the optic disc, in posterior pole, or if there is intense vitritis, may add oral steroid (prednisone 20–80 mg PO qd for 1 week, then taper) 24 hours *after* starting antimicrobial therapy (never start steroids alone); check PPD, blood glucose, and chest radiographs before starting systemic steroids.
- Add H_2-blocker (ranitidine [Zantac] 150 mg PO bid) when giving systemic steroids

Tuberculosis: Multifocal (may be focal), light-colored choroidal granulomas caused by the bacilli *Mycobacterium tuberculosis*; may present as endophthalmitis; usually associated with constitutional symptoms including malaise, night sweats, and pulmonary symptoms.

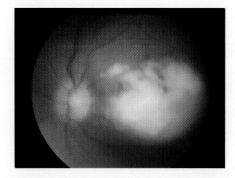

Figure 10–83 Tuberculosis with choroidal tubercle.

■ Lab tests: positive purified protein derivative (PPD) skin test and chest radiographs
■ Isoniazid (INH, 300 mg PO qd) and rifampin (600 mg PO qd) for 6–9 months; follow liver function tests for toxicity
■ Consider adding pyrazinamide (25–35 mg/kg PO qd) for first 2 months
■ Medical consultation for systemic evaluation

Posterior Uveitis

White Dot Syndromes: Group of inflammatory disorders that produce discrete yellow-white retinal lesions mainly in young adults; differentiated by history, appearance, laterality, and fluorescein angiogram findings.

Acute Macular Neuroretinopathy: Acute onset of paracentral scotomas usually in 20- to 30-year-old females (89%) following a viral prodrome (68%). Vision is often normal but may be decreased. Usually presents with bilateral (68%) cloverleaf or wedge-shaped, brown-red lesions in the posterior pole with no vitreous cells. Recovery of visual field defect is rare.

■ Check Amsler grid
■ Fluorescein angiogram: minimal hypofluorescence of the lesions
■ No effective treatment

Acute Posterior Multifocal Placoid Pigment Epitheliopathy (APMPPE): Rapid loss of central or paracentral vision in 20- to 30-year-old, healthy adults after a viral prodrome; no sex predilection; usually bilateral; multiple, round, discrete, large, flat gray-yellow lesions scattered throughout the posterior pole at the level of retinal pigment epithelium that later develop into well-demarcated retinal pigment epithelium scars; minimal vitreous cell; may have associated disc edema, cerebral vasculitis, headache, dysacousia, and tinnitus. Spontaneous resolution with visual recovery within 1–6 months (80% regain >20/40 vision); placoid lesions residue leaving irregular hyperpigmented scars; recurrences rare.

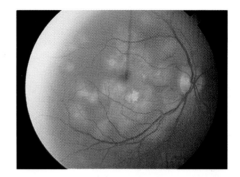

Figure 10–84 Acute posterior multifocal placoid pigment epitheliopathy.

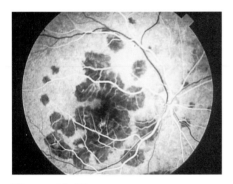

Figure 10–85 Same patient as shown in Figure 10-84 demonstrating hypofluorescence corresponding to the lesions in the early fluorescein angiogram.

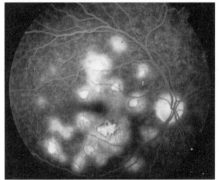

Figure 10–86 Same patient as shown in Figure 10-84 demonstrating late staining of the lesions on fluorescein angiogram.

- ICG: hypofluorescence of lesions
- Fluorescein angiogram: characteristic early blockage and late staining of the lesions
- No treatment necessary

Acute Retinal Pigment Epitheliitis/Krill Disease: Rare cause of acute, moderate, visual loss in young adults; no sex predilection; no viral prodrome. Discrete clusters of hyperpigmented spots (300–400 μm) with hypopigmented halos at the level of the retinal pigment epithelium in the perifoveal region. Usually unilateral with no vitritis. Spontaneous resolution with recovery of visual acuity within 7–10 weeks; recurrences possible.

- Fluorescein angiogram: blockage from the central spot and hyperfluorescence corresponding to the halo
- No effective treatment

Birdshot Choroidopathy/Vitiliginous Chorioretinitis: Multiple, small, discrete, ovoid, creamy yellow-white spots scattered like a birdshot blast from a shotgun in the midperiphery (spares macula); often in a vascular distribution; associated with mild vitritis, mild anterior chamber cell/flare, cystoid macular edema, vascular sheathing, and disc edema; usually bilateral; occurs in 50- to 60-year-old females (70%) and almost exclusively in Caucasians. Patients have mild blurring of vision, photopsias, night blindness, floaters. Chronic, slowly progressive, recurring disease with variable visual prognosis; subretinal neovascular membranes, epiretinal membranes, and macular cysts/holes are late complications; associated with HLA-A29 (90–98%).

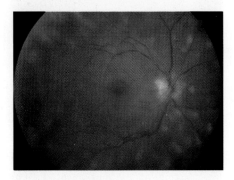

Figure 10–87 Birdshot choroidopathy/vitiliginous chorioretinitis.

- Fluorescein angiogram: mild hyperfluorescence, early and late staining of lesions; active lesions may hypofluoresce early. Late views show profuse vascular incompetence with leakage and secondary retinal staining
- Electroretinogram (ERG; subnormal) and electro-oculogram (EOG; subnormal); can monitor course of disease with serial ERG
- Treatment is reserved for patients with decreased visual acuity, significant inflammation, or complications including cystoid macular edema
- Despite historically poor responses to steroids, initial improvement can be seen with oral steroids (prednisone 60–100 mg PO qd); consider sub-Tenon's steroid injection (triamcinolone acetonide 40 mg/mL) in patients with severe inflammation or cystoid macular edema. Check PPD, blood glucose, and chest radiographs before starting systemic steroids
- Add H_2-blocker (ranitidine [Zantac] 150 mg PO bid) when taking systemic steroids
- Cyclosporine (2–7 mg/kg/d) can dramatically improve vitritis and cystoid macular edema; should be administered by a specialist trained in inflammatory diseases

Multifocal Choroiditis/Punctate Inner Choroidopathy (PIC)/Subretinal Fibrosis and Uveitis Syndrome: Spectrum of disorders causing blurred vision, metamorphopsia, paracentral scotomas, and photopsias; mainly occurs in 20- to 30-year-old, healthy, myopic females (3:1). Usually unilateral symptoms with bilateral fundus findings including small (100–200 μm), round, discrete, yellow-white spots and minimal signs of intraocular inflammation. Lesions develop into punched out, atrophic scars or subretinal fibrosis; choroidal neovascular membranes and macular edema are late complications (very common in PIC); poor visual prognosis; recurrences common.

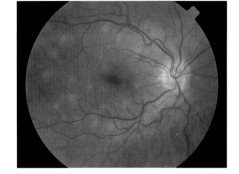

Figure 10–88 Multifocal choroiditis.

- ICG: multiple areas of hypofluorescence
- Fluorescein angiogram: early hyperfluorescence and late staining of the lesions
- Treatment with steroids is controversial

Multiple Evanescent White Dot Syndrome (MEWDS): Sudden, unilateral, blurred vision with paracentral/central scotomas and photopsias mainly occurs in 20- to 30-year-old, healthy females (4:1) after a viral prodrome. Multiple, small (100–200 μm), discrete, gray-white spots at the level of the retinal pigment epithelium in the posterior pole sparing the fovea (spots appear and disappear quickly). May have positive relative afferent pupillary defect (RAPD), foveal granularity, mild vitritis, mild anterior chamber cell/flare, optic disc edema, and an enlarged blind spot. Spontaneous resolution with recovery of vision in 3–10 weeks; recurrences rare (10%).

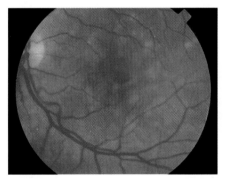

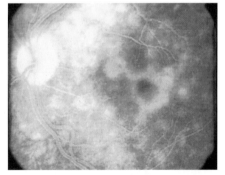

Figure 10–89 Multiple evanescent white dot syndrome.

Figure 10–90 Same patient as shown in Figure 10–89 demonstrating late fluorescein angiogram appearance.

- ICG: lesions are hypofluorescent
- Check Amsler grid or visual fields (central 10 degrees)
- Fluorescein angiogram: early, punctate hyperfluorescence in a wreath-like pattern and late staining of the lesions
- ERG subnormal in acute stages, returns to normal with recovery
- No treatment recommended

Acute Idiopathic Blind Spot Enlargement Syndrome (AIBSE): Subset of MEWDS (see above) seen in young females with enlargement of the blind spot and no optic disc edema and no visible fundus lesions; may represent MEWDS after lesions have faded; usually no RAPD exists.

■ Check Amsler grid or visual fields (central 10 degrees)
■ No treatment recommended

Other Inflammatory Syndromes:

Behçet's Disease: Triad of aphthous oral ulcers, genital ulcers, and bilateral nongranulomatous uveitis; also associated with erythema nodosum, arthritis, vascular lesions, HLA-B5 (subtypes Bw51 and B52) and HLA-B12. The uveitis (see Chap. 6) is severe and recurring, causing hypopyon, iris atrophy, posterior synechiae, optic disc edema, attenuation of arterioles, severe vitritis, cystoid macular edema, and an occlusive retinal vasculitis with retinal hemorrhages and edema. Patients have photophobia, pain, red eye, and decreased vision. Lab tests are positive for antinuclear antibody (ANA), elevated erythrocyte sedimentation rate (ESR)/C-reactive protein/ acute phase reactants/serum proteins, but are not diagnostic. Visual prognosis is poor; frequent relapses are common; ischemic optic neuropathy is a late complication.

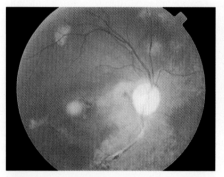

Figure 10–91 Behçet's disease demonstrating old vasculitis with sclerosed vessels and chorioretinal atrophy.

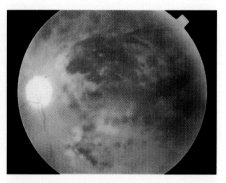

Figure 10–92 Behçet's disease demonstrating acute vasculitis with hemorrhage.

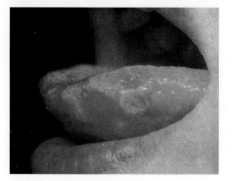

Figure 10–93 Behçet's disease demonstrating aphthous oral ulcers on tongue.

- Fluorescein angiogram: extensive vascular leakage early with late staining of vessel walls
- Lab tests: Behçetine skin test (prick skin with sterile needle, the formation of a pustule within a few minutes is a positive result), ESR, ANA, C-reactive protein, serum haplotyping
- Topical steroid (prednisolone acetate 1% q2–6h)
- Colchicine (600 mg PO bid) is controversial
- **Mild:** oral steroid (prednisone 60–100 mg PO qd); check PPD, blood glucose, and chest radiographs before starting systemic steroids
- Add H_2-blocker (ranitidine [Zantac] 150 mg PO bid) when taking systemic steroids
- **Severe:** sub-Tenon's steroid injection (triamcinolone acetonide 40 mg/mL), oral steroid (prednisone 60–100 mg PO qd), and either chlorambucil (2–8 mg/d) cyclophosphamide (1–2 mg/kg/d IV) *or* cyclosporine (2–7 mg/kg/d); should be administered by a specialist trained in inflammatory diseases
- Medical consultation

Posterior Scleritis: Orange-red elevation of choroid and retinal pigment epithelium by the thickened choroid with overlying serous retinal detachments, choroidal folds, vitritis, and optic disc edema; scleral thickening can cause induced hyperopia, proptosis, limitation of ocular motility, and angle-closure glaucoma (anterior rotation of ciliary body with forward displacement of the lens-iris diaphragm); usually occurs in 20- to 30-year-old females; 20–30% bilateral; patients have pain, photophobia, and decreased vision; associated with collagen vascular diseases, rheumatoid arthritis, relapsing polychondritis, inflammatory bowel disease, Wegener's granulomatosis, and syphilis.

- B-scan ultrasonography: diffuse scleral thickening (echolucent space between choroid and Tenon's capsule), and edema with medium reflectivity in Tenon's space, T-sign in the peripapillary region from scleral thickening around echolucent optic nerve
- Fluorescein angiogram: punctate hyperfluorescence early with pooling late within serous retinal detachments
- Oral steroid (prednisone 60–100 mg PO qd); if severe, consider high-dose IV steroids; check PPD, blood glucose, and chest radiographs before starting systemic steroids
- Oral nonsteroidal anti-inflammatory drugs (NSAIDs; indomethacin 25–50 mg PO tid)
- Add H_2-blocker (ranitidine [Zantac] 150 mg PO bid) when taking systemic steroids or NSAIDs
- Sub-Tenon's steroid injection (triamcinolone acetonide 40 mg/mL) sometimes required
- Consider immunosuppressive therapy (azathioprine, cyclosporine) in refractory cases; should be administered by a specialist trained in inflammatory diseases
- Medical consultation

Sarcoidosis: Granulomatous panuveitis with retinal vasculitis, vascular sheathing, periphlebitis (candle wax drippings), vitreous snowballs or string of pearls, yellow-white retinal/choroidal granulomas, anterior chamber cell/flare, mutton fat keratic precipitates, Koeppe/Busacca iris nodules, and macular edema. Disc/retinal neovascularization (often in sea-fan configuration) and epiretinal membranes are late complications. Occurs in young African Americans. Chronic, relapsing course (72%).

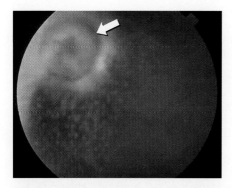

Figure 10–94 Sarcoidosis demonstrating peripheral granuloma (arrow) with overlying vitritis (scattered white spots).

- Fluorescein angiogram: early hyperfluorescence and late leakage from vascular permeability and macular edema
- Lab tests: angiotensin converting enzyme (ACE), chest radiographs, serum lysozyme, sickle cell prep/hemoglobin electrophoresis (to rule out sickle cell anemia); consider upper body gallium scan
- Oral steroid (prednisone 60–100 mg PO qd); check PPD, blood glucose, and chest radiographs before starting systemic steroids
- Add H_2-blocker (ranitidine [Zantac] 150 mg PO bid) when giving systemic steroids
- Sub-Tenon's steroid injection (triamcinolone acetonide 40 mg/mL) when macular edema is severe
- Laser photocoagulation to areas of capillary nonperfusion when neovascularization persists or progresses after steroid treatment
- Medical consultation

Serpiginous Choroidopathy/Geographic Helicoid Peripapillary Choroidopathy (GHPC): Active lesions appear as peripapillary, well-circumscribed, gray-white lesions with mild vitritis. The lesions extend from the disc in a pseudopodal, serpiginous pattern leaving chorioretinal scars and extensive RPE atrophy in areas of previous infection; skip lesions common; may develop subretinal neovascular membranes (25%); usually bilateral, slight male predilection, and occurs in the 5–7th decades. Patients are often asymptomatic until macular involvement occurs, causing paracentral scotomas and decreased vision; chronic, recurrent disease with good visual prognosis (severe visual loss rare); associated with HLA-B7.

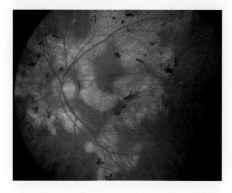

Figure 10–95 Serpiginous choroidopathy.

- Fluorescein angiogram: in acute episodes, lesions show hypofluorescence early and stain late, beginning at the borders of the lesion and spreading centrally; healed lesions appear as window defects
- Oral steroids (prednisone 60–100 mg PO qd) and sub-Tenon's steroid injection (triamcinolone acetonide 40 mg/mL) are controversial (consider when macula threatened)
- Consider immunosuppressive therapy (azathioprine, cyclosporine) in refractory cases; should be administered by a specialist trained in inflammatory diseases
- Laser photocoagulation for SRNVM

Sympathetic Ophthalmia (SO): Rare, bilateral, immune-mediated, mild to severe granulomatous uveitis seen 2 weeks to 3 months (80%) after penetrating trauma or surgery. Scattered, multifocal, yellow-white subretinal infiltrates (Dalen-Fuchs' nodules, 50%) with overlying serous retinal detachments, vitritis, and papillitis. Associated with inflammation in sympathizing (fellow) eye and worsened inflammation in exciting (injured) eye (keratic precipitates are an ominous sign); may have meningeal signs, poliosis, and alopecia (as in Vogt-Koyanagi-Harada syndrome). Patients have transient obscuration of vision, photophobia, pain, and blurred vision. Male predilection (probably reflects increased incidence of trauma in this group); chronic, recurring course; prognosis good (65% achieve >20/60 vision after treatment); associated with HLA-A11.

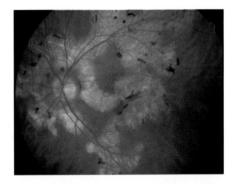

Figure 10–96 Sympathetic ophthalmia demonstrating Dalen-Fuchs nodules (arrow).

- Check for previous history of penetrating surgery or trauma
- Fluorescein angiogram: pinpoint areas of hyperfluorescence with central hypofluorescence and patchy areas of choriocapillaris hypoperfusion, leakage late from optic nerve
- Moderate to high-dose oral steroids (prednisone 60–200 mg PO qd); check PPD, blood glucose, and chest radiographs before starting systemic steroids
- Add H_2-blocker (ranitidine [Zantac] 150 mg PO bid) when giving systemic steroids
- Sub-Tenon's steroid injection (triamcinolone acetonide 40 mg/mL)
- Topical steroids (prednisolone acetate 1% q2–6h) and cycloplegic (scopolamine 0.25% bid to qid)
- Consider immunosuppressive therapy (azathioprine, methotrexate, chlorambucil); should be administered by a specialist trained in inflammatory diseases

■ No proven benefit in enucleating exciting eye, but this option should be considered in eyes with no light perception (NLP) vision, since removal of the eye within 2 weeks of injury may prevent sympathetic ophthalmia

Uveal Effusion Syndrome: Bullous serous retinal detachment (with shifting fluid), serous choroidal and ciliary body detachments, mild vitritis, leopard spot retinal pigment epithelium pigmentation, and dilated conjunctival vessels. Patients have decreased vision, metamorphopsia, and scotomas. Occurs in healthy, middle-aged males. Chronic, recurrent course.

■ B-scan ultrasonography: thickening of the sclera
■ Fluorescein angiogram: no discrete leak under serous retinal detachment
■ Steroids and antimetabolites are not effective
■ Consider decompression of vortex veins and scleral resection in nanophthalmic eyes
■ Surgery to create partial-thickness scleral windows is controversial

Vogt-Koyanagi-Harada Syndrome (VKH)/Harada's Disease: Bilateral inflammatory disorder with yellow-white exudates at the level of the retinal pigment epithelium, bullous serous retinal detachments (75%, shifting fluid often present) and focal retinal pigment epithelial detachments; associated with anterior chambers cell/flare, mutton fat keratic precipitates, posterior synechiae, vitritis, choroidal folds, choroidal thickening, Dalen-Fuchs–like nodules, optic disc hyperemia, and systemic manifestations including meningeal signs (headache, nausea, stiff neck, deafness, tinnitus), poliosis, alopecia, dysacousis, and vitiligo (Vogt-Koyanagi-Harada syndrome); late retinal pigment epithelial changes result in yellow-orange ("sunset glow") fundus. Occurs in pigmented individuals (Native Americans, African Americans, Asians, and Hispanics) 20–40 years old; slight female predilection (60%); patients have decreased vision and photophobia; associated with HLA-DR4, HLA-DRw53, HLA-DQw7, HLA-DQw3, and HLA-Bw54; recurrences common; visual prognosis good.

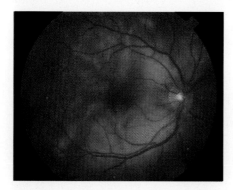

Figure 10–97 Vogt-Koyanagi-Harada syndrome with multiple serous retinal detachments.

■ B-scan ultrasonography: low reflectivity and choroidal thickening with overlying serous retinal detachment
■ Fluorescein angiogram: pinpoint areas of hyperfluorescence and delayed choroidal fluorescence

- Moderate- to high-dose oral steroids (prednisone 60–200 mg PO qd, then taper slowly); check PPD, blood glucose, and chest radiographs before starting systemic steroids
- Add H_2-blocker (ranitidine [Zantac] 150 mg PO bid) when giving systemic steroids
- Topical steroid (prednisolone acetate 1% q2–6h) and cycloplegic (scopolamine 0.25% bid to qid) if anterior uveitis present
- Sub-Tenon's steroid injection (triamcinolone acetonide 40 mg/mL) sometimes required
- Cyclosporine (2–7 mg/kg/d) or immunosuppressive agents for refractory cases; should be administered by a specialist trained in inflammatory diseases

Intermediate Uveitis/Pars Planitis

Definition

Uveitis of unknown etiology involving pars plana of ciliary body.

Epidemiology

Occurs in children and young adults; 70–80% bilateral; associated with multiple sclerosis (up to 15%) and sarcoidosis; rare in African Americans and Asians.

Symptoms

Decreased vision, floaters; no red eye, pain, or photophobia.

Signs

Decreased visual acuity, fibrovascular exudates especially along the inferior pars plana ("snow-banking"), extensive vitreous cells, vitreous cellular aggregates ("snowballs") inferiorly, minimal anterior chamber cell/flare, posterior vitreous detachment, and cystoid macular edema; may develop neovascularization in the pars plana exudate.

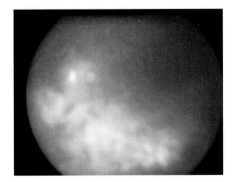

Figure 10–98 Pars planitis demonstrating snowballs.

Differential Diagnosis

Sarcoidosis, Behçet's disease, masquerade syndromes, syphilis, vitritis, posterior uveitis, amyloidosis, familial exudative vitreoretinopathy, Irvine-Gass syndrome (cystoid macular edema after cataract extraction), toxocariasis, retinoblastoma.

Evaluation

- Complete ophthalmic history and eye exam with attention to anterior chamber, anterior vitreous, 78/90 diopter or contact lens fundus exam, and ophthalmoscopy (cystoid macular edema and retinal periphery)
- Fluorescein angiogram: petaloid cystoid macular edema pattern seen in late views
- Lab tests: ACE, chest radiographs, and serum lysozyme to rule out sarcoidosis, and VDRL, FTA-ABS to rule out syphilis

Management

- Sub-Tenon's steroid injection (triamcinolone acetonide 40 mg/mL) when vision is affected by cystoid macular edema or severe inflammation
- Oral steroids (prednisone 60–100 mg PO qd) if unable to tolerate injections. Check PPD, blood glucose, and chest radiographs before starting systemic steroids
- Add H_2-blocker (ranitidine [Zantac] 150 mg PO bid) when taking systemic steroids
- Consider topical steroids (prednisolone acetate 1% q2–6h) and cycloplegic (scopolamine 0.25% bid to qid) if severe inflammation or macular edema exists
- Cryotherapy to the peripheral retina for snow-banking is controversial
- Consider immunosuppressive agents including alkylating agents (cyclophosphamide 1–2 mg/kg/d, chlorambucil 2–8 mg/d), antimetabolites (azathioprine 50–150 mg/d, methotrexate 7.5–25 mg/week), or T-cell suppressors (cyclosporine 5 mg/kg/d) for vision threatening inflammation and/or refractory cases unresponsive to steroids; should be administered by a specialist trained in inflammatory diseases

Prognosis

Usually good (51% achieve >20/30 vision); may have self-limited (10–20%) or chronic course (40–60%).

Hereditary Chorioretinal Dystrophies

Central Areolar Choroidal Dystrophy (Autosomal Dominant [AD]): Starts as mild retinal pigment epithelial granularity and mottling in the macula, progresses to a round, well-defined area of geographic atrophy with loss of the choriocapillaris; the area of atrophy slowly enlarges with large choroidal vessels visible underneath. Usually bilateral and symmetric; decreased vision occurs in 4th decade.

- Check color vision (protan-deutan defect) and visual fields (central scotoma)
- Fluorescein angiogram: well-circumscribed, hyperfluorescent window defects corresponding to the area of atrophy; late fading of lesions
- ERG (normal to subnormal), EOG (normal), and dark adaptation (normal)
- No effective treatment

Choroideremia (X-Linked): Progressive, bilateral, diffuse atrophy of the choriocapillaris and overlying retinal pigment epithelium with scalloped edges and large choroidal vessels visible underneath; spares macula until late. Affected males have nyctalopia, photophobia, and constricted visual fields in late childhood. Female carriers have normal vision, visual fields, color vision, and ERG, but may show pigmentary retinal changes; poor prognosis with legal blindness by 50–60 years of age. Mapped to chromosome Xq.

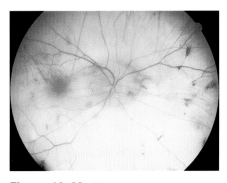

Figure 10–99 Choroideremia.

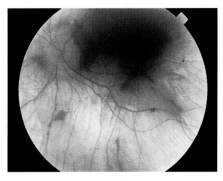

Figure 10–100 Choroideremia.

- Check color vision and visual fields (constricted)
- Fluorescein angiogram: absent choroidal flush with large choroidal vessels visible underneath with scalloped borders
- ERG (markedly reduced)
- No effective treatment

Congenital Stationary Night Blindness (CSNB): Group of bilateral, nonprogressive disorders with reduced night vision (rods) and normal day vision (cones). Patients usually have normal acuity, color vision, and full visual fields, but have reduced acuity with low light levels (nyctalopia), paradoxical pupillary response, absent Purkinje shift, and reduced rod ERG by 1st decade. Two categories:

(1) **Without fundus changes:**
- *Nougaret's Disease (AD):* No rod function (ERG with no scotopic a-wave), no myopia
- *Riggs' Type (AR):* Rare; some residual rod function, no myopia (ERG with some scotopic a-wave detectable)

■ *Schubert-Bornschein Type (X-linked/AR):* May have some residual rod function (incomplete form) or no rod function (complete form); associated with myopia. Carriers are asymptomatic. Negative ERG pattern (scotopic a-wave amplitude larger than b-wave)

(2) **With fundus changes:**
  ■ *Fundus albipunctatus (AR):* Yellow-white (50 μm) deep spots located in the midperipheral retina, sparing the macula. Not all lesions fluoresce on fluorescein angiogram (unlike drusen); nonprogressive, unlike retinitis punctata albescens

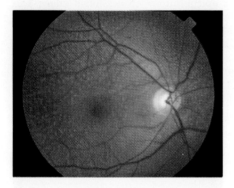

Figure 10–101 Fundus albipunctatus.

  ■ *Kandori's Flecked Retina Syndrome (AR):* Irregularly shaped, deep yellow spots usually seen in the equatorial region. Fewer and larger spots than fundus albipunctatus (may be variant).
  ■ *Oguchi's Disease (AR):* Golden brown-gray retinal discoloration in light that returns to normal retinal color (orange-red) with prolonged (2–12 hours) dark adaptation (Mizuo-Nakamura phenomenon)

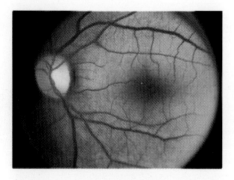

Figure 10–102 Oguchi's disease.

■ Check color vision and visual fields
■ Photopic ERG (normal or selective reduction in b-wave amplitude), scotopic ERG (reduced), and dark adaptation (no rod phase)
■ No effective treatment

Crystalline Retinopathy of Bietti (AR): Glittering, yellow-white, refractile spots scattered throughout fundus (located in inner and outer layers of retina) with multiple areas of geographic atrophy. Associated with crystals in the perilimbal anterior corneal stroma. Patients have slowly progressive decreased vision beginning in 5th decade.

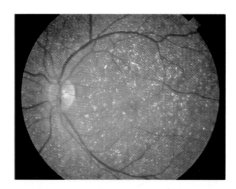

Figure 10–103 Crystalline retinopathy of Bietti.

- Check color vision and visual fields
- Fluorescein angiogram: patchy areas of blocked fluorescence and window defects corresponding to the areas of atrophy; crystals hyperfluoresce early
- ERG (reduced)
- No effective treatment

Gyrate Atrophy (AR): Progressive, bilateral retinal degeneration with well-circumscribed, scalloped areas of chorioretinal atrophy that enlarge and coalesce starting anteriorly and spreading posteriorly. Patients develop nyctalopia, constricted visual fields, and decreased vision by the 2nd decade. Abnormal laboratory studies including hypolysinemia, hyperornithinuria, and increased plasma ornithine levels (10–20 times normal) due to deficiency of the mitochondrial matrix enzyme, ornithine aminotransferase. Associated with posterior subcapsular cataracts and high myopia. Mapped to chromosome 10.

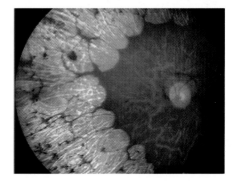

Figure 10–104 Gyrate atrophy.

- Lab tests: plasma ornithine levels, also consider urine ornithine levels and plasma lysine levels
- Check color vision and visual fields

- Fluorescein angiogram: window defects corresponding to the areas of atrophy
- ERG (reduced) and dark adaptation (prolonged)
- Restrict dietary arginine and protein
- Vitamin B_6 (pyridoxine 300–500 mg PO qd) therapy may be helpful

Progressive Cone Dystrophy (AD>X-Linked): Profound cone dysfunction with normal rod function. Often develop bull's eye macular pigment changes, patchy atrophy in the posterior pole, vascular attenuation, and temporal pallor or optic atrophy. Patients have slowly progressive loss of central vision (worse during day), dyschromatopsia, and photophobia that develops in the 1st–3rd decades. Called cone degeneration when not inherited. Poor prognosis with vision deteriorating to the 20/200 level by 4th decade.

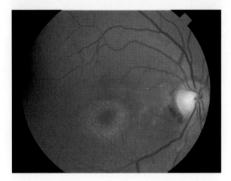

Figure 10–105 Progressive cone dystrophy.

- Check color vision, Amsler grid, visual fields (central scotomas, periphery intact)
- Fluorescein angiogram: hypofluorescence with ring of hyperfluorescence corresponding to the bull's eye lesion
- Photopic ERG (markedly reduced), scotopic ERG (normal), and EOG (normal)
- No effective treatment; dark glasses may help photophobia

Rod Monochromatism (Achromatopsia) (AR): Absence of cone function with normal rod function may be incomplete (not as severe) or complete; patients have poor central vision, achromatopsia, nystagmus, and photophobia from birth. Similar pigmentary changes as progressive cone dystrophy with granular changes and bull's eye maculopathy; poor prognosis with vision deteriorating to the 20/200 level by 4th decade.

- Check color vision (absent, all appears gray), Amsler grid, visual fields (central scotomas, periphery intact)
- Photopic ERG (absent), scotopic ERG (normal), EOG (normal), dark adaptation (rod phase only)
- No effective treatment; dark glasses may help photophobia

Hereditary Macular Dystrophies

Adult Foveomacular Vitelliform Dystrophy (AD): Bilateral, symmetric, round, slightly elevated, yellow-orange lesions with surrounding darker border and pigment clumping. Onset between 30 and 50 years of age with minimally affected vision and metamorphopsia (often unilateral symptoms, but bilateral disease). Smaller lesions than Best's disease, no disruption or layering of the yellow pigment, and seen in older patients; good prognosis.

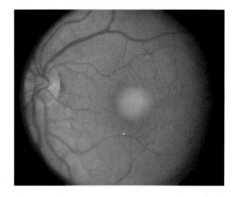

Figure 10–106 Adult foveomacular vitelliform dystrophy.

- Check color vision (mild tritan defect), Amsler grid, visual fields (may have small central scotoma)
- Fluorescein angiogram: central hypofluorescence with surrounding ring of hyperfluorescence
- ERG (normal) and EOG (normal to slightly subnormal; differentiates from Best's disease)
- No effective treatment

Best's Disease (AD): Second most common hereditary macular dystrophy. Starts as asymptomatic, yellow, round, subretinal vitelliform macular lesion ("sunny-side up" egg-yolk lesion) in childhood (first decade). Progresses to the "scrambled-egg" stage with irregular subretinal spots, then the pseudohypopyon stage with retinal pigment epithelium atrophy, and finally leaves a round atrophic scar. Usually bilateral and seen in Caucasians who are slightly hyperopic; good prognosis, vision deteriorates slowly (75–88% have >20/40 vision); may develop choroidal neovascular membrane; good prognosis with vision ranging from 20/30 to 20/100; mapped to chromosome 11q.

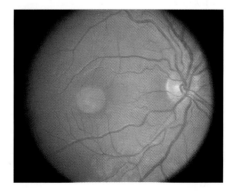

Figure 10–107 Best's disease demonstrating egg-yolk stage.

- Check color vision (abnormal, proportional to degree of visual loss), Amsler grid, visual fields (may have small central scotoma)
- Fluorescein angiogram: egg-yolk lesion hypofluorescent early, with surrounding hyperfluorescence, window defects seen in the areas of atrophy and pigment changes
- ERG (normal), EOG (markedly abnormal, reduced light-to-dark ratio [Arden ratio <1.6], even subnormal in carriers who have no fundus changes), and dark adaptation (normal)
- No effective treatment

Butterfly-Shaped Pigment Dystrophy (?AD): Bilateral, symmetric, gray-yellow, butterfly-shaped lesions in central macula with surrounding halo of depigmentation. Onset between 20 and 50 years of age with mild decrease in vision and slow progression.

- Check color vision (normal), Amsler grid, visual fields (may have small central scotoma)
- Fluorescein angiogram: reticular hypofluorescence corresponding to areas of pigmentation
- ERG (normal), EOG (markedly subnormal), and dark adaptation (normal)
- No effective treatment

Dominant Drusen/Doyne's Honeycomb Dystrophy (AD): Asymptomatic, bilateral, symmetric, yellow-white drusen (nodular thickening of the retinal pigment epithelium basement membrane) scattered throughout the posterior pole and nasal to the optic disc. Seen by age 20–30 years. The lesions coalesce (forming a honeycomb appearance), enlarge, or disappear. Associated with pigment clumping, chorioretinal atrophy, and choroidal neovascular membranes.

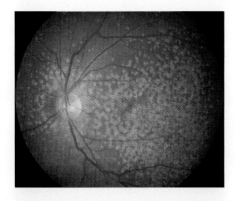

Figure 10–108   Dominant drusen.

- Check color vision (normal), Amsler grid, visual fields (normal)
- Fluorescein angiogram: early blockage, late staining of drusen
- ERG (normal), EOG (subnormal in late stages), and dark adaptation (normal)
- No effective treatment

North Carolina Macular Dystrophy (AD): Yellow spots (drusen) appear in early childhood (first decade) and progress to chorioretinal atrophy, macular staphyloma, and peripheral drusen. May develop choroidal neovascular membranes. Mapped to chromosome 6q.

- Check color vision (normal), Amsler grid, visual fields (may have central scotoma)
- Fluorescein angiogram: hyperfluorescent window defects early, late staining of drusen; may have areas of capillary nonperfusion
- ERG (normal), EOG (normal), and dark adaptation (normal)
- No effective treatment

Pseudoinflammatory Macular Dystrophy (Sorsby's Syndrome) (AD): Bilateral, symmetric, diffuse choroidal atrophy, macular edema, hemorrhage, and exudate with decreased vision and tritone dyschromatopsia; seen in 40- to 50-year-old patients.

- Check color vision, Amsler grid, and visual fields
- ERG (subnormal in advanced stages), EOG (subnormal in advanced stages), and dark adaptation (delayed)
- No effective treatment

Sjögren's Reticular Pigment Dystrophy (AR): Hyperpigmented fishnet/reticular pattern at the level of the retinal pigment epithelium that starts centrally and spreads peripherally. Usually asymptomatic with good vision.

- Check color vision (normal), Amsler grid, and visual fields (normal)
- Fluorescein angiogram: hypofluorescence of the fishnet-reticulum over normal background fluorescence in early views
- ERG (normal), EOG (lower limit of normal), and dark adaptation (normal to subnormal)
- No effective treatment

Stargardt's Disease/Fundus Flavimaculatus (AR>AD): Most common hereditary macular dystrophy. Bilateral, deep, symmetric, yellow pisciform (fishtail-shaped) flecks composed of lipofuscin in the retinal pigment epithelium and scattered throughout the posterior pole. Onset in first to second decade; spectrum of disease: fundus flavimaculatus (no macular dystrophy; extensive fundus flecks) to Stargardt's disease ("bull's eye" atrophic maculopathy with "beaten bronze" appearance; limited fundus flecks). Salt-and-pepper pigmentary changes in periphery may develop late; no sex predilection; patients have bilateral decreased vision even before fundus changes appear; poor prognosis with vision deteriorating to the 20/200 level by 3rd decade. Mapped to chromosome 1p.

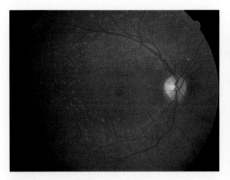

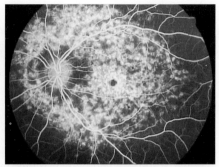

Figure 10–109 Stargardt's disease.

Figure 10–110 Fluorescein angiogram of patient shown in Figure 10–109 demonstrating hyperfluorescence of the lesions and the characteristic "silent" choroid.

- Check color vision (normal to deutan-tritan defect), Amsler grid, and visual fields (may have central scotoma)
- Fluorescein angiogram: dark or "silent" choroid, hyperfluorescent spots that do not correspond to the flecks seen clinically, and window defects corresponding to the areas of the maculopathy
- ERG (normal to subnormal), EOG (normal to subnormal), and dark adaptation (mildly elevated in late stages)
- No effective treatment

Hereditary Vitreoretinal Degenerations

Familial Exudative Vitreoretinopathy (FEVR) (AD): Rare, slowly progressive, bilateral, peripheral vascular developmental disorder; similar in appearance to retinopathy of prematurity, but without premature birth and supplemental oxygen.

Stage 1: Starts with peripheral avascularity, white without pressure, vitreous bands, peripheral cystoid degeneration, microaneurysms, telangiectasia, straightened vessels, and vascular engorgement especially in the temporal periphery; asymptomatic in 73% of cases, but may have strabismus and nystagmus. Progression to stage 2 may or may not occur.

Stage 2: Neovascularization, fibrovascular proliferation, subretinal/intraretinal exudation, dragging of disc and macula, falciform retinal folds, and localized retinal detachments. Visual loss after 2nd–3rd decade is rare unless degeneration progresses to stage 3.

Stage 3: Cicatrization causes traction (rare) and/or rhegmatogenous retinal detachments (10–20%); retinal detachments common in 3rd–4th decade; retinal detachments difficult to repair (recurrent retinal detachments and proliferative vitreoretinopathy).

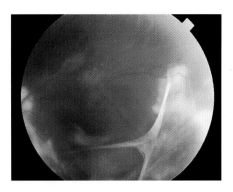

Figure 10–111 Familial exudative vitreoretinopathy.

- Fluorescein angiogram: peripheral nonperfusion past vascularized retina; at border area, arteriovenous anastomoses form and leak fluorescein
- Prophylactic treatment of the avascular retina is controversial
- Retinal surgery for retinal detachments; should be performed by a retina specialist

Goldmann-Favre Vitreotapetoretinal Degeneration (AR): Rare, bilateral vitreotapetoretinal degeneration with foveal and peripheral retinoschisis, optically empty vitreous cavity, condensed vitreous veils, attenuation of retinal vessels, peripheral pigmentary (bone spicules) changes, lattice degeneration, progressive cataracts, and waxy optic disc pallor. No sex predilection (unlike juvenile retinoschisis). Patients have nyctalopia and constricted visual fields.

- Fluorescein angiogram: no leakage from foveal schisis
- ERG (markedly reduced) and EOG (abnormal; differentiates from juvenile retinoschisis)
- Consider prophylactic treatment of any retinal breaks/tears
- Retinal surgery for retinal detachments

Snowflake Degeneration (AD): Rare degeneration with yellow-white deposits in peripheral retina associated with white without pressure, sheathing of retinal vessels, vitreous degeneration, and cataracts. Increased risk of retinal detachments.

- No treatment recommended
- Retinal surgery for retinal detachments

Wagner's/Jansen's/Stickler's Vitreoretinal Dystrophies (AD): All have optically empty vitreous cavity with thick, transvitreal and preretinal membranes/strands, retinal perivascular pigmentary changes, and lattice degeneration; associated with myopia, glaucoma, and posterior subcapsular cataracts.

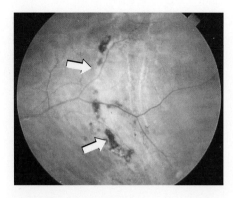

Figure 10–112 Stickler's vitreoretinal dystrophy with pigmented demarcation lines (arrows) from a chronic retinal detachment.

- **Wagner's Disease:** No systemic associations and no increased risk of retinal detachments

- **Jansen's Disease:** No systemic associations, but patients do have an increased risk of retinal detachments; often bilateral retinal detachments

- **Stickler's Syndrome:** Associated with systemic abnormalities including marfanoid habitus, facial hypoplasia, cleft palate, neurosensory hearing loss, skeletal abnormalities, and arthritis; patients have increased risk of retinal breaks (75%) and bilateral detachments (42%); mapped to chromosome 12q
- ERG (reduced) and EOG (normal)
- No treatment recommended
- Retinal surgery for retinal detachments

Leber's Congenital Amaurosis (AR)

Group of disorders with onset in infancy or early childhood of severe visual impairment, sluggish pupils, nyctalopia, and nystagmus. May have range of fundus abnormalities from no fundus changes (most common) to retinal pigment epithelial granularity, vascular attenuation, tapetal sheen, yellow flecks, salt-and-pepper fundus, chorioretinal atrophy, or a retinitis pigmentosa appearance. Associated with hyperopia, mental retardation (37%), deafness, seizures, skeletal abnormalities, posterior subcapsular cataracts, keratoconus, and renal/muscular abnormalities. Mapped to chromosome 17p.

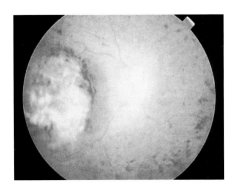

Figure 10–113 Leber's congenital amaurosis.

- ERG (markedly reduced to absent), visual fields (constricted)
- No effective treatment

Retinitis Pigmentosa (RP)

Definition

Group of hereditary, progressive retinal degenerations (rod-cone dystrophies) that result from abnormal production of photoreceptor proteins.

Several atypical forms exist:

Retinitis Pigmentosa Inversus: Macula and posterior pole are affected rather than midperiphery; confused with hereditary macular disorders; central and color vision are reduced earlier than normal; pericentral ring/central scotomas can occur.

Retinitis Pigmentosa Sine Pigmento: Descriptive term for condition in patients with symptoms of retinitis pigmentosa who fail to show pigmentary fundus changes; seen in up to 20% of cases; associated with more pronounced cone dysfunction.

Retinitis Punctata Albescens (AR): Multiple, punctate white (50–100 μm) spots at the level of the retinal pigment epithelium scattered in the midperiphery with attenuated vessels and bone spicules. Slowly progressive disease (differentiates from fundus albipunctatus).

Sector Retinitis Pigmentosa: Pigmentary changes are limited to one retinal area; generally do not enlarge; usually inferonasal quadrant; relatively good electroretinographic responses (normal cone and rod implicit times).

Several forms are associated with systemic abnormalities:

Abetalipoproteinemia (Bassen-Kornzweig Syndrome) (AR): Associated with ataxia, steatorrhea, erythrocyte acanthocytosis, growth retardation, neuropathy, and lack of serum beta-lipoprotein causing intestinal malabsorption of fat-soluble vitamins (A, D, E, K), triglycerides, and cholesterol; minimal pigmentary changes early.

- Treat with Vitamin A (15,000 IU PO qd), Vitamin E (100 IU/kg PO qd), Vitamin K (0.15 mg/kg PO qd), omega-3 fatty acids (0.10 g/kg PO qd), and dietary fat restriction.

Alström's Disease (AR): Associated with cataracts, deafness, obesity, renal failure, acanthosis nigricans, baldness, and hypogenitalism. Early and profound visual loss.

Cockayne's Syndrome: Associated with band keratopathy, cataracts, dwarfism, deafness, intracranial calcifications, and psychosis.

Kearns-Sayre Syndrome (AR): Associated with chronic progressive external ophthalmoplegia, ptosis, cardiac conduction defects (arrhythmias, heart block, cardiomyopathy), and other abnormalities (see Chap. 2). Ragged red fibers seen histologically on muscle biopsy.

Laurence-Moon/Bardet-Biedl Syndromes (AR): *Bardet-Biedl:* polydactyly in 75% and syndactyly in 14%; *Laurence-Moon:* spastic paraplegia, no polydactyly/syndactyly. Both include short stature, congenital obesity, hypogenitalism (50%), partial deafness (5%), renal abnormalities, and mental retardation (85%). Minimal pigmentary changes early.

Neuronal Ceroid Lipofuscinosis (Batten's Disease) (AR): Associated with seizures, dementia, ataxia, and mental retardation; can have infantile (Hagberg-Santavuori syndrome), juvenile, or adult onset; conjunctival biopsy shows granular inclusions with autofluorescent lipopigments that also accumulate in neurons causing retinal and central nervous system (CNS) degeneration.

Refsum's Disease (AR): Associated with ichthyosis, electrocardiographic abnormalities, anosmia, deafness, progressive peripheral neuropathy, cerebellar ataxia, hypotonia, hepatomegaly, mental retardation, and elevated cerebrospinal fluid (CSF) protein; minimal pigmentary changes and enlarged corneal nerves early. Defect in fatty acid metabolism due to phytanic acid oxidase deficiency; causes elevated plasma phytanic acid, pipecolic acid, and very long-chain fatty acid levels.

- Treat by restricting dietary phytanic acid (animal fats and milk products) and phytol (leafy green vegetables); follow serum phytanic acid levels.

Usher's Syndrome (AR): Associated with congenital, neurosensory hearing loss. Most common syndrome associated with retinitis pigmentosa (5%). Type I (total deafness with no vestibular function), Type II (partial deafness with normal vestibular function, most common type [67%], better vision), Type III (Hallgren's syndrome: deafness, vestibular ataxia, psychosis), Type IV (deafness and mental retardation). *Note:* Controversy over whether Types III and IV are forms of Usher's syndrome or separate genetic entities.

- Protect ears from loud noises; avoid ototoxic medications

Epidemiology

Most common hereditary degeneration (1:5000); can have any inheritance pattern: AR (25%), AD (20%, usually with variable penetrance, later onset, milder course), X-linked (9%, more severe, carriers also affected), isolated (38%), and undetermined (8%).

Symptoms

Nyctalopia, dark adaptation problems, photophobia, progressive constriction of visual fields (tunnel vision), dyschromatopsia, photopsias, and slowly progressive, decreased central vision starting at approximately 20 years of age.

Signs

Decreased visual acuity, constricted visual fields, dyschromatopsia (tritanopic); classic fundus appearance with dark pigmentary clumps in the midperiphery and perivenous areas (bone spicules), attenuated retinal vessels, cystoid macular edema, fine pigmented vitreous cells, and waxy optic disc pallor; associated with posterior subcapsular cataracts (39–72%), high myopia, astigmatism, keratoconus, and mild hearing loss (30%, excluding Usher's patients). 50% of female carriers with X-linked form have golden reflex in posterior pole.

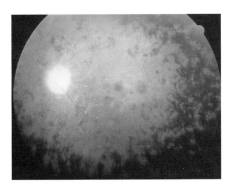

Figure 10–114 Retinitis pigmentosa.   **Figure 10–115** Retinitis pigmentosa.

Differential Diagnosis

Congenital rubella syndrome, syphilis, thioridazine/chloroquine drug toxicity, carcinoma-associated retinopathy, congenital stationary night blindness, Vitamin A deficiency, atypical cytomegalovirus or herpes virus chorioretinitis, trauma, diffuse unilateral subacute neuroretinitis, gyrate atrophy, bear tracks, congenital hypertrophy of the retinal pigment epithelium (CHRPE).

Evaluation

- Complete ophthalmic history with attention to consanguinity, family history, and hearing

- Complete eye exam with attention to refraction, pupils, cornea, lens, vitreous cells, and ophthalmoscopy
- Check color vision (Farnsworth panel D15) and visual fields (constricted, ring scotoma)
- ERG (markedly reduced/absent; decreases 10% per year; abnormal in 90% of female carriers with X-linked form), EOG (abnormal), dark adaptation (prolonged)
- Lab tests: plasma ornithine levels, fat-soluble vitamin levels (especially vitamin A), serum lipoprotein electrophoresis (Bassen-Kornzweig), serum cholesterol/triglycerides, VDRL, FTA-ABS, peripheral blood smears (acanthocytosis), serum phytanic acid levels (Refsum's)

Management

- No effective treatment except in forms with treatable systemic diseases (abetalipoproteinemia, Refsum's disease)
- Correct any refractive error; prescribe dark glasses
- Low vision consultation for visual aids
- For common forms of retinitis pigmentosa (>18 years of age): Vitamin A (15,000 IU PO qd of palmitate form) slows reduction of ERG amplitudes; avoid Vitamin E; follow liver function tests and serum retinol levels annually. *Note:* Controversial and not tested in atypical forms of RP
- Treatment of cystoid macular edema controversial
- Cataract surgery may be indicated depending on retinal function; check potential acuity meter (PAM) when considering cataract extraction

Prognosis

Poor, usually legally blind by 4th decade.

Albinism

Two types:

Ocular Albinism (X-linked/AR): Congenital disorder of melanogenesis limited to the eye; decreased number of melanosomes (although each melanosome is fully pigmented). Patients have decreased vision and photophobia; signs include nystagmus, strabismus, high myopia, diffuse iris transillumination, foveal hypoplasia, and fundus hypopigmentation.

Oculocutaneous Albinism (AR>AD): Systemic problem with decreased melanin in all melanosomes; two forms: tyrosinase-positive (some pigmentation) and tyrosinase-negative (no pigmentation). These patients lack pigmentation of the hair, skin, and eyes. Potentially lethal variants include:

- **Chédiak-Higashi syndrome (AR):** Reticuloendothelial incompetence with neutropenia, anemia, thrombocytopenia, recurrent infections, leukemia, and lymphoma

■ **Hermansky-Pudlak syndrome (AR):** Clotting disorder and bleeding tendency secondary to platelet abnormalities.

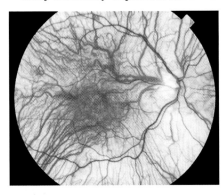

Figure 10–116 Fundus hypopigmentation in a patient with albinism.

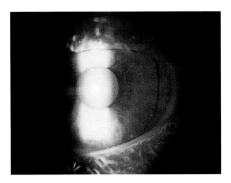

Figure 10–117 Albinism demonstrating diffuse iris transillumination; note that equator of lens is visible.

■ ERG and EOG (supranormal)
■ No effective treatment
■ Medical and hematology consultation to rule out potentially lethal variants

Phakomatoses

Group of congenital, mainly heritable, syndromes with multiple ocular and systemic hamartomas; commonly have incomplete penetrance and variable expressivity. Phako = "motherspot" (birthmark).

Angiomatosis Retinae (von Hippel-Lindau Disease) (AD): Bilateral retinal capillary hemangiomas (40–60%), cystic cerebellar hemangioblastoma (60%, most common cause of death), renal cell carcinoma, pheochromocytoma, liver, pancreas, and epididymis cysts (if only retinal findings = von Hippel disease). Mapped to chromosome 3p.

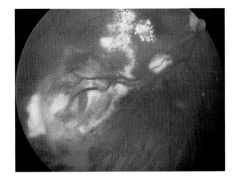

Figure 10–118 Angiomatosis retinae (von Hippel-Lindau disease) demonstrating retinal capillary hemangioma with feeder and draining vessels, and surrounding exudates.

- Head, upper cervical spinal cord, and abdominal CT scan or MRI
- Medical consultation if intracranial or systemic lesions exist

Ataxia-Telangiectasia (Louis-Bar Syndrome) (AR): Progressive cerebellar ataxia (first symptom), telangiectasia of the skin (especially around face, ears, and neck) and bulbar conjunctiva, and ocular motility abnormalities; also associated with seborrheic dermatitis, mental retardation, thymus gland hypoplasia with reduced T-cell immunity, high incidence of malignancies (33%) including lymphoma and leukemia, and humoral/cellular immunodeficiency with increased risk of infections, especially chronic respiratory infections. Mapped to chromosome 11q; poor prognosis with death by adolescence.

- Medical consultation

Encephalotrigeminal Angiomatosis (Sturge-Weber Syndrome): Diffuse, flat, dark red, "tomato-catsup" choroidal hemangioma (40–50%), congenital facial hemangioma (nevus flammeus or "port wine stain"), ipsilateral intracranial hemangioma, nevus flammeus involving the eyelid (suspect glaucoma if upper eyelid involved), large anomalous blood vessels in the conjunctiva and episclera, and congenital, ipsilateral glaucoma (30%). May have mental retardation, convulsions, and cerebral calcifications. No hereditary pattern. Variable prognosis depending on CNS involvement.

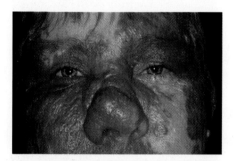

Figure 10–119 Encephalotrigeminal angiomatosis (Sturge-Weber syndrome) demonstrating nevus flammeus.

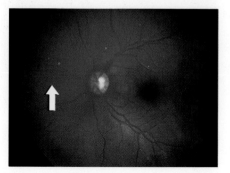

Figure 10–120 Encephalotrigeminal angiomatosis demonstrating tomato-catsup fundus appearance of a diffuse choroidal hemangioma (arrow).

- Head and orbital CT scan
- May require treatment of increased intraocular pressure (see Chap. 11)
- Neurology consultation if intracranial lesions exist

Neurofibromatosis (von Recklinghausen's Disease) (AD): Disorder of the neuroectodermal system. Two forms (see Chap. 3 for descriptions).

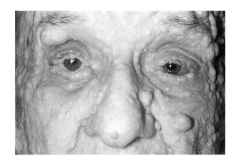

Figure 10–121 Neurofibromatosis (von Recklinghausen's disease) demonstrating facial neurofibromas.

Racemose Hemangiomatosis (Wyburn-Mason Syndrome): Anomalous anastomosis between the arterial and venous systems of the retina, brain (20–30% have intracranial arteriovenous malformations causing mental status changes or hemiparesis; 30% cause visual field defects including homonymous hemianopsia), orbit, and facial bones (pterygoid fossa, mandible, and maxilla). Usually unilateral (96%); appears as intertwined tangles of dilated vessels; may cause visual loss due to retinal or vitreous hemorrhage. No hereditary pattern. Early mortality due to intracranial arteriovenous malformations.

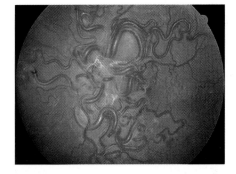

Figure 10–122 Racemose hemangiomatosis (Wyburn-Mason syndrome) demonstrating retinal vascular arteriovenous malformation (AVM) with dilated, tortuous vessels.

- Head and orbital CT scan
- Neurology consultation if intracranial lesions exist
- Asymptomatic retinal lesions do not require treatment
- Consider laser photocoagulation around lesions (direct treatment is dangerous) if symptomatic

Tuberous Sclerosis (Bourneville's Disease) (AD): Triad of seizures (infantile spasms, 80–93%), mental retardation (50–60%), and adenoma sebaceum (85%, a misnomer for angiofibromas, appearing as a red-brown papular malar rash). Primary criteria include: facial angiofibromas (adenoma sebaceum), subungual angiofibromas, subependymal hamartomas and multiple retinal hamartomas. Secondary criteria include: cutaneous shagreen patch (fibromatous skin infiltration especially on lower back and forehead; 25%), ash-leaf spots (hypopigmented skin macules seen best with ultraviolet Wood's lamp; 80%), skin tags (molluscum fibrosum pendulum), bilateral renal angiomyolipomata or cysts (80%), cystic lung disease, cardiac rhabdomyoma, calcified central nervous system (CNS) astrocytic hamartomas (brain stones in cerebellum, basal ganglia, and posterior fossa), or a first degree relative with tuberous sclerosis. Mapped to chromosome 9q. Poor prognosis, with 75% mortality prior to 20 years of age.

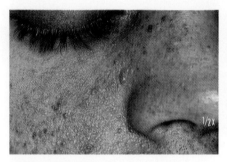

Figure 10–123 Tuberous sclerosis (Bourneville's disease) demonstrating adenoma sebaceum.

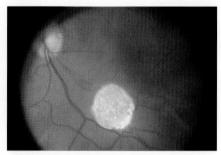

Figure 10–124 Tuberous sclerosis demonstrating astrocytic hamartoma with mulberry appearance.

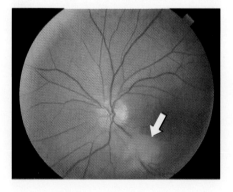

Figure 10–125 Tuberous sclerosis demonstrating astrocytic hamartoma with smooth appearance (arrow).

■ Medical and neurology consultation

Benign Choroidal Tumors

Choroidal Hemangioma: Vascular tumor; two forms:

(1) Usually unilateral, well-circumscribed, solitary; round, slightly elevated (<3 mm), orange-red lesion located in the posterior pole often with an overlying serous retinal detachment. Occurs in 4th decade.

(2) Diffuse, reddish, choroidal thickening described as "tomato-catsup" fundus (reddish thickening overlying dark fundus). Occurs in children with Sturge-Weber syndrome (see Fig. 10–120).

Usually asymptomatic, but both types can cause exudative retinal detachments (50%).

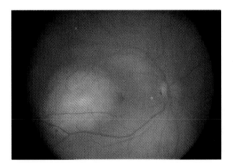

Figure 10–126 Choroidal hemangioma (discrete type).

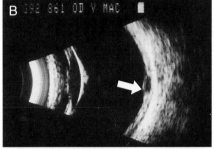

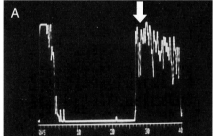

Figure 10–127 Same patient as shown in Figure 10–126, demonstrating B-scan and A-scan appearance with high internal reflectivity (arrow).

- B-scan ultrasonography: mass with moderate elevation, thickened choroid, and high internal reflectivity, often with overlying serous retinal detachment
- Fluorescein angiogram: early filling of the tumor vessels, progressive hyperfluorescence during the transit views, and late leakage (multiloculated pattern)
- Observe if asymptomatic
- Treat tumor directly with grid laser photocoagulation (moderately intense, white reaction on the tumor surface) if serous retinal detachment threatens fovea; goal of laser treatment is to decrease serous fluid, not obliterate tumor

Choroidal Nevus: Dark gray-brown pigmented, flat or slightly elevated lesion (<2 mm); often with overlying drusen and a hypopigmented ring around the base.

Usually nonprogressive, but can grow during puberty. Growth in an adult should be watched carefully. Subretinal neovascular membrane and serous retinal detachments (sign of growth potential) can occur adjacent to the nevus. Multiple nevi are seen in patients with neurofibromatosis. 10% of suspicious nevi progress to malignant melanoma.

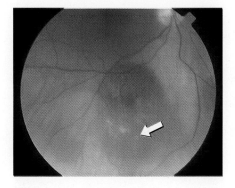

Figure 10–128 Large choroidal nevus (nevoma) with overlying drusen (arrow).

■ B-scan ultrasonography: flat to slightly elevated lesion, choroidal discontinuity, and medium to high internal reflectivity
■ Follow with serial photographs, ultrasonography, and clinical examination for any growth that would be suspicious for malignant melanoma

Choroidal Osteoma: Slighly elevated, well-circumscribed, peripapillary, orange-red (early) to cream-colored (late) benign tumor with small vascular spiders on the surface. 80–90% unilateral; occurs in young patients who may be asymptomatic or have decreased vision, paracentral scotomas, and metamorphopsia; slight female predilection; consists of mature cancellous bone and may spontaneously resolve; subretinal neovascular membrane common at tumor margins; variable prognosis.

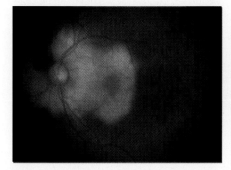

Figure 10–129 Choroidal osteoma with orange, placoid appearance.

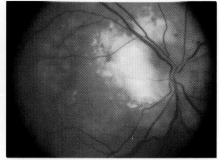

Figure 10–130 Choroidal osteoma with calcification.

- B-scan ultrasonography: calcification, orbital shadowing, and a high reflective spike from the tumor surface
- Fluorescein angiogram: irregular hyperfluorescence and late staining of the tumor; the vascular spiders appear hypofluorescent against the hyperfluorescent tumor
- Orbital radiographs and CT scan show the calcifications within the tumor
- Treat SRNVM with laser photocoagulation; often requires multiple sessions

Benign Retinal Tumors

Astrocytic Hamartoma: Yellow-white, well-circumscribed, elevated lesion that may contain nodular areas of calcification and/or clear cystic spaces; classically has mulberry appearance but may have softer, smooth appearance. Multiple lesions common in tuberous sclerosis. Usually do not grow (see Figs. 10–124 and 10–125).

- Fluorescein angiogram: variable vascularization within tumor that leaks in late views
- No treatment necessary

Capillary Hemangioma: Benign vascular tumor arising from the inner retina and extending toward the retinal surface.

Two forms of capillary hemangioma:

(1) Sporadic, nonhereditary, and unilateral; no systemic associations; usually no feeder vessels
(2) Hereditary, bilateral (50%), multifocal, and associated with multiple systemic abnormalities (von Hippel-Lindau syndrome). Classically has dilated feeder and draining vessels.

Both forms initially appear as a red, pink, or gray lesion that later grows as proliferation of capillary channels within the tumor progresses. These new capillaries leak fluid, leading to exudates and often serous retinal detachments. Associated with preretinal membranes.

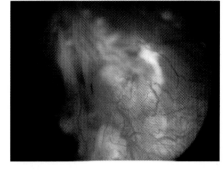

Figure 10–131 Capillary hemangioma in a patient with von Hippel disease.

- Fluorescein angiogram: early filling of tumor in arterial phase with late leakage
- No treatment recommended for sporadic tumor unless vision is affected

- Consider cryotherapy, photocoagulation, surgery, and radiation therapy for hereditary tumors; should be performed by a tumor specialist
- Medical consultation for hereditary form

Cavernous Hemangioma: Rare, vascular tumor composed of clumps of saccular, intraretinal aneurysms filled with dark venous blood ("cluster-of-grapes" appearance). Fine, gray epiretinal membranes may cover the tumor. Usually unilateral; occurs in 2nd–3rd decade with slight female predilection (60%). Usually no exudation seen; retinal/vitreous hemorrhages rare. Commonly asymptomatic and nonprogressive.

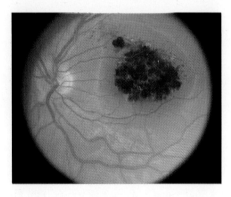

Figure 10–132 Cavernous hemangioma with "cluster-of-grapes" appearance.

- Fluorescein angiogram: hyperfluorescent saccules with fluid levels
- No treatment necessary

Congenital Hypertrophy of the Retinal Pigment Epithelium (CHRPE): Flat or slightly elevated, round, solitary, dark brown-black pigmented lesion with sharp borders, scalloped edges, and central hypopigmented lacunae. Nonprogressive, rarely enlarges. Bilateral, multifocal CHRPE lesions (>4 lesions) seen in familial adenomatous polyposis (Gardner's syndrome [AD]: triad of multiple intestinal polyps, skeletal hamartomas, and soft tissue tumors).

- No treatment necessary

Figure 10–133 Congenital hypertrophy of the retinal pigment epithelium with hypopigmented lacunae.

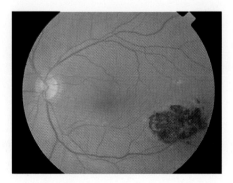

Bear Tracks: Multifocal variant of CHRPE clustered in one quadrant with appearance of animal tracks. Polar bear tracks are another variant in which the lesions are hypopigmented. Familial cases have been reported.

- No treatment necessary

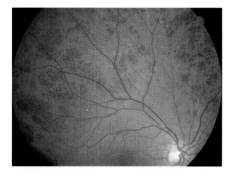

Figure 10–134 Bear tracks.   **Figure 10–135** Polar bear tracks.

Combined Hamartoma of Retinal Pigment Epithelium and Retina: Slightly elevated, dark gray (variable pigmentation) lesion with poorly defined, feathery borders often associated with a fine glial membrane on the surface of the tumor; dilated, tortuous retinal vessels common. Can occur in a peripapillary location (46%) or in the posterior pole; causes decreased vision, metamorphopsia, and strabismus in children and young adults. Subretinal neovascular membrane and subretinal exudation are late complications. Bilateral cases associated with neurofibromatosis type 2 (NF-2); variable prognosis.

Figure 10–136 Combined hamartoma of retinal pigment epithelium (RPE) and retina.

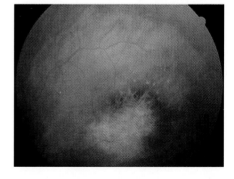

- Fluorescein angiogram: early filling of the dilated, tortuous retinal vessels with late leakage
- Consider retinal surgery with membrane peel if epiretinal membrane results in significant visual distortion
- Laser photocoagulation if SRNVM develops

Malignant Tumors

Note: Treatment and work-up for tumors of the retina and choroid should be per-formed by a multidisciplinary team composed of an internist, an oncologist, and an ocular tumor specialist. Therefore, in-depth discussions of management for these tumors is beyond the scope of this book, and treatment is best relegated to the physicians caring for the patient.

Choroidal Malignant Melanoma: Focal, darkly pigmented (amelanotic lesions lack pigmentation), dome- or collar-button–shaped (break through Bruch's mem-brane) tumor associated with overlying serous retinal detachment and lipofuscin (orange spots); commonly have episcleral sentinel vessels. Classified by size: small (<10 mm diameter, 2–3 mm height), medium (<15 mm diameter, <5 mm height), and large (>15 mm diameter, >5 mm height). Factors predictive of metastasis include epithelioid cells (Callender cytologic classification), high num-ber of mitoses, extrascleral extension, larger tumor size (57% die within 5 years), ciliary body involvement, and greater tumor pigmentation; poor prognosis.

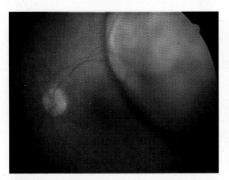

Figure 10–137 Choroidal malignant melanoma.

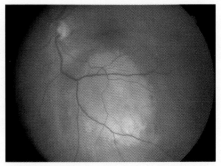

Figure 10–138 Choroidal amelanotic melanoma.

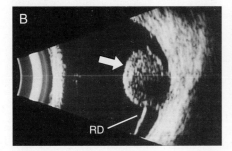

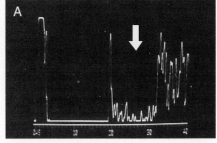

Figure 10–139 B-scan and A-scan appearance of choroidal melanoma demonstrating low internal reflectivity (arrow) and an exudative retinal detachment (RD).

- Intraocular shadow with transillumination
- B-scan ultrasonography: collar-button–shaped or dome-shaped mass >2.5 mm (95%), acoustically silent zone within the tumor, orbital shadowing, and choroidal excavation; low to medium internal reflectivity
- Fluorescein angiogram: double circulation due to intrinsic tumor circulation in large tumors, late staining of lesion with multiple pinpoint hyperfluorescent hot spots
- Enucleation, cryotherapy, laser photocoagulation, radiation therapy, brachytherapy, and chemotherapy are all used based largely on the results of the Collaborative Ocular Melanoma Study (COMS); should be performed by an experienced tumor specialist
- Medical and oncology consultation for systemic work-up

Choroidal Metastasis: Most common intraocular malignancy in adults; creamy yellow-white lesions with mottled pigment clumping (leopard spots); low to medium elevation; often with overlying serous retinal detachment; predilection for posterior pole; may be multifocal and bilateral (20%). Most common primary tumors are breast (females, metastasis late), lung (males, metastasis early), and unknown primary; also prostate, renal cell, and cutaneous melanoma; ocular involvement by hematogenous spread; rapid growth; very poor prognosis (median survival is 8.5 months from the time of diagnosis).

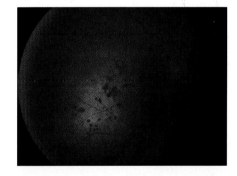

Figure 10–140 Choroidal metastasis with leopard-spot appearance (lung carcinoma).

- B-scan ultrasonography: flat or mildly elevated mass with irregular surface, medium to high internal reflectivity, serous retinal detachment usually visible, no orbital shadowing or acoustically silent zone
- Fluorescein angiogram: early hypofluorescence with pinpoint hyperfluorescence in the venous phase that increases in later views
- Lab tests: liver enzymes and chest radiographs
- Enucleation, laser photocoagulation, radiation therapy, brachytherapy, and chemotherapy are all used; should be performed by an experienced tumor specialist
- Oncology consultation for metastatic work-up if no known primary site

Primary Intraocular Lymphoma (Reticulum Cell Sarcoma): Bilateral (80%) anterior uveitis, vitritis, retinal vasculitis, cystoid macular edema, creamy yellow pigment epithelial detachments, hypopigmented retinal pigment epithelial lesions with overlying serous retinal detachments, and disc edema; occurs in 6th to 7th decade; patients have decreased vision and floaters; associated with central nervous system involvement and dementia; poor prognosis, with death within 2 years of diagnosis.

- Fluorescein angiogram: early staining of pigment epithelial detachments with late pooling; window defects seen in areas of atrophy
- Consider diagnostic pars plana vitrectomy to obtain vitreous biopsy for histopathologic and cytologic analysis
- Lumbar puncture for cytology
- Head MRI
- Treatment with chemotherapy and radiation should be performed by a tumor specialist
- Medical and oncology consultation

Retinoblastoma (RB): Globular, white-yellow, elevated mass with calcifications that may grow toward the vitreous (endophytic), causing vitreous seeding, or toward the choroid (exophytic) causing retinal detachment. Most common (1 in 20,000 live births) intraocular malignancy in children (90% diagnosed by 5 years of age). 20–35% bilateral, diagnosed earlier than unilateral (15 versus 24 months). 40% heritable, 95% sporadic (25% germinal, 75% somatic), 5% familial (AD). Mapped to chromosome 13q14. Children present with leukocoria (50%), strabismus (18%), intraocular inflammation, and decreased vision. Risk factors for poor prognosis include optic nerve invasion, extraocular extension, bilaterality, and delay in diagnosis. Prognosis good, with long-term survival approaching 85–90%; 25–30% of children with heritable retinoblastoma may develop a secondary malignancy.

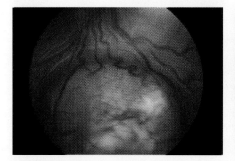

Figure 10–141 Retinoblastoma.

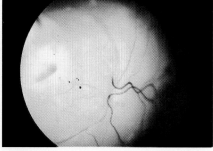

Figure 10–142 Retinoblastoma demonstrating exophytic growth with a serous retinal detachment.

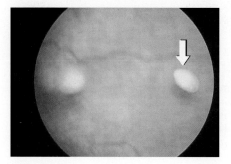

Figure 10–143 Retinoblastoma demonstrating endophytic growth with vitreous seeding (arrow).

- Examination under anesthesia (EUA) required for ophthalmoscopy and treatment
- B-scan ultrasonography and CT scan to detect calcifications (80%)
- Head and orbital MRI to evaluate for extraocular extension and trilateral retinoblastoma (bilateral with pinealblastoma or parasellar mass)
- Enucleation, cryotherapy, laser photocoagulation, radiation therapy, brachytherapy, and chemotherapy are all used to treat retinoblastoma; should be performed by an experienced tumor specialist
- Oncology consultation

Paraneoplastic Syndromes

Bilateral Diffuse Uveal Melanocytic Proliferation Syndrome (BDUMPS): Rare paraneoplastic disorder consisting of diffuse uveal thickening with multiple, faint, yellow-orange spots or slightly elevated, pigmented lesions scattered throughout the fundus ("giraffe-skin" fundus). Occurs in elderly patients with a systemic malignancy who have progressive decreased vision; retinal detachment may occur late; poor prognosis, with death within 2 years of diagnosis.

- B-scan ultrasonography: diffuse uveal thickening
- Fluorescein angiogram: orange spots appear hyperfluorescent
- ERG (markedly reduced)
- No effective treatment
- Oncology consultation

Carcinoma-Associated Retinopathy (CAR): Sudden onset of nyctalopia, decreased vision (can progress to no light perception [NLP] over months to years), dyschromatopsia, and visual field changes in patients >50 years old who have a systemic malignancy (notably small-cell lung carcinoma). Patients develop a retinal pigment degeneration with narrowed retinal vessels and vitreous cells; poor prognosis.

- ERG (markedly reduced)
- No effective treatment
- Oncology consultation

Cutaneous Melanoma-Associated Retinopathy (MAR): Subset of CAR with similar symptoms and fundus findings; paraneoplastic syndrome associated with cutaneous melanoma; antibodies to bipolar cells causes a selective loss of b-wave on ERG.

- ERG (markedly reduced with selective loss of b-wave)
- No effective treatment
- Oncology consultation

Optic Nerve / Glaucoma

Papilledema

Definition

Optic disc swelling caused by increased intracranial pressure.

Symptoms

Asymptomatic; may have headache, nausea, emesis, transient visual obscurations (lasting seconds), diplopia, altered mental status, or other neurologic deficits.

Signs

Normal visual acuity and color vision, transient obscurations of vision, enlarged blind spot, bilateral (rarely unilateral) optic disc edema with blurred disc margins, disc hyperemia, loss of physiologic cup, thickened nerve fiber layer obscuring retinal vessels, peripapillary nerve fiber layer hemorrhages, cotton-wool spots, exudates, and retinal folds (Paton's lines); may have absent venous pulsations (found in 20% of normal individuals) and cranial nerve VI palsy; optic atrophy, visual field defects, dyschromatopsia, vascular attenuation, and decreased visual acuity seen late.

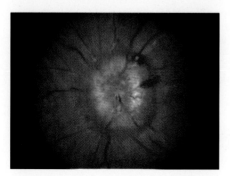

Figure 11–1 Papilledema due to an intracranial tumor.

Differential Diagnosis

Intracranial mass, neoplasm, infection (meningitis, encephalitis), or infiltration; subdural or subarachnoid hemorrhage; other causes of optic disc edema including malignant hypertension, idiopathic intracranial hypertension, diabetes mellitus, anemia, central retinal vein occlusion, neuroretinitis, uveitis, optic neuritis (papillitis), anterior ischemic optic neuropathy, Leber's optic neuropathy, hypotony, lymphoma, leukemia, optic nerve mass, Foster-Kennedy syndrome; pseudopapilledema (eg, optic nerve drusen).

Evaluation

- Complete ophthalmic history, neurologic exam, and eye exam with attention to color vision, pupils, and ophthalmoscopy
- Check visual fields (enlarged blind spot)
- Emergent head and orbital computed tomography (CT) or magnetic resonance imaging (MRI) to rule out intracranial processes
- Lumbar puncture to check opening pressure and rule out other intracranial processes
- Lab tests: fasting blood sugar (diabetes mellitus), complete blood count (CBC; anemia, leukemia, infection), erythrocyte sedimentation rate (ESR)
- Check blood pressure
- Neurology consultation

Management

- Treat underlying cause

Prognosis

Depends on etiology.

Idiopathic Intracranial Hypertension (Pseudotumor Cerebri)

Definition

Disorder of unknown etiology that meets four criteria: papilledema, increased intracranial pressure (>250 mm H_2O), normal cerebrospinal fluid (CSF) composition, and normal neuroimaging studies.

Etiology

Idiopathic; may be associated with vitamin A intoxication, tetracycline, oral contraceptive pills, nalidixic acid, lithium, or steroid use/withdrawal; also associated with dural sinus thrombosis, radical neck surgery, middle ear disease, obesity, chronic obstructive pulmonary disease, and pregnancy. Idiopathic intracranial hypertension is a diagnosis of exclusion.

Epidemiology

Usually occurs in obese 20- to 30-year-old females (2:1).

Symptoms

Asymptomatic; patient may have headache, transient visual obscurations (lasting seconds), diplopia, tinnitus, dizziness, nausea, and emesis.

Signs

Normal or decreased visual acuity, color vision, and contrast sensitivity; bilateral optic disc edema; may have cranial nerve (CN) VI palsy (30%) and/or visual field defect.

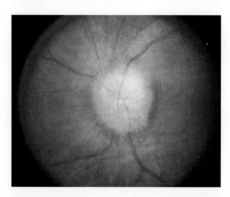

Figure 11–2   Idiopathic intracranial hypertension demonstrating papilledema.

Differential Diagnosis

Rule out other causes of papilledema and optic disc edema (see Papilledema section).

Evaluation

- Complete ophthalmic history, neurologic exam, and eye exam with attention to color vision, pupils, motility, and ophthalmoscopy
- Check visual fields (enlarged blind spot, generalized constriction)
- Emergent head and orbital CT scan or MRI to rule out intracranial processes
- Lumbar puncture to check opening pressure (>250 mm H_2O is abnormal) and composition of cerebrospinal fluid
- Check blood pressure
- Neurology consultation

Management

- If the patient is obese, initiate a weight-loss program
- Discontinue vitamin A, tetracycline, oral contraceptive pills, nalidixic acid, lithium, or steroid use
- No further treatment recommended unless patient exhibits progressive visual loss, visual field defects, or intractable headaches
- Systemic acetazolamide (Diamox; 500–2000 mg PO qd)
- Consider systemic diuretics (furosemide [Lasix] 60–120 mg PO qd), serial lumbar punctures; follow visual field, visual acuity, and color vision
- Systemic steroids (prednisone 60–100 mg PO qd) are controversial; check purified protein derivative (PPD), blood glucose, and chest radiographs before starting systemic steroids
- Add H_2-blocker (ranitidine [Zantac] 150 mg PO bid) when giving systemic steroids
- Consider surgery for progressive visual loss despite maximal medical therapy (optic nerve sheath fenestration, lumboperitoneal shunt)

Prognosis

Usually self-limited over 3–6 months; poor if visual loss has occurred.

Optic Neuritis

Definition

Primary inflammation of the optic nerve; two types depending on location:

Papillitis: Optic disc swelling present.

Retrobulbar: No optic disc swelling, the inflammation is behind the globe.

Devic's syndrome is bilateral optic neuritis with transverse myelitis.

Epidemiology

Usually seen in 15- to 45-year-old females; 55% of patients with multiple sclerosis (MS) develop optic neuritis; presenting diagnosis in 20% of multiple sclerosis cases; 74% of women and 34% of men will develop multiple sclerosis in 15 years. *Note:* optic neuritis in children is usually bilateral, post-viral, and not associated with multiple sclerosis.

Symptoms

Acute visual loss (may progress for up to 10 days, then stabilizes and improves), pain on eye movement, dyschromatopsia, decreased brightness sense; may have previous viral syndrome, or phosphenes on eye movement or with loud noises.

Signs

Decreased visual acuity ranging from 20/20 to no light perception (NLP); decreased color vision and contrast sensitivity; positive relative afferent pupillary defect (RAPD), central or paracentral scotoma; may have optic disc swelling (65%), mild vitritis, altered depth perception (Pulfrich phenomenon), and increased latency and decreased amplitude of visual evoked response (VER).

Differential Diagnosis

Idiopathic, viral infection (mumps, measles), intraocular inflammation, malignant hypertension, diabetes mellitus, sarcoidosis, syphilis, tuberculosis, collagen vascular disease, Leber's optic neuropathy, optic nerve glioma, orbital tumor, anterior ischemic optic neuropathy (AION), central serous retinopathy (CSR), multiple evanescent white dot syndrome (MEWDS), acute idiopathic blind spot enlargement syndrome (AIBSE).

Evaluation

- Complete ophthalmic history, neurologic exam, and eye exam with attention to color vision, Amsler grid, contrast sensitivity, pupils, motility, and ophthalmoscopy
- Check visual fields
- If patient does not carry the diagnosis of multiple sclerosis, then obtain an MRI of the head and orbits to evaluate for periventricular white matter demyelinating lesions or plaques (≥3 plaques is considered positive) and other intracranial processes
- Lab tests: fasting blood glucose, CBC, antinuclear antibody (ANA), angiotensin converting enzyme (ACE), Veneral Disease Research Laboratory (VDRL), fluorescent treponemal antibody absorption test (FTA-ABS), erythrocyte sedimentation rate (ESR)
- Check blood pressure
- Consider lumbar puncture to rule out intracranial processes
- Neurology consultation

Management

- If MRI is positive, treat with systemic IV steroids (methylprednisolone 1 g IV qd in divided doses for first 72 hours, then prednisone 1 mg/kg/day tapered over 11 days). The Optic Neuritis Treatment Trial (ONTT) showed that this regimen led to visual recovery 2 weeks faster than other treatments, no difference in final visual acuity, and a decreased incidence of multiple sclerosis over the ensuing 2 years (no difference after 3 years). *Note:* Do not use oral steroids alone, since this led to an increased risk of recurrent optic neuritis (ONTT conclusion)
- Check PPD, blood glucose, and chest radiographs before starting systemic steroids
- Add H_2-blocker (ranitidine [Zantac] 150 mg PO bid) when taking systemic steroids

Prognosis

Good; visual acuity improves over months; final acuity depends on severity of initial visual loss; 70% of patients will recover 20/20 vision; permanent subtle color vision and contrast sensitivity deficits are common; after recovery, patient may have blurred vision with increased body temperature or exercise (Uhthoff's symptom).

Anterior Ischemic Optic Neuropathy (AION)

Definition

Ischemic infarction of anterior optic nerve due to occlusion of posterior ciliary circulation just behind lamina cribrosa; two types:

Arteritic: Giant cell arteritis (GCA)/temporal arteritis.

Nonarteritic/Idiopathic: Associated with hypertension (40%) and diabetes mellitus (20%); arteriosclerotic changes are seen in optic disc vessels.

Epidemiology

Arteritic: Usually seen in patients >55 years old, fellow eye involved in 75% of cases within 2 weeks without treatment; associated with polymyalgia rheumatica (PMR).

Nonarteritic/Idiopathic: Usually seen in younger patients; fellow eye involved in 25–40% of cases; associated with hypertension and diabetes mellitus.

Symptoms

Acute visual loss (arteritic > nonarteritic) and dyschromatopsia.

Arteritic: May also have headache, fever, malaise, weight loss, scalp tenderness, jaw claudication, amaurosis fugax, diplopia, polymyalgia rheumatica symptoms (joint pain), and eye pain.

Signs

Sudden, unilateral, decreased visual acuity and color vision (bilateral later), positive relative afferent pupillary defect (RAPD), altitudinal visual field defect (usually inferior and large), swollen optic disc (pallor/atrophy after 6–8 weeks), fellow nerve often crowded with a small or absent cup, fellow nerve may be pale from prior episode (pseudo Foster-Kennedy syndrome; more common than true Foster-Kennedy, which is a rare syndrome due to frontal lobe tumor causing ipsilateral optic atrophy and contralateral disc swelling secondary to increased intracranial pressure).

Arteritic: May also have swollen, tender, temporal artery, cotton-wool spots, central retinal artery occlusion, ophthalmic artery occlusion, anterior segment ischemia, cranial nerve palsy (especially CN VI); optic disc cupping is seen late.

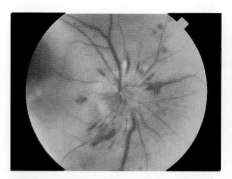

Figure 11–3 Anterior ischemic optic neuropathy with disc edema and flame hemorrhages.

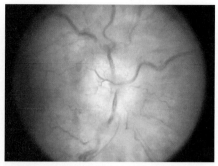

Figure 11–4 Anterior ischemic optic neuropathy with disc edema.

Differential Diagnosis

Malignant hypertension, diabetes mellitus, retinal vascular occlusion, compressive lesion, collagen vascular disease, syphilis, herpes zoster; also migraine, postoperative, massive blood loss, normal (low) tension glaucoma.

Evaluation

- Complete ophthalmic history and eye exam with attention to color vision, Amsler grid, pupils, and ophthalmoscopy
- Check visual fields
- Lab tests: **STAT** erythrocyte sedimentation rate (ESR) (to rule out arteritic form; ESR > [age/2] in men and > [(age+10)/2] in women is abnormal), CBC (low hematocrit), fasting blood glucose, C-reactive protein, VDRL, FTA-ABS, ANA
- Check blood pressure
- **Arteritic:** Temporal artery biopsy (beware; can get false negative results from skip lesions); can perform up to 1 week after starting systemic steroids
- Fluorescein angiogram: choroidal nonperfusion in arteritic form
- Medical consultation

Management

- **Arteritic:** Systemic steroids (methylprednisolone 1 g IV qd in divided doses for 72 hours, then prednisone 60–100 mg PO qd with a slow taper; decrease by no more than 2.5–5.0 mg/wk) started before results of biopsy known to prevent ischemic optic neuropathy in fellow eye; follow ESR and symptoms carefully
- Check PPD, blood glucose, and chest radiographs before starting systemic steroids
- Add H$_2$-blocker (ranitidine [Zantac] 150 mg PO bid) when giving systemic steroids
- **Nonarteritic/Idiopathic:** Treat underlying medical condition

Prognosis

Poor; visual loss is usually permanent.

Other Optic Neuropathies

Definition

Variety of processes that cause unilateral or bilateral optic nerve damage and subsequent optic atrophy. Atrophy of axons with resultant disc pallor occurs 6–8 weeks after injury anterior to lateral geniculate nucleus.

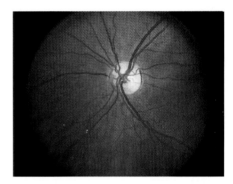

Figure 11–5 Optic atrophy demonstrating pale nerve.

Etiology

Compressive: Meningioma, glioma, thyroid ophthalmopathy, idiopathic intracranial hypertension, and other primary or metastatic orbital tumors.

Hereditary:

■ **Behr's (autosomal recessive [AR]):** Occurs between 1 and 9 years of age; male predilection; moderate to severe visual loss; no progression; associated with severe dyschromatopsis, nystagmus in 50%, increased deep tendon reflexes, hypotonia, cerebellar ataxia, and mental retardation.

■ **Kjer's (autosomal dominant [AD]):** Most common hereditary optic neuropathy; occurs between 4 and 8 years of age; mild, insidious loss of vision, tritanopic dyschromatopsia; slight progression; nystagmus rare.

■ **Leber's optic neuropathy (mitochondrial DNA):** Typically occurs in 10- to 30-year-old males (9:1); rapid, severe visual loss that starts unilaterally, but sequentially involves fellow eye usually within 1 year but can be within days to weeks; optic nerve hyperemia and swollen nerve fiber layer with small, peripapillary, telangiectatic blood vessels that do not leak on fluorescein angiography (optic nerve also does not stain); mothers transmit defect to all sons (50% affected) and all daughters are carriers (10% affected).

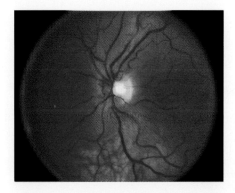

Figure 11-6 Leber's optic neuropathy.

Infiltrative: May be infectious/inflammatory from sarcoidosis, toxoplasmosis, toxocariasis, cytomegalovirus, and tuberculosis; or from malignancies including lymphoma, leukemia, carcinoma, plasmacytoma, and metastasis.

Toxic/Nutritional: Radiation, tobacco-alcohol amblyopia, ethambutol, isoniazid, chloramphenicol, streptomycin, arsenic, lead, methanol, digitalis, chloroquine, quinine, and various vitamin deficiencies including B_1 (thiamine), B_2 (riboflavin), B_6 (pyridoxine), B_{12} (cobalamin), and folic acid.

Traumatic: Optic nerve avulsion, canalicular compression, hematoma.

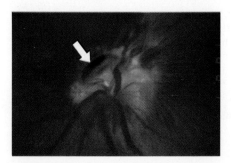

Figure 11-7 Traumatic optic nerve avulsion; arrow indicates site of avulsion.

Symptoms

Decreased vision, dyschromatopsia, central scotoma.

Signs

Unilateral or bilateral decreased visual acuity ranging from 20/20 to 20/400, dyschromatopsia, and decreased contrast sensitivity; positive relative afferent pupillary defect (RAPD) if optic nerve damage is asymmetric (if symmetric damage, RAPD may be absent); optic disc pallor, retinal nerve fiber layer defects, central or centrocecal visual field defects; abnormal visual evoked response; retro-bulbar mass lesions may cause proptosis and motility deficits; optociliary shunt vessels in meningioma or glioma.

Differential Diagnosis

As above.

Evaluation

- Complete ophthalmic history, neurologic exam, and eye exam with attention to color vision, pupils, motility, Hertel exophthalmometry, and ophthalmoscopy
- Check visual fields
- Head and orbital CT scan and/or MRI to rule out intracranial processes or mass lesion
- Lab tests: CBC, vitamin B_1, B_2, B_6, and B_{12} levels
- Consider medical consultation

Management

- **Compressive:** Systemic steroids (prednisone 60–200 mg PO qd) and surgical decompression for thyroid ophthalmopathy; consider surgical resection for some tumors
- **Hereditary:** Genetic counseling; no effective treatment
- **Infiltrative:** Leukemic optic nerve infiltration occurs in children and is an OCULAR EMERGENCY that requires radiation therapy to salvage vision
- **Toxic/Nutritional:** Discontinue offending toxic agent; consider vitamin B_1 (thiamine 100 mg PO bid), vitamin B_{12} (vitamin B_{12} 1 mg IM q month), folate (0.1 mg PO qd), or multivitamin (qd) supplementation
- **Traumatic:** Consider high-dose IV steroids (controversial)

Prognosis

Poor; visual loss is permanent once atrophy has occurred.

Congenital Anomalies

Definition

Variety of developmental optic nerve anomalies:

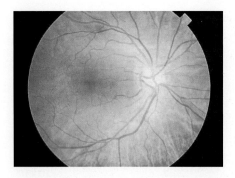

Figure 11–8 Anomalous optic nerve.

Aplasia: Very rare, no optic nerve or retinal vessels present.

Dysplasias:

■ **Coloboma:** Spectrum of large, abnormal-appearing optic discs due to incomplete closure of the embryonic fissure; usually located inferonasally; associated with other ocular colobomata. May be associated with systemic defects including congenital heart defects, double aortic arch, transposition of the great vessels, coarctation of the aorta, and intracranial carotid anomalies.

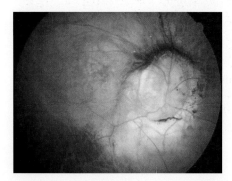

Figure 11–9 Optic nerve coloboma.

■ **Hypoplasia:** Small discs, "double ring" sign (peripapillary ring of pigmentary changes); unilateral cases usually idiopathic; bilateral cases associated with midline abnormalities, endocrine dysfunction, and maternal history of diabetes mellitus or drug use (Dilantin, quinine, alcohol, LSD) during pregnancy.

■ **Morning Glory Syndrome:** Large, unilateral, excavated disc with central, white, glial tissue surrounded by elevated pigment ring; may represent a form of optic nerve coloboma; involves entire peripapillary region; female predilection (2:1); usually severe visual loss; may develop a localized serous retinal detachment; associated with midline facial defects and forebrain anomalies.

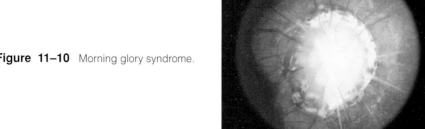

Figure 11–10 Morning glory syndrome.

■ **Pit:** 0.1–0.7 disc diameter depression in optic disc usually located temporally; appears gray-white; 85% unilateral; peripapillary retinal pigment epithelium (RPE) changes in 95%; 40% develop localized serous retinal detachment in teardrop configuration extending from the pit into papillomacular retina; source of subretinal fluid (CSF vs. liquefied vitreous) still controversial; retinal detachments often spontaneously resolve.

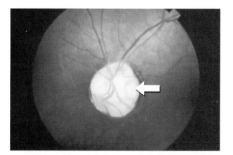

Figure 11–11 Optic nerve pit (arrow).

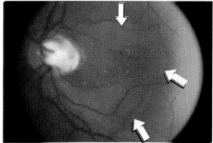

Figure 11–12 Optic nerve pit with serous retinal detachment (arrows).

■ **Septo-optic Dysplasia (de Morsier):** Syndrome of optic disc hypoplasia, absence of septum pellucidum, agenesis of corpus callosum, and endocrine problems; may have see-saw nystagmus.

■ **Tilted Optic Disc:** Displacement of one side of optic disc peripherally with oblique insertion of retinal vessels; associated with high myopia; can cause bitemporal visual field defects that do not respect midline.

Optic Nerve Drusen: Superficial or buried hyaline-like material in the substance of the nerve anterior to the lamina cribrosa; may calcify; 75% bilateral; may be hereditary (AD); associated with retinitis pigmentosa; may develop visual field defects usually inferonasal and/or arcuate (50%); subretinal neovascular membranes are late complications.

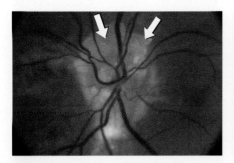

Figure 11–13 Optic nerve drusen (arrows).

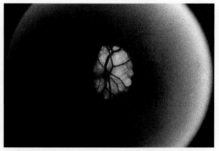

Figure 11–14 Optic nerve drusen demonstrating autofluorescence.

Symptoms

Asymptomatic; may have decreased vision, metamorphopsia, scotomas, or visual field defects.

Signs

Normal or decreased visual acuity, abnormal-appearing optic disc, variety of visual field defects, may have positive relative afferent pupillary defect (RAPD); calcified drusen appear on B-scan ultrasonogram and CT scan.

Differential Diagnosis

See above; optic disc drusen may give appearance of papilledema (pseudo-papilledema).

Evaluation

- Complete ophthalmic history and eye exam with attention to color vision, pupils, 78/90 diopter or contact lens fundus exam, and ophthalmoscopy
- Consider visual fields
- Fluorescein angiogram: serous retinal detachment with early punctate fluorescence and late filling may be seen with optic pits; optic nerve drusen autofluoresce with only filter in place before any fluorescein administration
- Consider B-scan ultrasonography to identify buried drusen
- Head and orbital CT scan for dysplasias
- Endocrine consultation for hypoplasia

Management

- No treatment usually required
- May require polycarbonate protective lenses if amblyopia or decreased visual acuity present
- Consider laser photocoagulation to demarcate serous retinal detachments associated with optic pits (controversial); may also consider pars plana vitrectomy, peeling of posterior hyaloid, air fluid exchange, and long-acting gas tamponade if laser fails (controversial)
- Treat any underlying endocrine abnormalities

Prognosis

Stable; decreased vision from compression, subretinal neovascularization, or central retinal artery occlusion can rarely occur with optic nerve drusen; basal encephalocele can occur in any of the dysplasias.

Optic Nerve Tumors

Definition

Variety of neoplasms (benign and malignant) that may affect optic nerve anywhere along its course.

Angioma (von Hippel Lesion): Retinal capillary hemangioma (see Chap. 10); benign lesion that may involve the optic nerve; may be associated with intracranial (especially cerebellar) hemangiomas (von Hippel-Lindau syndrome) (see Figs. 10–118 & 10–131).

Astrocytic Hamartoma: Benign, yellow-white, nodular, glistening, "mulberry-like" lesion seen in tuberous sclerosis and neurofibromatosis (see Chap. 10); may be isolated, multiple, unilateral, or bilateral (see Fig. 10–124 & 10–125).

Combined Hamartoma of Retina and RPE: Rare, peripapillary tumor composed of retinal, retinal pigment epithelial, vascular, and glial tissue; may cause epiretinal membranes with macular traction or edema (see Chap. 10; Fig. 10–136).

Glioma: Two types:

- **Glioblastoma Multiforme:** Rare, malignant tumor seen in adults who develop rapid, painful visual loss in one eye with fellow eye involvement over the ensuing weeks; aggressive tumor with blindness in months and death within 6–9 months; may have central retinal artery and/or central retinal vein occlusion as tumor compromises blood supply; enlargement of optic canal present on CT scan; endocrine or neurologic deficits may appear if tumor invades other structures.

- **Juvenile Pilocytic Astrocytoma:** Uncommon, benign, neural tumor seen in children; 90% occur in 1st–2nd decade with peak between 2 and 6 years of age;

presents with gradual, unilateral, progressive, painless proptosis, decreased vision, positive relative afferent pupillary defect (RAPD), and optic disc edema; optic atrophy or strabismus may develop later; chiasmal involvement in 50% of cases; orbital CT scan shows fusiform enlargement of the optic nerve; histologically characterized by Rosenthal fibers, pilocytic astrocytes, and myxomatous differentiation; associated with neurofibromatosis (NF-1) in 25–50% of cases.

Melanocytoma: Benign, darkly pigmented tumor that lies over or adjacent to the optic disc, usually jet black with fuzzy borders; rarely increases in size; more common in African Americans; malignant transformation is exceedingly rare.

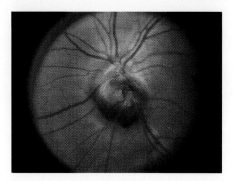

Figure 11–15 Melanocytoma.

Meningioma: Rare (3–5% of all orbital tumors), histologically benign tumor arising from optic nerve sheath arachnoid tissue or from adjacent meninges; usually seen in middle-aged females (3:1) in the 3rd–5th decade; signs include unilateral proptosis, painless, decreased visual acuity and color vision, positive relative afferent pupillary defect (RAPD), optociliary shunt vessels, and optic nerve edema or atrophy; may grow rapidly during pregnancy and involute after delivery; optic nerve pallor and optociliary shunt vessels occur later; orbital CT scan demonstrates tubular enlargement of the optic nerve and hyperostosis; "railroad-track" sign seen on axial views and "double ring" appearance seen on coronal views; histologic features include whorl pattern and Psammoma bodies.

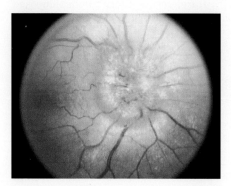

Figure 11–16 Meningioma producing optic disc edema.

Symptoms

Asymptomatic; may have decreased vision, dyschromatopsia, metamorphopsia, or pain.

Signs

Normal or decreased visual acuity and dyschromatopsia, positive relative afferent pupillary defect (RAPD), proptosis, motility disturbances, increased intraocular pressure (IOP), optic nerve or peripapillary lesion, optic disc swelling or pallor, visual field defect; optociliary shunt vessels in meningioma or glioma; angiomas may rarely cause vitreous or retinal hemorrhage.

Differential Diagnosis

See above.

Evaluation

- Complete ophthalmic history, neurologic exam, and eye exam with attention to color vision, pupils, tonometry, and ophthalmoscopy
- Check visual fields
- B-scan ultrasonography to evaluate course of optic nerve
- Fluorescein angiogram to rule out retinal angiomas
- Head and orbital CT scan or MRI to rule out intracranial lesions

Management

- Treatment depends on etiology
- May require treatment of increased intraocular pressure (see Primary Open-Angle Glaucoma section)
- Consider laser photocoagulation of angiomas (see Chap. 10)
- Treatment of malignant tumors with chemotherapy, radiation, or surgery should be performed by a tumor specialist

Prognosis

Good for benign lesions, variable for meningiomas, and poor for malignant lesions.

Chiasmal Syndromes

Definition

Variety of optic chiasm disorders that cause visual field defects.

Epidemiology

Mass lesions in 95% of cases; most lesions are large, since chiasm is 10 mm above sella (microadenomas do not cause field defects); may present acutely with pituitary apoplexy secondary to hemorrhage or necrosis.

Symptoms

Asymptomatic; patient may have headache, decreased vision, visual field defects, diplopia, or vague visual complaints.

Signs

Normal or decreased visual acuity and dyschromatopsia; may have positive relative afferent pupillary defect (RAPD), optic atrophy (often in bow-tie configuration), visual field defect (junctional scotoma, bitemporal hemianopia, incongruous homonymous hemianopia), or signs of pituitary apoplexy (severe headache, ophthalmoplegia, and decreased visual acuity).

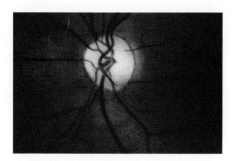

Figure 11–17 Optic atrophy demonstrating "bow-tie" appearance.

Differential Diagnosis

Pituitary tumor, pituitary apoplexy, meningioma, aneurysm, trauma, sarcoidosis, craniopharyngioma, multiple sclerosis, glioma.

Evaluation

- Complete ophthalmic history, endocrine history, and eye exam with attention to visual acuity, color vision, pupils, and ophthalmoscopy
- Check visual fields with attention to vertical midline
- Head and orbital CT scan or MRI (**EMERGENT** if pituitary apoplexy suspected)
- Lab tests: consider checking hormone levels

Management

- Treatment depends on etiology
- Pituitary lesions that require surgery, radiation therapy, bromocriptine, hormone replacement should be managed by a neurosurgeon and/or internist
- Systemic steroids and surgical decompression for pituitary apoplexy

Prognosis

Generally poor; depends on etiology.

Congenital Glaucoma

Definition

Congenital = onset of glaucoma from birth to 3 months of age (infantile = 3 months to 3 years; juvenile = 3 to 35 years).

Epidemiology

Incidence of 1 in 10,000 births; three forms: approximately one third primary, one third secondary, one third associated with systemic syndromes or anomalies.

Primary: 70% bilateral, 65% male, usually recessive with incomplete penetrance, 40% at birth, 85% by 1 year of age.

Secondary: Inflammation, steroid induced, trauma, tumors.

Associated Syndromes: Mesodermal dysgenesis syndromes, aniridia, lens-induced, persistent hyperplastic primary vitreous (PHPV), nanophthalmos, rubella, nevus of Ota, Sturge-Weber syndrome, neurofibromatosis, Marfan's syndrome, Weill-Marchesani syndrome, Lowe's syndrome, mucopolysaccharidoses.

Mechanism

Primary: Developmental abnormality of the angle (goniodysgenesis) with faulty cleavage and abnormal insertion of ciliary muscle.

Symptoms

Epiphora, photophobia, blepharospasm.

Signs

Decreased visual acuity, myopia, amblyopia, increased intraocular pressure, corneal diameter > 12 mm by 1 year of age, corneal edema, Haab's striae (breaks in Descemet's membrane horizontal or concentric to limbus), optic nerve cupping (may reverse with treatment), buphthalmos (enlarged eye).

Differential Diagnosis

Nasolacrimal duct obstruction, megalocornea, high myopia, proptosis, birth trauma, congenital hereditary endothelial dystrophy of the cornea, sclerocornea, metabolic diseases.

Evaluation

- Complete ophthalmic history and eye exam with attention to retinoscopy, tonometry, corneal diameter, gonioscopy, and ophthalmoscopy
- Complete evaluation may require examination under anesthesia (EUA); *Note:* Intraocular pressure affected by anesthetic agents (transiently increased by ketamine; decreased by inhalants)
- Check visual fields in older children

Management

- Treatment is primarily surgical, but depends on the type of glaucoma, intraocular pressure level and control, and amount and progression of optic nerve cupping and visual field defects (older children); should be performed by a glaucoma specialist; treatment options include:
- **Medical** (temporize prior to surgery): Topical beta-blocker (timolol maleate [Timoptic] or betaxolol [Betoptic S] bid) and/or carbonic anhydrase inhibitor (dorzolamide [Trusopt] tid or acetazolamide [Diamox] 15 mg/kg/d PO)
- **Surgical:** Goniotomy, trabeculotomy; also trabeculectomy, glaucoma drainage implant, cycloablation
- Correct any refractive error (myopia)
- Patching/occlusion therapy for amblyopia (see Chap. 12)

Prognosis

Usually poor; best for primary congenital form and onset between 1 and 24 months of age.

Primary Open-Angle Glaucoma (POAG)

Definition

Progressive, bilateral, optic neuropathy with open angles, typical pattern of nerve fiber bundle visual field loss, and increased intraocular pressure (IOP > 21 mm Hg) not caused by another systemic or local disease (see Secondary Glaucoma section).

Epidemiology

Occurs in 0.5–2.1% of population >40 years old; risk increases with age; 60–70% of all glaucomas; no sex predilection; African Americans are 3–6 times more likely to develop POAG than Caucasians; POAG also occurs earlier, is 6 times more likely to cause blindness, and is the leading cause of blindness in African Americans; in addition to level of IOP, race, and age, other risk factors include positive family history of POAG (first-degree relatives), myopia, diabetes mellitus, hypertension, and cardiovascular disease.

Mechanism

Various theories of optic nerve damage:

Mechanical: Resistance to outflow (at juxtacanalicular meshwork), disturbance of trabecular meshwork collagen, trabecular meshwork endothelial cell dysfunction, basement membrane thickening, glycosaminoglycan deposition, narrowed intertrabecular spaces, collapse of Schlemm's canal.

Vascular: Poor optic nerve perfusion.

Apoptosis: Programmed cell death secondary to intercellular communication breakdown.

Glutamate Toxicity: Increased levels of glutamate in vitreous.

Symptoms

Asymptomatic; may have decreased vision or constricted visual fields in late stages.

Signs

Normal or decreased visual acuity, increased intraocular pressure, cupping of optic nerve, retinal nerve fiber layer defects, visual field defects.

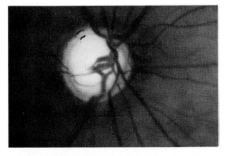

Figure 11–18 Optic nerve cupping due to primary open-angle glaucoma.

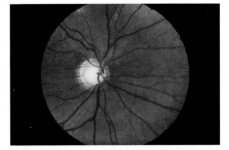

Figure 11–19 Physiologic cupping.

Differential Diagnosis

Secondary open-angle glaucoma, normal tension glaucoma, ocular hypertension, optic neuropathy, physiologic cupping.

Evaluation

- Complete ophthalmic history and eye exam with attention to cornea, tonometry, anterior chamber gonioscopy, iris, lens, and ophthalmoscopy
- Check visual fields
- Stereo optic nerve photos are useful for comparison at subsequent evaluations

Management

Choice and order of treatment modality depend on many factors, including patient's age, intraocular pressure level and control, and amount and progression of optic nerve cupping and visual field defects. Treatment options include:

- **Observation:** Intraocular pressure checks every 3–6 months, visual field examination every 6–12 months, gonioscopy and optic nerve evaluation yearly
- **Medical:** Classically, topical β-blockers are the first line of treatment. If intraocular pressure is not controlled, additional medications can be added. Follow-up (after intraocular pressure stabilization) at 3–4 weeks after changing treatment to evaluate efficacy. (*Note:* Brand names are used in this section; for generic names, please consult the Appendix); treatment options include single or combinations of the following medications:
    - Topical β-blocker (Timoptic, Betoptic S (selective β$_1$-blocker), Betagan, OptiPranolol, or Ocupress bid); decreases aqueous production; check for history of cardiac and pulmonary disease before prescribing
    - Topical α-adrenergic agonist (Iopidine tid, Alphagan bid, or Propine bid); decreases aqueous production
    - Topical cholinergic (Pilocarpine qid, Ocusert, carbachol tid, Phospholine Iodide bid); increases outflow through trabecular meshwork
    - Topical prostaglandin analogue (Xalatan qd); increases uveoscleral outflow
    - Topical carbonic anhydrase inhibitor (Trusopt tid); decreases aqueous production
    - Systemic carbonic anhydrase inhibitor (Diamox or Neptazane qd to qid); decreases aqueous production
- **Laser:** Trabeculoplasty, sclerostomy, cyclophotocoagulation
- **Surgical:** Trabeculectomy, glaucoma drainage implant, cycloablation

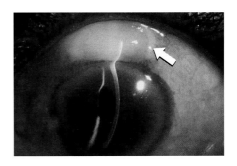

Figure 11–20 Conjunctival filtering bleb following glaucoma surgery (arrow) (trabeculectomy).

Prognosis

Usually good if intraocular pressure is adequately controlled; worse prognosis in African Americans; visual loss is permanent.

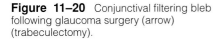
Secondary Open-Angle Glaucoma

Definition

Open-angle glaucoma caused by a variety of local or systemic disorders.

Etiology

Pseudoexfoliation syndrome (see Chap. 8), pigment dispersion syndrome (see Chap. 7), ocular inflammation, lens-induced (see Chap. 8), intraocular tumors, trauma, and drugs; also elevated episcleral venous pressure (orbital mass, thyroid ophthalmopathy, arteriovenous fistulas, orbital varices, superior vena cava syndrome, Sturge-Weber syndrome, idiopathic), retinal disease (retinal detachment, retinitis pigmentosa, Stickler's syndrome), systemic disease (pituitary tumors, Cushing's syndrome, thyroid disease, renal disease), postoperative (laser and surgical procedures), and UGH syndrome (see Chap. 6).

Drug-Induced:

Epidemiology

Steroid-related intraocular pressure elevation correlates with potency and duration of use; 30% of population develop increased intraocular pressure after 4–6 weeks of topical steroid use, intraocular pressure >30 mm Hg in 4%; 95% of primary open-angle glaucoma patients are steroid responders; increased incidence of steroid response in patients with diabetes mellitus, high myopia, connective tissue disease, and family history of glaucoma.

Mechanism

Alpha-Chymotrypsin: Zonular debris blocks trabecular meshwork.

Steroids: Unknown, possibly due to increased trabecular meshwork glycosaminoglycans.

Viscoelastic: Viscous substance injected during ophthalmic surgery obstructs trabecular meshwork, self-limited (1–2 days).

Management

- Treatment of increased intraocular pressure (see Primary Open-Angle Glaucoma section)
- Taper, change, or stop steroids
- Consider releasing viscoelastic through paracentesis site on first postoperative day if intraocular pressure >30 mm Hg

Intraocular Tumors:

Mechanism

Hemorrhage, angle neovascularization, direct tumor infiltration of the angle, or trabecular meshwork obstruction by tumor, inflammatory, or red blood cells.

Symptoms

Asymptomatic; may have decreased vision, pain, or systemic symptoms.

Signs

Normal or decreased visual acuity, increased intraocular pressure, iris mass, focal iris elevation, hyphema, hypopyon, anterior chamber cell/flare, pseudohypopyon, leukocoria, segmental cataract, invasion of angle, extrascleral extension, sentinel episcleral vessels.

Evaluation

- Complete ophthalmic history and eye exam with attention to cornea, tonometry, anterior chamber, gonioscopy, iris, lens, and ophthalmoscopy
- B-scan ultrasonography if unable to visualize the fundus; consider ultrasound biomicroscopy (UBM) to evaluate angle and ciliary body
- Check visual fields
- Medical or oncology consultation for metastatic work-up

Management

- Treatment of increased intraocular pressure (see Primary Open-Angle Glaucoma section)
- Treatment for tumor with radiation, chemotherapy, or surgery should be performed by a tumor specialist

Ocular Inflammation:

Epidemiology

Fuchs' Heterochromic Iridocyclitis: Usually unilateral (90%), low-grade iritis affecting lighter colored eye with stellate, white keratic precipitates (KP), fine branching angle vessels, and no posterior or peripheral anterior synechiae, poor response to steroids; associated with glaucoma (15%) and cataracts (70%) (see Chap. 6).

Glaucomatocyclitic Crisis (Posner-Schlossman Syndrome): Usually unilateral, recurrent, spontaneously resolving episodes of elevated intraocular pressure and corneal edema with minimal inflammation and symptoms, normal discs and visual fields, no posterior or peripheral anterior synechiae; crisis episodes can last hours to days (see Chap. 6).

Interstitial Keratitis: Associated with open-angle and angle-closure glaucoma.

Iridocyclitis: May be viral (eg, herpes, rubella, mumps), idiopathic, traumatic, or autoimmune (eg, sarcoidosis, juvenile rheumatoid arthritis).

Mechanism

Outflow obstruction due to inflammatory cells, trabeculitis, scarring of trabecular meshwork, and/or increased aqueous viscosity.

Symptoms

Asymptomatic; patient may have pain, photophobia, red eye, decreased vision.

Signs

Normal or decreased visual acuity, increased intraocular pressure (may be complicated by steroid response), ciliary injection, anterior chamber cell/flare, keratic precipitates, miotic pupil, peripheral anterior synechiae, posterior synechiae, iris heterochromia, iris atrophy, fine angle vessels, decreased corneal sensation, corneal edema, corneal scarring, ghost vessels, cataract; may have low intraocular pressure due to decreased aqueous production.

Evaluation

- Complete ophthalmic history and eye exam with attention to cornea, tonometry, anterior chamber, gonioscopy, iris, lens, and ophthalmoscopy
- Check visual fields
- Consider uveitis work-up

Management

- Treatment of increased intraocular pressure (see Primary Open-Angle Glaucoma section); do not use pilocarpine

Management *Continued*

- Treat anterior uveitis with topical cycloplegic (cyclopentolate 1% or scopolamine 0.25% tid) and topical steroid (prednisolone acetate 1%, rimexolone [Vexol], or fluorometholone [FML] qd to q1h depending on the amount of inflammation; beware of increased intraocular pressure with steroid use due to steroid response or recovery of ciliary body to normal aqueous production; consider tapering or changing steroid if steroid response exists); steroids are not effective in Fuchs' heterochromic iridocyclitis

Trauma:

Mechanism

Angle Recession: If more than two thirds of angle is involved, 10% of patients develop glaucoma from scarring of angle structures.

Chemical Injury: Toxicity to angle structures from direct or indirect (prostaglandin, ischemia-mediated) damage.

Hemorrhage: Red blood cells, ghost cells (degenerated red blood cells), or macrophages that have ingested red blood cells (hemolytic glaucoma) obstruct the trabecular meshwork; increased incidence in patients with sickle cell disease.

Siderosis/Chalcosis: Toxicity to angle structures from iron or copper intraocular foreign body.

Symptoms

Asymptomatic; may have decreased vision, pain, red eye.

Signs

Normal or decreased visual acuity, increased intraocular pressure, anterior chamber cell/flare; may have other signs of trauma including red blood cells in anterior chamber and/or vitreous, angle recession, iridodialysis, cyclodialysis, sphincter tears, iridodonesis, phacodonesis, cataract, corneal blood staining, corneal scarring, scleral blanching/ischemia, intraocular foreign body, iris heterochromia, retinal tears, choroidal rupture.

Evaluation

- Complete ophthalmic history and eye exam with attention to cornea, tonometry, anterior chamber, gonioscopy, iris, lens, and ophthalmoscopy
- Consider B-scan ultrasonography if unable to visualize the fundus
- Consider orbital radiographs or head and orbital CT scan to rule out intraocular foreign body
- Check visual fields

Management

- Treatment of increased intraocular pressure (see Primary Open-Angle Glaucoma section)
- Laser trabeculoplasty is usually not effective
- May require anterior chamber washout and/or pars plana vitrectomy for hemorrhage-related, uncontrolled elevation of intraocular pressure

Normal (Low) Tension Glaucoma

Definition

Similar optic nerve and visual field damage as in primary open-angle glaucoma (POAG), but with normal intraocular pressure (≤21 mm Hg).

Epidemiology

Higher prevalence of vasospastic disorders including migraine, Raynaud's phenomenon, ischemic vascular disease, autoimmune disease, and coagulopathies; also associated with history of poor perfusion of the optic nerve from hypotension, shock, myocardial infarction, or massive hemorrhage.

Symptoms

Asymptomatic; may have decreased vision or constricted visual fields in late stages.

Signs

Normal or decreased visual acuity, normal intraocular pressure (≤21 mm Hg), cupping of optic nerve, splinter hemorrhages at optic disc (more common than in POAG), peripapillary atrophy, nerve fiber layer defects, visual field defects.

Differential Diagnosis

Primary open-angle glaucoma, secondary glaucoma (steroid-induced, "burned out" pigmentary or post-inflammatory glaucoma), intermittent angle-closure glaucoma, optic neuropathy, optic nerve anomalies, glaucomatocyclitic crisis (Posner-Schlossman syndrome).

Evaluation

- Complete ophthalmic history and eye exam with attention to cornea, tonometry, anterior chamber, gonioscopy, iris, lens, and ophthalmoscopy
- Check visual fields

- Consider diurnal curve (eg, IOP measurement q2h for 10–24 hours) and tonography
- For neuroretinal rim pallor, check color vision and lab tests (CBC, ESR, VDRL, FTA-ABS, ANA), neuroimaging, and cardiovascular evaluation

Management

- Choice and order of topical glaucoma medications depend on many factors, including patient's age, intraocular pressure level and control, and amount and progression of optic nerve cupping and visual field defects. Treatment options are presented in the Primary Open-Angle Glaucoma section

Prognosis

Worse than that for POAG.

Chapter 12

Visual Acuity / Refractive / Sudden Visual Loss

Refractive Error

Definition

The state of an eye in which light rays are not properly focused on the retina and therefore images are blurred. As a result, uncorrected visual acuity is decreased. Visual acuity measures the ability to see an object at a certain distance. It is frequently recorded as a ratio comparing an individual's results to a standard. Snellen acuity (a measure of central acuity) is the most common method to test vision (Table 12–1). For children and illiterate adults, other tests may be used, including the "E" game, Landolt "C" chart, HOTV match test, and Allen pictures.

Ametropia: Refers to a refractive error (eg, myopia, hyperopia, or astigmatism).

Anisometropia: Refers to a difference in refractive error between the two eyes; usually ≥2 diopters.

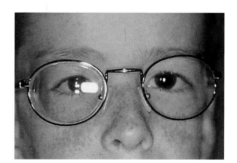

Figure 12–1 Anisometropia with myopia in the right eye (OD) (note minification from spectacle lens) and hyperopia in the left eye (OS) (note magnification from spectacle lens).

Table 12–1   Measures of Visual Acuity

Central Visual Acuity Notations

Distance Acuity Notations

Snellen, English Distance (ft)	Snellen, Metric Distance (m)	Loss of Central Vision (%)
20/15	6/5	0
20/20	6/6	0
20/25	6/7.5	5
20/30	6/10	10
20/40	6/12	15
20/50	6/15	25
20/60	6/20	35
20/70	6/22	40
20/80	6/24	45
20/100	6/30	50
20/125	6/38	60
20/150	6/50	70
20/200	6/60	80
20/300	6/90	85
20/400	6/120	90
20/800	6/240	95

Near Acuity Notations

Near Snellen Inches	cm	Jaeger Standard	American Point-Type	Distance Snellen Equivalent	Loss (%)
14/14	35/35	1	3	20/20	0
14/18	35/45	2	4	20/25	0
14/21	35/53	3	5	20/30	5
14/24	35/50	4	6	20/40	7
14/28	35/70	5	7	20/45	10
14/35	35/88	6	8	20/50	50
14/40	35/100	7	9	20/60	55
14/45	35/113	8	10	20/70	60
14/60	35/150	9	11	—	80
14/70	35/175	10	12	—	85
14/80	35/200	11	13	—	87
14/88	35/220	12	14	20/100	90
14/112	35/280	13	21	—	95
14/140	35/350	14	23	—	98

Astigmatism: The curvature of the cornea or, less commonly, the curvature of the lens varies in different meridians. If the cornea is steeper in the vertical meridian, it is referred to as *with-the-rule* astigmatism; if it is steeper in the horizontal meridian, it is called *against-the-rule* astigmatism. Astigmatism can also be designated as regular or irregular. A cylindrical lens corrects regular astigmatism.

Emmetropia: No refractive error exists and thus no corrective lens is required to achieve good distance vision. In the emmetropic eye, parallel rays of light are brought to focus on the retina, and the far point is infinity, which is conjugate with the retina.

Hyperopia ("Farsightedness"): Light rays are focused behind the retina. A "plus" lens is used to correct this refractive error.

Myopia ("Nearsightedness"): Light rays from a distant object are focused in front of the retina and those from a near object are focused on the retina; therefore, distant objects are blurry and near objects are clear. A "minus" lens is used to correct this refractive error.

Presbyopia: Loss of accommodative response resulting from loss of lens elasticity or possible anatomic change in lens equator to ciliary body position. Average age of onset is 40 years old. A "plus" lens is used to correct this problem (bifocal "add").

Symptoms

Decreased vision when not wearing corrective lenses, distant objects are blurry and near objects are clear (myopia), distant and near objects are blurry (hyperopia), or near objects that are blurry become clearer when held further away (presbyopia).

Signs

Decreased visual acuity that improves with pinhole testing, glasses, or contact lenses.

Differential Diagnosis

Normal eye exam in presence of decreased vision: amblyopia, retrobulbar optic neuropathy, other optic neuropathies (toxic, nutritional), nonorganic (functional) visual loss, rod monochromatism, cone degeneration, retinitis pigmentosa sine pigmento, cortical blindness.

Evaluation

- Complete ophthalmic history and eye exam with attention to pinhole acuity (corrects most low to moderate refractive errors to the 20/25 to 20/30 level), manifest (undilated) and cycloplegic (dilated) refraction, retinoscopy, pupils, keratometry, cornea, lens, and ophthalmoscopy
- Consider potential acuity meter (PAM) testing, rigid contact lens over-refraction, and corneal topography (computerized videokeratography) if irregular astigmatism is suspected

Management

- Glasses are the first line of treatment and can correct virtually all refractive errors with the exception of high or irregular astigmatism
- Contact lenses (soft or rigid). Numerous styles of contact lenses are available to correct almost any refractive error

Management Continued

- Consider incisional refractive surgery: radial keratotomy (RK) for the correction of low myopia, and astigmatic keratotomy (AK) for the correction of astigmatism (see below)
- Consider laser refractive surgery: photorefractive keratectomy (PRK), or laser in situ keratomileusis (LASIK)

Prognosis

Good.

Corneal Refractive Procedures

Definition

Astigmatic Keratotomy (AK): An incisional refractive surgical procedure using a diamond knife in which midperipheral arcuate or straight incisions are made in the steep corneal meridian causing flattening of the cornea and reduced astigmatism.

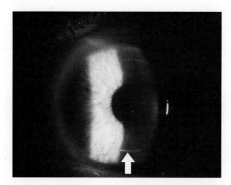

Figure 12–2 Astigmatic keratotomy demonstrating a pair of arcuate incisions in the vertical meridian (arrow).

Automated Lamellar Keratoplasty (ALK): A lamellar refractive surgical procedure to correct either myopia or hyperopia. A mechanical device (keratome) is used to cut a partial-thickness flap in the cornea. For myopia, a second cut is made with the keratome in the corneal stromal bed. For hyperopia, one deep stromal cut is made to weaken the cornea. The corneal flap is then replaced.

Laser In Situ Keratomileusis (LASIK): This method employs a combination of ALK and photorefractive keratectomy (PRK) techniques. The keratome is first used to cut a hinged partial-thickness corneal flap which is then folded back.

Laser energy is applied to the underlying stromal bed, and the flap is replaced. This technique can correct large refractive errors.

Photorefractive Keratectomy (PRK): A laser refractive surgical procedure that utilizes excimer laser surface ablation to correct myopia (central ablation), hyperopia (peripheral ablation), and/or astigmatism (toric ablation).

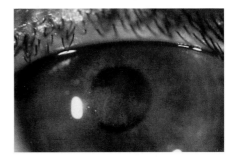

Figure 12–3 Photorefractive keratectomy demonstrating mild central haze.

Radial Keratotomy (RK): An incisional refractive surgical procedure performed with a diamond knife using deep radial incisions in the cornea to centrally flatten the cornea for the correction of low to moderate myopia. This method can be combined with AK for compound myopia (myopia with astigmatism).

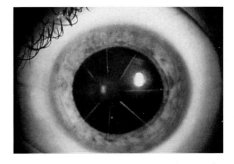

Figure 12–4 Radial keratotomy demonstrating eight incisions.

Symptoms

Postoperatively, patient may have: decreased vision (due to undercorrection, overcorrection, or irregular astigmatism), fluctuating vision, difficulty with night vision, halos, glare, starbursts, ghost images, double vision, or foreign body sensation.

Signs

Corneal incisional scarring (RK, AK), minimal to severe anterior corneal stromal haze (PRK), corneal ectasia (ALK, lost cap), or evidence of a circular lamellar flap with or without haze, cap wrinkling, or epithelial ingrowth (ALK, LASIK); may have residual refractive error.

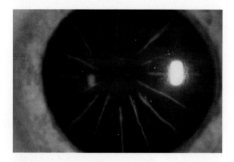

Figure 12–5 Radial keratotomy demonstrating 16 irregular incisions with hypertrophic scarring and varying optical zones.

Differential Diagnosis

Corneal scarring from previous trauma, infection, or inflammation.

Evaluation

- Complete ophthalmic history and eye exam with attention to pinhole acuity, manifest and cycloplegic refractions, pupil size, keratometry, cornea, lens, and ophthalmoscopy
- Corneal topography (computerized videokeratography)
- Consider rigid contact lens over-refraction

Management

- No treatment recommended unless patient is symptomatic and vision is decreased. Choice of treatment depends on type of refractive surgery performed.
- **Undercorrections/overcorrections:** Modification of topical medication regimen, spectacles or contact lens, consider retreatment after corneal stabilization and failure of conservative management. Specific treatment must be tailored on an individual basis and is beyond the scope of this book, but should be performed by a cornea/refractive specialist.
- **Halo/glare/starbursts:** Consider topical miotic (pilocarpine 0.5%–1% qd to bid), polarized sunglasses
- Topical artificial tears (see Appendix) up to q1h or a bandage contact lens for corneal surface irregularities

Prognosis

Usually good; depends on specific surgical technique and attempted correction.

Vertebrobasilar Artery Insufficiency

Definition

Impaired vertebrobasilar circulation produces neurologic deficits referable to the brainstem or occipital lobe.

Etiology

Hypertensive vascular disease, atheromatous occlusion, microembolization (heart), or changes in cardiac output.

Symptoms

Transient visual blurring (seconds to minutes), photopsias (flashes of light), diplopia, unilateral weakness, sensory loss, ataxia, nystagmus, dysarthria, hoarseness, dysphagia, hearing loss, and vertigo; history of drop attacks.

Signs

Small, paracentral, congruous, homonymous visual field defects.

Differential Diagnosis

Amaurosis fugax, migraine, papilledema, temporal arteritis.

Evaluation

- Complete ophthalmic history, neurologic exam and eye exam with attention to extraocular motility, pupils, and ophthalmoscopy
- Check visual fields
- Lab tests: complete blood count (CBC), erythrocyte sedimentation rate (ESR), and blood glucose (hypoglycemia)
- Check blood pressure
- Head and orbital computed tomography (CT) or magnetic resonance imaging (MRI)
- Cervical spine radiographs (cervical spondylosis)
- Medical consultation for complete cardiovascular evaluation, including electrocardiogram, echocardiogram, duplex and Doppler scans of carotid and vertebral arteries

Management

- No effective treatment
- Aspirin (325 mg PO qd)
- Medical or neurology consultation, as long-term anticoagulation may be required

Prognosis

Usually poor

Migraine

Definition

From the Greek *hemikranos* = half skull. A neurologic disorder caused by changes in intracranial vasomotor control. Often with headache, but not a necessary feature. Typically classified as classic, common, or complicated.

Classic Migraine (10–20%): Well-defined prodrome or aura (10–40 minutes); usually visual or other fleeting neurologic signs including visual scintillations, dazzling zig zag lines (fortification phenomenon), photophobia, spreading scotomas, dizziness, and tinnitus followed by unilateral throbbing head pain, nausea, and/or emesis. Patients may have premonitory symptoms including hunger, thirst, elation, excessive energy, drowsiness, depression, and/or a feeling of impending doom. Strong family history.

Common Migraine (70–80%): Poorly defined prodrome with mood fluctuations, fatigue, and gastrointestinal disturbances (anorexia, nausea, and emesis). Headache may occur without prodrome.

Complicated Migraine: Persistent neurologic deficits beyond headache including numbness/tingling, paralysis, aphasia, weakness that eventually resolve over minutes to hours; includes basilar artery migraine (mimics vertebrobasilar artery insufficiency), retinal migraine (monocular visual loss), ophthalmoplegic migraine (children, cranial nerve [CN] paresis [CN III > CN VI]), and cerebral migraine (motor/sensory defect).

Acephalgic Migraine: Visual aura without headache. Visual symptoms described as fortification phenomenon, scintillating scotoma, tunnel vision, double vision, amaurosis fugax, and altitudinal field loss; 25% have family history of migraine.

Epidemiology

Affects 15% of men and 25% of women; can occur at any age; family history of migraine 60%, or a history of motion sickness or cyclic vomiting as a child is common. In women, increased incidence during premenstrual tension and pregnancy.

Symptoms

Aura (see above), photophobia, headache, nausea, emesis.

Signs

None; may have visual field defect, cranial nerve palsy, or other neurologic deficits.

Differential Diagnosis

Serious: Meningitis, subarachnoid hemorrhage, temporal arteritis, malignant hypertension, intracranial tumor, arteriovenous malformation, vertebrobasilar artery insufficiency, aneurysm, subdural hematoma, or cerebral ischemia.

Others: Tension or cluster headaches, trigeminal neuralgia, temporomandibular joint (TMJ) syndrome, cervical spondylosis, herpes zoster ophthalmicus, sinus or dental pathology, uveitis, angle-closure glaucoma, post-lumbar puncture, nonorganic, caffeine withdrawal, carbon monoxide inhalation, and nitrite exposure.

Evaluation

- Careful headache history (eg, precipitating factors, location, frequency)
- Complete ophthalmic history, neurologic exam, and eye exam with attention to motility, pupils, tonometry, and ophthalmoscopy
- Check visual fields
- Check blood pressure and temperature
- Consider lumbar puncture for suspected meningitis
- Neuroimaging for complicated migraines or migraines with atypical features
- Medical or neurology consultation

Management

- Place patient in dark, low-noise surroundings; encourage rest
- Aspirin (325–500 mg PO qd) or nonsteroidal anti-inflammatory drugs (ibuprofen 600 mg PO qd)
- Patients who have > 3 attacks per month:
  - At first sign of aura give ergotamine (1–3 mg PO 1 tablet at onset of headache, 1 more 15-20 minutes later); consider adding caffeine 100 mg/ergotamine 1 mg [Cafergot] PO 2 tablets at onset of headache, 1 more 30 minutes later)
  - Consider sumatriptan (Imitrex IM) or oral narcotic medications (codeine, oxycodone PRN) if headache severe
  - **Prophylaxis:** Systemic β-blocker (propranolol 20-40 mg PO bid to tid initially), tricyclic antidepressant (amitriptyline 25-75 mg PO qd to bid initially), or calcium-channel blocker (nifedipine 10-40 mg PO tid or verapamil 80 mg PO tid); avoid precipitating agents (eg, alcohol [especially red wine], foods, medications, stress)
  - Treatment should be monitored by an internist or neurologist

Prognosis

Good.

Convergence Insufficiency

Definition

Decreased fusional convergence with near fixation and a remote near point of convergence.

Epidemiology

Typically occurs in teenagers and young adults, rare before 10 years of age; slight female predilection; usually idiopathic; common cause of asthenopia (eye strain); aggravated by anxiety, illness, or lack of sleep.

Symptoms

Eye strain (asthenopia), crossed diplopia, blurred vision, headaches, difficulty reading.

Signs

Inability to maintain fusion at near (patient closes one eye while reading to relieve visual fatigue), distant near point of convergence, reduced fusional convergence amplitudes; possible exophoria at near without exotropia (especially after prolonged reading).

Differential Diagnosis

Presbyopia, uncorrected refractive error (hyperopia), accommodative insufficiency.

Evaluation

- Complete ophthalmic history and eye exam with attention to manifest and cycloplegic refractions, motility (cover and alternate cover tests [exophoria at near]), near point of accommodation (normal is 5–10 cm, abnormal is 10–30 cm), and fusional convergence amplitudes (normal is 30–35 prism diopters, base-out causes diplopia; abnormal is <20 PD)

Management

- Correct any refractive error (undercorrect hyperopes, fully correct myopes)
- **Orthoptic exercises:** Training of fusional convergence with pencil push-ups (bring pencil in from arms length toward nose while focusing on eraser. When diplopia [break point] develops, the exercise is repeated. Each attempt is designed to bring the pencil closer without

diplopia) or using base-out prisms (increase amount of prism diopters until blur point is reached, usually 4–6 PD, then increase further until break point is reached); exercises are repeated 15 times, five times a day; can also use major amblyoscope (stereograms).

- When no improvement is noted with exercises, base-in prism reading glasses are helpful
- Very rarely, muscle surgery with bimedial rectus muscle resection

Prognosis

Usually good.

Accommodative Excess

Definition

A clinical state of excessive accommodation (lens focusing) due to medications, uncorrected refractive errors, or ocular disease. Spasm of the near reflex is the triad of excess accommodation, excess convergence, and miosis.

Symptoms

Headache, browache, and variable blurring of distance vision.

Signs

Abnormally close near point and miosis; relief of symptoms with cycloplegia.

Differential Diagnosis

Iridocyclitis, uncorrected refractive errors (usually hyperopes, but also astigmats and myopes), hyperglycemia (lens swells), use of anticholinesterases or sulfa-containing drugs.

Evaluation

- Complete ophthalmic history and eye exam with attention to manifest, cyclo-plegic, and post-cycloplegic refractions, and pupils.

Management

- Stop offending medication if applicable
- Correct any refractive error including prescribing a reading add if esotropic at near
- Consider cycloplegic (scopolamine 0.25% qd to qid) to break spasm (only occasionally needed)
- Teach patient to intermittently focus at distance during periods of prolonged near work

Prognosis

Good.

Functional Visual Loss (Malingering, Hysteria)

Definition

Visual abnormality not attributable to any organic disease process (nonphysiologic).

Malingering: Fabrication of existence or extent of disorder for secondary gain; usually involved in legal action or compensation claim.

Hysteria: Subconscious (not willful) expression of symptoms.

Symptoms

Decreased vision (mild [20/20^{-1}] to no light perception [NLP], monocular or binocular), diplopia, metamorphopsia, oscillopsia.

Signs

Decreased visual acuity, abnormal visual field (usually inconsistent or has characteristic pattern); may have voluntary nystagmus, gaze palsy, or blepharospasm; malingerer often uncooperative and combative, hysteric often indifferent but cooperative; otherwise normal exam (especially pupils, optokinetic nystagmus [OKN] response, fundus).

Differential Diagnosis

Organic disease especially amblyopia, early keratoconus, anterior basement membrane dystrophy, early cataracts, central serous retinopathy, early Stargardt's disease, retinitis pigmentosa sine pigmento, rod monochromatism, cone degeneration, retrobulbar optic neuropathy, other optic neuropathies [toxic, nutritional], and cortical blindness.

Evaluation

- Complete ophthalmic history and eye exam with attention to vision (distance and near, monocular and binocular, varying distance, fogging, red-green, prism dissociation, stereopsis, startle reflex, proprioception, signing name, mirror tracking, OKN response), retinoscopy, motility, pupils, and ophthalmoscopy
- Check visual fields (monocular and binocular); beware tunnel vision, spiraling fields, crossing isopters
- Consider electroretinogram (ERG), visual evoked response (VER), fluorescein angiogram, or neuroimaging in difficult cases

Management

- Reassurance
- Consider psychiatric consultation

Prognosis

No improvement in up to 30%; may have coexistent organic disease in 20%.

Transient Visual Loss (Amaurosis Fugax)

Definition

Unilateral or bilateral transient visual loss.

Etiology

Carotid disease, vertebrobasilar artery insufficiency, arrhythmias, cardiac valvular disease, coagulation disorders, vasospasm, migraine, orbital mass, anterior ischemic optic neuropathy, pseudopapilledema (optic nerve drusen), papilledema.

Symptoms

Brief (2–30 minutes), reversible dimming or loss of vision.

Signs

Asymptomatic; may have intravascular emboli in retinal vessels.

Evaluation

- Complete ophthalmic history, neurologic exam, and eye exam with attention to pupils and ophthalmoscopy
- Check visual fields
- Medical consultation for complete cardiovascular evaluation including electrocardiogram, echocardiogram, and carotid Doppler studies

Management

- No treatment recommended
- Treat underlying disease

Prognosis

Depends on etiology; 1-year risk of cerebrovascular accident is 2%.

Amblyopia

Definition

Decreased vision in an otherwise anatomically normal eye.

Epidemiology

Present in approximately 2% of general population.

Etiology

Deprivation due to obstruction of visual axis (eg, cataract, corneal opacity, ptosis, patching), refractive (anisometropia [>1.5 diopter for hyperopia, >3 D for myopia, >1.5 D for astigmatism] or high ametropia), strabismic, organic (eg, toxic, alcohol, nutritional).

Symptoms

Asymptomatic; may have decreased vision; may notice eye turn, droopy eyelid, or white pupil.

Signs

Decreased visual acuity (unilateral or bilateral), visual acuity often improves with neutral density filter; may have strabismus, nystagmus, ptosis, cataract, corneal opacity, small relative afferent pupillary defect (RAPD).

Differential Diagnosis

Functional visual loss, optic neuropathy.

Evaluation

- Complete ophthalmic history and eye exam with attention to vision with neutral density filters (worsens in organic amblyopia) and single letters (improves acuity), cycloplegic refraction, retinoscopy, pupils, and ophthalmoscopy

Management

- Correct any refractive error
- Patching/occlusion therapy for children <10 years old (full-time occlusion of preferred eye for no more than 1 week per year of age of child before re-examination) and continue until vision stabilizes. Discontinue if no improvement after 2–3 months of compliant, full-time patching. May require part-time occlusion to maintain visual level.
- Protective eyewear with polycarbonate lenses if significant amblyopia exists after 10 years of age to protect fellow eye
- Consider surgery in cases of deprivation (eg, cataract extraction), or strabismus

Prognosis

Depends on extent and duration of amblyopia and age at which appropriate corrective therapy is initiated (the earlier the better, must be prior to 9 years of age); poor prognosis in deprivation amblyopia, good in strabismic amblyopia.

Cortical Blindness (Cortical Visual Impairment)

Definition

Rare syndrome of bilateral blindness due to widespread damage to occipital lobes.

Etiology

Cerebrovascular accident (bilateral occipital lobe infarction), rarely neoplasia.

Symptoms

Complete visual loss; rarely, denies blindness (Anton's syndrome).

Signs

Normal ocular exam (including pupillary response) except no light perception (NLP) vision in both eyes; patient may demonstrate the Riddoch phenomenon (ability to perceive moving, but not static, objects) and "blindsight" (intact primitive mechanism that may allow navigation around objects).

Differential Diagnosis

Functional visual loss.

Evaluation

- Complete ophthalmic history, neurologic exam, and eye exam with attention to vision, pupils, and ophthalmoscopy

- Head and orbital CT scan and/or MRI
- Medical and neurology consultation

Management

- No treatment recommended
- Treat underlying condition

Prognosis

Poor.

Appendices

Common Ophthalmic Medications and Dosages

acetazolamide (Diamox; 250 mg, 500 mg sequels) up to 1 g PO qd in divided doses

acetylcholine (Miochol; 1:100 [20 mg]) for miosis during surgery

acetylcysteine (Mucomyst) 10–20% up to q4h

acyclovir (Zovirax; 200–800 mg) for herpes simplex virus: 200–400 mg PO bid to qid; for herpes zoster virus: 800 mg PO five times a day for 10 days

aminocaproic acid (Amicar) 50–100 mg/kg q4h

amphotericin B 0.1–0.25% qd to q1h

apraclonidine (Iopidine) 0.5%, 1.0% tid

artificial tears (*preserved:* GenTeal, HypoTears, Murine, Ocucoat, Tears Naturale II; *nonpreserved:* AquaSite, Bion Tears, Cellufresh, Celluvisc, HypoTears PF, Refresh Plus, Tears Naturale Free, TheraTears; *ointments:* Lacri-Lube, Refresh P.M.) up to qid (preserved) or q1h (nonpreserved)

atropine 0.5%, 1% qd to qid

azathioprine (Imuran) 50–150 mg/d

bacitracin (AK-Tracin) qd to qid

betaxolol (Betoptic S 0.25%, Betoptic 0.5%) bid

bromonidine (Alphagan) 0.2% bid

carbachol (Isopto Carbachol, Miostat [intraocular 0.01%]) 0.75%, 1.5%, 2.25%, 3% tid

carteolol (Ocupress) 1.5%, 3% bid

chlorambucil (Leukeran) 2–8 mg/d

chloramphenicol (Chloroptic, AK-Chlor, Ocuchlor, Chloromycetin) 0.5% gtts, 1.0% ung qd to q4h

chlorhexidine 0.02% qd to q1h

ciprofloxacin (Ciloxan) 0.3% qd to q1h

clotrimazole 1% qd to q1h

cocaine 4% for anesthesia, pupil testing (Horner's syndrome)

cromolyn sodium (Crolom) 4% qd to q4h

cyclopentolate (Cyclogyl) 0.5%, 1%, 2% qd to qid

cyclophosphamide (Cytoxan) 1–2 mg/kg/d

cyclosporine (Sandimmune) 5 mg/kg/d

dapiprazole (Rēv-Eyes) 0.5% for reversing pupillary dilation

dexamethasone alcohol (Maxidex) 0.1% qd to q1h

dexamethasone phosphate (Decadron) 0.1% qd to q1h

diclofenac (Voltaren) 0.1% qd to qid
dipivefrin (Propine) 0.1% bid
dorzolamide (Trusopt) 2% tid
echothiophate (Phospholine Iodide) 0.03%, 0.0625%, 0.125%, 0.25% bid
emedastine (Emadine) 0.05% qd to qid
epinephrine (Glaucon, Epifrin, Epitrate) 0.25%, 0.5%, 1%, 2% bid
erythromycin (Ilotycin, AK-Mycin) 0.5% qd to qid
famciclovir (Famvir) 500 mg q8h for 7–10 days
fluorescein (Fluress [with benoxinate 0.4% anesthetic]) 0.25%–2% for examination of conjunctiva, cornea, and intraocular pressure
fluorometholone acetate (Flarex) qd to q1h
fluorometholone alcohol (Fluor-Op, FML, FML Forte) 0.1%, 0.25% qd to q1h
flurbiprofen (Ocufen) 0.03% for prevention of intraoperative miosis
fortified cefazolin 50–100 mg/mL up to q1h
fortified ceftazidime 50–100 mg/mL up to q1h
fortified tobramycin 13.6 mg/mL up to q1h
fortified vancomycin 25–50 mg/mL up to q1h
foscarnet (Foscavir) induction: 90–120 mg/kg IV bid for 14–21 days; maintenance: 90–120 mg/kg IV qd
ganciclovir (Cytovene) induction: 5 mg/kg IV bid for 14–21 days; maintenance: 5 mg/kg IV qd
gentamicin (Genoptic, Gentak, Gentacidin, Garamycin) 0.3% qd to qid
gentamicin-prednisolone acetate (Pred-G) qd to q2h
hexamidine (Desomedine) 0.1% qd to q1h
homatropine 2%, 5% qd to qid
hydroxyamphetamine (Paredrine) 1% for pupil testing (Horner's syndrome)
idoxuridine (Herplex, Stoxil) 0.5% ointment, 0.1% solution qd to 5 times a day
isosorbide (Ismotic) up to 2 g/kg PO of 45% solution
ketorolac (Acular) 0.5% qd to qid
latanoprost (Xalatan) 0.005% qd
levobunolol (Betagan) 0.3% bid
levocarbastine (Livostin) 0.05% qd to tid
lodoxamide (Alomide) 0.1% qd to qid
loteprednol etabonate (Lotemax) 0.5% qd to q1h
loteprednol etabonate (Alrex) 0.2% qd to q1h
mannitol (Osmitrol) up to 2 g/kg IV of 20% solution over 30–60 minutes
methacholine (Mecholyl) 2.5% for pupil testing (Adie's pupil)
methazolamide (Neptazane 25–50 mg) up to 50 mg PO tid
methotrexate (MTX) 7.5–25 mg q week
metipranolol (OptiPranolol) 0.3% bid
miconazole 1% qd to q1h
naphazoline (Naphcon, Vasocon) qd to qid
naphazoline-antazoline (Vasocon A) qd to qid
naphazoline-pheniramine (Naphcon-A, Opcon-A) qd to qid
natamycin (Natacyn) 5% qd to q1h
neomycin–polysporin B–gramicidin (Neosporin) qd to q1h
neomycin–polymyxin B–dexamethasone (Maxitrol, Dexacidin) qd to q2h
norfloxacin (Chibroxin) 0.3% qd to q1h
ofloxacin (Ocuflox) 0.3% qd to q1h
olopatadine (Patanol) 0.1% bid
paromomycin (Humatin) 10 mg/mL qd to q1h
phenylephrine (Neo-Synephrine, Mydfrin) 2.5%, 5%, 10% for pupillary dilation

pilocarpine (Pilocar, Isopto Carpine, Pilopine HS gel) 0.5%, 1%, 2%, 3%, 4%, 6%
    qid (qhs for gel)
polyhexamethylene biguanide (PHBG, Baquacil) 0.02% qd to q1h
polymyxin B–bacitracin (Polysporin, AK-Poly Bac) qd to q4h
polymyxin B–neomycin–bacitracin (Neosporin, AK-Spore) qd to q4h
polymyxin B–trimethoprim (Polytrim) qd to q4h
prednisolone acetate (Pred Mild, Pred Forte, Econopred) 0.125%, 1% qd to q1h
prednisolone phosphate (Inflamase Mild) 0.125%, 1% qd to q1h
propamidine isethionate (Brolene) 0.1% qd to q1h
proparacaine (Ophthaine) 0.5% for anesthesia
rimexilone (Vexol) qd to q1h
scopolamine (or hyoscine) 0.25% qd to qid
sodium chloride solution/ointment (Adsorbonac, Muro 128) 2.5%, 5% qd to qid
sulfacetamide sodium (Bleph-10, AK-Sulf, Cetamide, Ophthacet, Sodium Sulamyd,
    Sulf–10) 10–30% gtts, 2.5-10% ung, qd to q2h
sulfacetamide-prednisolone (Blephamide) qd to q4h
sulfacetamide-prednisolone phosphate (Vasocidin) qd to q4h
suprofen (Profenal) 1% for prevention of intraoperative miosis
tetracaine (Pontocaine) 0.5% for anesthesia
tetracycline (Achromycin) 1% qd to q2h
timolol (Timoptic, Betimol) 0.25%, 0.5% bid
timolol gel (Timoptic-XE) 0.25%, 0.5% qd
tobramycin (Tobrex, AKtob) 0.3% qd to q1h
tobramycin-dexamethasone-chlorbutanol (TobraDex) qd to q2h
trifluridine (Viroptic) 0.1% qd to 9 times a day
tropicamide (Mydriacyl) 0.5%, 1% for pupillary dilation
vidarabine (Vira-A) 3% qd to 5 times a day

Color Codes for Topical Ocular Medication Caps

(based on the American Academy of Ophthalmology recommendations to the FDA
to aid patients in distinguishing among drops and thus minimize the chances of
using an incorrect medication)

Class	Color
Anti-infectives	Tan
Anti-inflammatories/steroids	Pink
Mydriatics/cycloplegics	Red
Nonsteroidal anti-inflammatories	Gray
Miotics	Green
Beta-blockers	Yellow or blue
Adrenergic agonists	Purple
Carbonic anhydrase inhibitors	Orange
Prostaglandin analogues	Turquoise

List of Important Ocular Measurements

Volumes: Orbit = 30 mL
Globe = 6.5 mL
Vitreous = 4.5 mL
Anterior chamber = 250 μL

Densities: Rods = 120 million
Cones = 6 million
Retinal ganglion cells = 1.2 million

Distances: Corneal thickness (central) = 0.5–0.6 mm
Anterior chamber depth = 3.0 mm
Diameter of . . .
  Cornea (horizontal) = 10 mm (infant), 11.5 mm (adult)
  Lens = 9.5 mm
  Capsular bag = 10.5 mm
  Ciliary sulcus = 11.0 mm
  Optic disc = 1.5 mm
  Macula = 5 mm
  Fovea = 1.5 mm
  Foveal avascular zone (FAZ) = 0.5 mm
  Foveola = 0.35 mm
Distance from limbus to . . .
  Ciliary body = 1 mm
  Ora serrata = 7–8 mm
  Rectus muscle insertions:
    Medial = 5.5 mm
    Inferior = 6.5 mm
    Lateral = 6.9 mm
    Superior = 7.7 mm
Length of . . .
  Pars plicata = 2 mm
  Pars plana = 4 mm
  Optic nerve = 46 mm
    Intraocular optic nerve = 1 mm
    Intraorbital optic nerve = 25 mm
    Intracanalicular optic nerve = 10 mm
    Intracranial optic nerve = 10 mm
Extent of monocular visual field . . .
  Nasal = 60 degrees
  Temporal = 100 degrees
  Superior = 60 degrees
  Inferior = 70 degrees

Miscellaneous: Visual field background illumination = 31.5 apostilb
Photopic maximum sensitivity = 555 nm
Scotopic maximum sensitivity = 507 nm
Fibers crossing in chiasm = 52% (nasal fibers)
Basal tear secretion = 2 µL/min

List of Eponyms

Adie's pupil: Tonic pupil that demonstrates cholinergic supersensitivity

Alexander's law: Jerk nystagmus, usually increases in amplitude with gaze in direction of the fast phase

Argyll Robertson pupil: Small, irregular pupils that do not react to light but do respond to accommodation; seen in syphilis

Arlt's line: Horizontal palpebral conjunctival scar in trachoma

Arlt's triangle: (Ehrlich-Türck line) base-down triangle of central keratic precipitates in uveitis

Bergmeister's papilla: Remnant of fetal glial tissue at optic disc

Berlin's edema: (Commotio retinae) whitening of retina in the posterior pole from disruption of photoreceptors after blunt trauma

Bielschowsky phenomenon: Downdrift of occluded eye as increasing neutral density filters are placed over fixating eye in dissociated vertical deviation (DVD)

Bitot's spot: White, foamy-appearing area of keratinizing squamous metaplasia of bulbar conjunctiva in vitamin A deficiency

Bonnet's sign: Hemorrhage at arteriovenous crossing in branch retinal vein occlusion

Boston's sign: Lid lag on downgaze in thyroid disease

Brushfield spots: White-gray spots on peripheral iris in Down's syndrome

Busacca nodules: Clumps of inflammatory cells on front surface of iris in granulomatous uveitis

Coats' ring: White granular corneal stromal opacity containing iron from previous metallic foreign body

Cogan's sign: Upper eyelid twitch when patient with ptosis refixates from downgaze to primary position; nonspecific finding seen in myasthenia gravis; also refers to venous engorgement over lateral rectus muscle in thyroid disease

Collier's sign: Bilateral eyelid retraction associated with midbrain lesions

Czarnecki's sign: Segmental pupillary constriction with eye movements due to aberrant regeneration of cranial nerve III

Dalen-Fuchs' nodules: Small, deep, yellow retinal lesions composed of inflammatory cells seen histologically between retinal pigment epithelium and Bruch's membrane in sympathetic ophthalmia (also in sarcoidosis, Vogt-Koyanagi-Harada syndrome)

Dalrymple's sign: Widened palpebral fissure secondary to upper eyelid retraction in thyroid disease

Depression sign of Goldberg: Focal loss of nerve fiber layer after resolution of cotton-wool spot

Ehrlich-Türck line: (See Arlt's triangle)

Elschnig pearls: Cystic proliferation of residual lens epithelial cells on capsule after cataract extraction

Elschnig spot: Yellow patches (early) of retinal pigment epithelium overlying area of choroidal infarction in hypertension, eventually becomes hyperpigmented scar with halo

Enroth's sign: Eyelid edema in thyroid disease

Ferry's line: Corneal epithelial iron line at edge of filtering bleb

Fleischer's ring: Corneal epithelial iron ring at base of cone in keratoconus

Fischer-Khunt spot: (Senile scleral plaque) blue-gray area of hyalinized sclera anterior to horizontal rectus muscle insertions in elderly individuals

Fuchs' spots: Pigmented macular lesions (retinal pigment epithelial hyperplasia) in pathologic myopia

Globe's sign: Lid lag on upgaze in thyroid disease

Guiat's sign: Tortuosity of retinal veins in arteriosclerosis

Gunn's dots: Light reflections from internal limiting membrane around disc and macula

Gunn's sign: Arteriovenous nicking in hypertensive retinopathy

Haab's striae: Breaks in Descemet's membrane (horizontal or concentric with limbus) in congenital glaucoma (versus vertical tears associated with birth trauma)

Hassall-Henle bodies: Peripheral hyaline excrescences on Descemet's membrane due to normal aging

Henle's layer: Obliquely oriented cone fibers in fovea

Herbert's pits: Scarred limbal follicles in trachoma

Hering's law: Equal and simultaneous innervation to yoke muscles during conjugate eye movements

Hirschberg's sign: Pale round spots (Koplik spots) on conjunctiva and caruncle in measles

Hollenhorst plaque: Cholesterol embolus usually seen at vessel bifurcations, associated with amaurosis fugax and retinal artery occlusions

Horner-Trantas dots: Collections of eosinophils at limbus in vernal conjunctivitis

Hudson-Stahli line: Horizontal corneal epithelial iron line at inferior one third of cornea due to normal aging

Hutchinson's pupil: Fixed, dilated pupil in comatose patient due to uncal herniation and compression of cranial nerve III

Hutchinson's sign: Involvement of tip of nose in herpes zoster ophthalmicus (nasociliary nerve involvement)

Hutchinson's triad: Three signs of congenital syphilis—interstitial keratitis, notched teeth, and deafness

Kayes' dots: Subepithelial infiltrates seen in corneal allograft rejection

Kayser-Fleischer ring: Limbal copper deposition in Descemet's membrane seen in Wilson's disease

Khodadoust line: Corneal graft endothelial rejection line composed of inflammatory cells

Klein's tags: Yellow spots at base of macular hole

Krukenberg spindle: Bilateral, central, vertical corneal endothelial pigment deposits in pigment dispersion syndrome

Koeppe nodules: Clumps of inflammatory cells at pupillary border in granulomatous uveitis

Kyreileis' plaques: White-yellow vascular plaques in toxoplasmosis

Lander's sign: Inferior preretinal nodules in sarcoidosis

Lisch nodules: Iris melanocytic hamartomas in neurofibromatosis

Loops of Axenfeld: Dark limbal spots representing scleral nerve loops

Mittendorf's dot: White spot (remnant of hyaloid artery) at posterior lens surface

Mizuo-Nakamura phenomenon: Loss of abnormal macular sheen with dark adaptation in Oguchi's disease

Morgagnian cataract: Hypermature cortical cataract in which liquified cortex allows nucleus to sink inferiorly

Munson's sign: Protrusion of lower lid with downgaze in keratoconus

Panum's area: Zone of single binocular vision around horopter

Parry's sign: Exophthalmos in thyroid disease

Paton's sign: Conjunctival microaneurysms in sickle cell disease

Paton's lines: Circumferential peripapillary retinal folds due to optic nerve edema

pseudo–von Graefe sign: Lid elevation on adduction or downgaze due to aberrant regeneration of cranial nerve III

Pulfrich phenomenon: Perception of stereopsis (elliptical motion of a pendulum) due to difference in nerve conduction times between eyes and cortex, seen in multiple sclerosis

Purkinje images: Reflected images from front and back surfaces of cornea and lens

Purkinje shift: Shift in peak spectral sensitivity from photopic (555 nm, cones) to scotopic (507 nm, rods) conditions

Riddoch phenomenon: Visual field anomaly in which a moving object can be seen whereas a static one cannot

Roth spots: Intraretinal hemorrhages with white center in subacute bacterial endocarditis, leukemia, severe anemia, collagen vascular diseases, diabetes mellitus, and multiple myeloma

Rizutti's sign: Triangle of light on iris from oblique penlight beam focused by cone in keratoconus

Salus' sign: Retinal vein angulation (90 degrees) at arteriovenous crossing in hypertension and arteriosclerosis

Sampaolesi's line: Increased pigmentation anterior to Schwalbe's line in pseudoexfoliation syndrome

Sattler's veil: Superficial corneal edema (bedewing) caused by hypoxia (contact lens)

Scheie's line: Pigment on lens equator and posterior capsule in pigment dispersion syndrome

Schwalbe's line: Angle structure representing peripheral edge of Descemet's membrane

Schwalbe's ring: Posterior embryotoxon (anteriorly displaced Schwalbe's line)

Seidel test: Method of detecting wound leak by observing aqueous dilute concentrated flourescein placed over the suspected leakage site

Shafer's sign: Anterior vitreous pigment cells (tobacco-dust) associated with retinal tear

Sherrington's law: Contraction of muscle causes relaxation of antagonist (reciprocal innervation)

Siegrist streak: Linear chain of hyperpigmented spots over sclerosed choroidal vessel in chronic hypertension or choroiditis

Soemmering's ring cataract: Residual peripheral cataractous lens material following capsular rupture and central lens resorption from trauma or surgery

Spiral of Tillaux: Imaginary line connecting insertions of rectus muscles

Stocker's line: Corneal epithelial iron line at edge of pterygium

Sugiura's sign: Perilimbal vitiligo associated with Vogt-Koyanagi-Harada syndrome

Tenon's capsule: Fascial covering of eye

Uhthoff's symptom: Decreased vision/diplopia secondary to increased body temperature (eg, exercise or hot shower) seen after recovery in optic neuritis

van Trigt's sign: Venous pulsations on optic disc (normal finding)

Vogt's sign: White anterior lens opacities (glaukomflecken) caused by ischemia of lens epithelial cells from previous attacks of angle-closure

Vogt's striae: Deep stromal vertical stress lines at apex of cone in keratoconus

Von Graefe's sign: Lid lag on downgaze in thyroid disease

Vossius ring: Ring of iris pigment from pupillary ruff deposited onto anterior lens capsule after blunt trauma

Watzke's sign: Patient with macular hole perceives break in light when a slit beam is focused on the fovea

Wessely ring: Corneal stromal infiltrate of antigen-antibody complexes

White lines of Vogt: Sheathed or sclerosed vessels seen in lattice degeneration

Wieger's ligament: Attachment of hyaloid face to back of lens

Weiss ring: Ring of adherent peripapillary glial tissue on posterior vitreous surface after posterior vitreous detachment

Willebrandt's knee: Inferonasal optic nerve fibers that decussate in chiasm and loop into contralateral optic nerve before travelling back to optic tract

Common Ophthalmic Abbreviations

(How to Read an Ophthalmology Chart)

AC	anterior chamber
AFX	air fluid exchange
AK	astigmatic keratotomy
ALT	argon laser trabeculoplasty
APD (RAPD)	(relative) afferent pupillary defect
ASC	anterior subcapsular cataract
AV	arteriovenous
BCVA (BSCVA)	best (spectacle) corrected visual acuity
CB	ciliary body
C/D	cup/disc ratio
CE (ECCE, ICCE, PE)	cataract extraction (extracapsular, intracapsular, phacoemulsification)
C/F	cell/flare
CF	count fingers
CL (DCL, SCL, EWCL)	contact lens (disposable, soft, extended wear)
CME	cystoid macular edema
CNVM	choroidal neovascular membrane
C_R	cycloplegic refraction
CRA	chorioretinal atrophy
C/S	conjunctiva/sclera
CS	cortical spoking (cataract)
CSME	clinically significant macular edema
CWS	cotton-wool spot
D	diopter(s)
DD	disc diameter(s)
DFE (NDFE)	(non)dilated fundus examination
DR (BDR, NPDR, PDR)	diabetic retinopathy (background, nonproliferative, proliferative)
E (ET)	esophoria (esotropia)
EL	endolaser
EOG	electro-oculogram
EOM	extraocular muscles/movements
ERG	electroretinogram
ERM	epiretinal membrane
FA	fluorescein angiogram
FAZ	foveal avascular zone
FB	foreign body
FBS	foreign body sensation or fasting blood sugar
GA	geographic atrophy

H	Hertel exophthalmometry measurement or hemorrhage
HM	hand motion
HT	hypertropia
I/L	iris/lens
ILM	internal limiting membrane
IO	inferior oblique muscle
IOFB (IOMFB)	intraocular (metallic) foreign body
IOL (ACIOL, PCIOL)	intraocular lens (anterior chamber, posterior chamber)
IOP	intraocular pressure
IR	inferior rectus muscle
IRMA	intraretinal microvascular abnormalities
K	keratometry
KP	keratic precipitates
L/L/L	lids/lashes/lacrimal
LF	levator function
LP	light perception/projection
LR	lateral rectus muscle
M_R	manifest refraction
MA	macro/micro aneurysm
MCE	microcystic corneal edema
MP	membrane peel
MR	medial rectus muscle
MRD	margin to reflex distance
NLP	no light perception
NS (NSC)	nuclear sclerosis (nuclear sclerotic cataract)
NV (NVD, NVE, NVI)	neovascularization (of the disc, elsewhere [retina], iris)
NVG	neovascular glaucoma
OD	right eye
ON	optic nerve
OS	left eye
OU	both eyes
P	pupil(s)
PC	posterior chamber/capsule
PCO	posterior capsular opacification
PD	prism diopters/pupillary distance
PERRL(A)	pupils equal round reactive to light (& accomodation)
PF	palpebral fissure
PH	pinhole vision
PI	peripheral iridectomy/iridotomy
PK or PKP	penetrating keratoplasty
PPV	pars plana vitrectomy
PRP	panretinal photocoagulation
PRK	photorefractive keratectomy
PSC	posterior subcapsular cataract
PVD	posterior vitreous detachment
R	retinoscopy
RD (RRD, TRD)	retinal detachment (rhegmatogenous, tractional)

RGP	rigid gas permeable contact lens
RK	radial keratotomy
RPE	retinal pigment epithelium
(R)PED	(retinal) pigment epithelial detachment
SB	scleral buckle
SLE	slit lamp examination
SO	superior oblique muscle
SPK (SPE)	superficial punctate keratopathy (epitheliopathy)
SR	superior rectus muscle
SRF	subretinal fluid
SRNVM	subretinal neovascular membrane
SS	scleral spur
T (Ta, Tp, Tt)	tonometry (applanation, palpation, Tonopen)
TH	macular thickening/edema
TM	trabecular meshwork
V (VA, Vcc, Vsc)	vision (visual acuity, with correction, without correction)
VH	vitreous hemorrhage
VF (GVF, HVF)	visual field (Goldmann, Humphrey)
W	wearing (refers to current glasses prescription)
X (XT)	exophoria (exotropia)

Common Spanish Phrases

Introduction:

I am doctor . . .	Yo soy el doctor/la doctora . . .
Ophthalmologist	Oftalmólogo/oculista
I don't speak Spanish	No hablo español
I speak a little Spanish	Hablo un poco de español
Please	Por favor
Come in, enter	Pase(n), entre
Come here	Venga acá
Sit down (here)	Siéntese (aquí)

History:

What is your name?	¿Cómo se llama usted?
Do you understand me?	¿Me comprende? *or* ¿Me entiende?
How are you?	¿Cómo está usted?
How old are you?	¿Cuántos años tiene usted?
Where do you live?	¿Dónde vive usted?
What is your telephone number?	¿Cuál es su número de teléfono?
Tell me	Dígame
Do you have?	¿Tiene usted? *or* ¿Tiene?
glasses	espejuelos/lentes/gafas
for distance	para ver de lejos
for reading	para leer
bifocals	bifocales
sunglasses	espejuelos obscuros/gafas de sol

contact lenses	lentes de contacto
prescription	receta/prescripción
insurance	seguro médico
allergies	alergias
Do you take?	¿Toma usted? *or* ¿Toma?
medications	medicinas
pills, tablets, capsules	pastillas/píldoras, tabletas, cápsulas
Do you use?	¿Usa usted? *or* ¿Usa?
drops	gotas
ointment	pomada
How much?	¿Cuánto?
Do you have problems?	¿Tiene problemas?
reading	al leer
with distance	al ver de lejos
with the cornea	con la cornea
with the retina	con la retina
Do you have?	¿Tiene usted? *or* ¿Tiene?
blurred vision	visión borrosa
diplopia	visión doble
excessive tearing	muchas lágrimas
How long?	¿Por cuánto tiempo?
How long ago?	¿Hace cuánto tiempo?
Does your eye hurt?	¿Le duele el ojo?
Never	Nunca
Once	Una vez
Many times	Muchas veces
What did you say?	¿Qué dijo? *or* ¿Cómo?
Please repeat	Repita, por favor
Again	Otra vez
Excuse me	Con permiso, dispénseme

Examination:

Cover one eye	Tápese un ojo
Can you read this?	¿Puede leer ésto?
the letters/numbers	las letras/números
Better or worse?	¿Mejor o peor?
Which is better, one or two?	¿Cuál es mejor, uno o dos?
Put your chin here	Ponga la barbilla aquí
Put your forehead against the bar	Ponga la frenta pegada a la barra
Look at the light	Mire la luz
Lie down	Acuéstese, boca arriba
Look up	Mire para arriba
Look down	Mire para abajo
Look to the right	Mire para la derecha
Look to the left	Mire para la izquierda

Diagnosis:

| You have . . . | Tiene . . . |
| normal eyes | ojos normales |

myopia	miopía
hyperopia	hiperopía
presbyopia	presbiopía
strabismus	estrabismo
cataracts	cataratas
glaucoma	glaucoma
infection	infección
inflammation	inflamación
a retinal detachment	un desprendimiento de retina

Treatment:

I'll be right back	Ahorita vengo **or** Regreso enseguida
I will put a patch/shield on the eye	Le voy a poner un parche/protector sobre el ojo
You need (do not need) . . .	Usted necesita (no necesita) . . .
an operation	una operación
new glasses	espejuelos nuevos
Don't worry	No se preocupe
Everything is OK (very good)	Toda está bien (muy bien)
I am giving you a prescription for drops/ointment	Le doy una prescripción para gotas/pomada
Take/put/use . . .	Tome/ponga/use . . .
one drop bid/tid/qid	una gota dos/tres/cuatro veces al día
ointment at bedtime	pomada por la noche antes de acostarse
in the right/left eye	en el ojo derecho/izquierdo
in both eyes	en los dos ojos
Do not bend over	No baje la cabeza
Do not strain	No haga fuerza
Do not touch/rub the eye	No se toque/frote el ojo
Do not get your eyes wet	No se moje los ojos
Do you understand the instructions?	¿Entiende las instrucciones?
I want to check your eye again tomorrow	Quiero examinarle el ojo otra vez mañana
I am giving you an appointment	le doy una cita
in one week	para dentro de una semana
in three months	para dentro de tres meses
Return when necessary	vuelva cuando lo necesite
Thank you	Gracias
Goodbye	Adiós

Suggested Readings

The following subspecialty textbooks can provide more detailed information regarding conditions discussed in this book, as well as less common entities:

Arffa RC: *Grayson's Diseases of the Cornea.* St. Louis: Mosby-Year Book; 1991.
Gass JDM: *Stereoscopic Atlas of Macular Diseases,* 4th ed. St. Louis: CV Mosby; 1997.

Grant WM, Schuman JS: *Toxicology of the Eye,* 4th ed. Springfield, IL: Charles C Thomas; 1993.

Kline LB, Bajandas F: *Neuro-Ophthalmology Review Manual,* 4th ed. Thoroughfare, NJ: SLACK; 1996.

Krachmer JH, Mannis MJ, Holland EJ: *Cornea.* St. Louis: CV Mosby; 1997.

Mannis MJ, Macsai MJ, Huntley AC: *Eye and Skin Disease.* Philadelphia: Lippincott-Raven; 1996.

Miller NR: *Walsh & Hoyt's Clinical Neuro-Ophthalmology,* 4th ed. Baltimore: Williams & Wilkins; 1995.

Nelson LB, Calhoun JH, Harley RD: *Pediatric Ophthalmology,* 3rd ed. Philadelphia: WB Saunders; 1991.

Nussenblatt RB, Whitcup SM, Palestine AG: *Uveitis: Fundamentals and Clinical Practice,* 2nd ed. St. Louis: CV Mosby; 1996.

Prepose JS, Holland GN, Wilhelmus KR: *Ocular Infection and Immunity.* St. Louis: CV Mosby; 1996.

Ritch R, Shields MB, Krupin T: *The Glaucomas,* 2nd ed. St. Louis: CV Mosby; 1996.

Rootman J: *Diseases of the Orbit.* Philadelphia: JB Lippincott; 1988.

Ryan SJ: *Retina,* 2nd ed. St. Louis: CV Mosby; 1994.

Shields JA, Shields CL: *Intraocular Tumors: A Text and Atlas.* Philadelphia: WB Saunders; 1992.

Smolin G, Thoft RA: *The Cornea: Scientific Foundations and Clinical Practice,* 3rd ed. Boston: Little, Brown & Co; 1994.

Spencer WH: *Ophthalmic Pathology: An Atlas and Textbook,* 4th ed. Philadelphia: WB Saunders; 1996.

Tabbara JH, Mannis MJ, Holland EJ: *Infections of the Eye,* 2nd ed. Boston: Little, Brown & Co; 1995.

von Noorden GK: *Atlas of Strabismus,* 4th ed. St. Louis: CV Mosby; 1983.

Walsh TJ: *Neuro-Ophthalmology: Clinical Signs and Symptoms,* 3rd ed. Philadelphia: Lea & Febiger; 1992.

Yanoff M, Fine BS: *Ocular Pathology: A Text and Atlas,* 3rd ed. Philadelphia: JB Lippincott; 1989.

Index

Note: Page numbers in *italics* refer to illustrations; page numbers followed by t refer to tables

A

Abbreviations, 394–396
Abetalipoproteinemia, 327–328
Accommodative excess, 381–382
Acetazolamide, 387
  for angle-closure glaucoma, 180
  for congenital glaucoma, 362
  for cystoid macular edema, 279
  for idiopathic intracranial
    hypertension, 347
  for orbital hemorrhage, 4
  for primary open-angle glaucoma, 364
  for retinal arterial occlusion, 252
Acetylcholine, 387
Acetylcysteine, 387
  for corneal burns, 123
  for dry eye syndrome, 95
  for peripheral ulcerative keratitis, 128
Achromatopsia, 320
Acne rosacea, 10–11, *11, 94*
  ectropion and, 52
  staphylococcal keratitis and, 127
  treatment of, 10–11, 95
Acquired immunodeficiency syndrome
    (AIDS). See also *Human
    immunodeficiency virus (HIV).*
  acute retinal necrosis treatment and,
    297
  cotton-wool spots and, 250, *301*
  cytomegalovirus and, 298
  Kaposi's sarcoma and, 75, 114
  microsporidium keratitis and, 142
  molluscum contagiosum and, 63
  retinal vein occlusion and, 253
Acute idiopathic blind spot enlargement
    syndrome (AIBSE), 310. See also
    *Multiple evanescent white dot
    syndrome (MEWDS).*
Acute posterior multifocal placoid
    pigment epitheliopathy (APMPPE),
    306–307, *307*
Acyclovir, 387
  for acute retinal necrosis, 297
  for corneal graft failure, 139
  for dacryoadenitis, 80
  for herpes simplex, 62, 80, 389
  for herpes zoster, 63, 80, 185, 387

Acyclovir *(Continued)*
  for herpetic keratitis, 139, 145
  for progressive outer retinal necrosis
    syndrome, 302
Adenocarcinoma, iris pigment epithelial
    tumors as, 215
  pleomorphic, 85, 86
Adenoma, cavernous sinus syndrome and,
    36–37
  oxyphilic, 115
  pleomorphic, 85, 86
Adenoma sebaceum, 333, *334*
Adie's tonic pupil, 201–202, 390
  anisocoria and, 199, 201
  evaluation of, 200, 202
α-Adrenergic agonist(s), for angle-closure
    glaucoma, 180
  for primary open-angle glaucoma, 364
β-Adrenergic blocker(s), for angle-closure
    glaucoma, 180
  for congenital glaucoma, 362
  for migraine, 379
  for orbital hemorrhage, 4
  for primary open-angle glaucoma, 364
  for retinal arterial occlusion, 252
Alagille's syndrome, 209
Albinism, 330–331, *331*
Alexander's law, 390
Alkaptonuria, 120
Alport's syndrome, 237, *237*
Alström's disease, 328
Amaurosis fugax, 383–384
Amblyopia, 384–385
American Academy of Ophthalmology,
    topical medication color code
    recommendations of, 389
Ametropia, 371
Amikacin, for endophthalmitis, 178
  maculopathy and, 284
Aminocaproic acid, 387
  for hyphema, 173
Aminoglycosides, maculopathy and, 284
Amitriptyline, for migraine, 379
  for post-herpetic neuralgia, 63
Amoxicillin, with clavulanate, antibiotic
    prophylaxis by, 1
  for dacryoadenitis, 81
  for dacryocystitis, 82

Bromonidine *(Continued)*
for primary open-angle glaucoma, 364
Brown's syndrome, 23, *24*
Brucellosis, granulomatous anterior
uveitis and, 183
Brushfield spots, 214, 393
Busacca nodules, 215, *215,* 391

C

C_3F_8 gas injection, for proliferative
vitreoretinopathy, 294
Calcium, corneal deposition of, 164
Canalicular laceration, 45
Canaliculitis, 78–79
Candidiasis, 297, *297*
Canthaxanthine, maculopathy and, 284,
284
Cantholysis, 5
Canthotomy, lateral, 5
Capsaicin, for post-herpetic neuralgia, 63
Capsulotomy, secondary cataract and,
225, *225*
Carbachol, 387
for primary open-angle glaucoma, 364
Carbogen treatment, for retinal arterial
occlusion, 252
Carbonic anhydrase inhibitor(s), for
glaucoma, 361, 364
hyphema and, 174
Carcinoma. See also *Adenocarcinoma;*
Tumor(s).
adenoid cystic, 85, 86
basal cell, 74–75, *74*
cranial nerve paresis and, 34, 35
Horner's syndrome and, 203
optic neuropathy and, 352
retinopathy of, 343
sebaceous cell, 76–77, *77*
chalazia and, 76
squamous cell, 77, *77*
conjunctival, 111, *111*
corneal, 168–169
Cardiovascular disease. See also
Atherosclerosis; Sickle cell disease;
Vascular occlusion.
age-related macular degeneration and,
271
capillary hemangioma and, 14
chronic progressive external
ophthalmoplegia and, 38
cotton-wool spots and, 250
glaucoma and, 363, 369
Kearns-Sayre syndrome and, 38, 327
lyme disease and, 182
ocular ischemic syndrome and, 256

Cardiovascular disease *(Continued)*
Peter's anomaly and, 210
retinal hemorrhage and, 248, 249
retinal ischemia and, 250
retinal vein occlusion and, 253
rubeosis iridis and, 195
transient visual loss and, 383
vertebrobasilar artery insufficiency
and, 377
Carotid cavernous fistula, 5, *5*
Horner's syndrome and, 203
Carteolol, 387
for primary open-angle glaucoma, 364
Caruncle, tumors in, 115–116, *116*
Cataract(s). See also *Posterior capsular*
opacification.
acquired, 220–225, *220–224*
Alström's disease and, 328
amblyopia and, 384
anterior chamber cell/flare and, 170
atrophia bulbi and, 6
capsular, 217
Cockayne's syndrome and, 328
congenital, 217–220, *218–219*
pediatric treatment of, 219–220
cortical degeneration, 220, *220*
diabetes mellitus and, 222, 264
galactosemia and, 218
glaucoma and, 223, 224, 366, 367
Goldmann-Favre vitreotapetoretinal
degeneration and, 325
gyrate atrophy and, 319
hypocalcemia and, 218, 222
hypopyon and, 174
lamellar, 217
Leber's congenital amaurosis and, 326
lens exfoliation and, 228
lens-induced glaucoma and, 232, 233
lenticonus and, 237, *238*
lenticular, 217
leukocoria and, 206
miotics and, 223
Morgagnian, 392
mucolipidosis and, 286
myopic degeneration and, 274
myotonic dystrophy and, 38, 222
nuclear, 217, *219*
nuclear sclerosis, 221, *221,* 224
persistent hyperplastic primary
vitreous and, 218
polar, 217
radiation and, 223
retinitis pigmentosa and, 223, 328,
330
rubella syndrome and, 217
seclusio pupillae and, 193
secondary, 225, *225*
snowflake degeneration and, 325